Translational Cancer Research for Surgeons

Editor

WILLIAM G. CANCE

SURGICAL ONCOLOGY CLINICS OF NORTH AMERICA

www.surgonc.theclinics.com

Consulting Editor
NICHOLAS J. PETRELLI

October 2013 • Volume 22 • Number 4

ELSEVIER

1600 John F. Kennedy Boulevard • Suite 1800 • Philadelphia, Pennsylvania, 19103-2899

http://www.theclinics.com

SURGICAL ONCOLOGY CLINICS OF NORTH AMERICA Volume 22, Number 4
October 2013 ISSN 1055-3207, ISBN-13: 978-0-323-22744-5

Editor: Jessica McCool
Developmental Editor: Susan Showalter

Surgical Oncology Clinics of North America (ISSN 1055-3207) is published quarterly by Elsevier Inc., 360 Park Avenue South, New York, NY 10010-1710. Months of publication are January, April, July, and October. Business and Editorial Offices: 1600 John F. Kennedy Blvd., Ste. 1800, Philadelphia, PA 19103-2899. Customer Service Office: 3251 Riverport Lane, Maryland Heights, MO 63043. Periodicals postage paid at New York, NY and additional mailing offices. Subscription prices are $274.00 per year (US individuals), $401.00 (US institutions) $135.00 (US student/resident), $314.00 (Canadian individuals), $498.00 (Canadian institutions), $193.00 (Canadian student/resident), $392.00 (foreign individuals), $498.00 (foreign institutions), and $193.00 (foreign student/resident). Foreign air speed delivery is included in all *Clinics* subscription prices. All prices are subject to change without notice. **POSTMASTER**: Send address changes to *Surgical Oncology Clinics of North America*, Elsevier Health Science Division, Subscription Customer Service, 3251 Riverport Lane, Maryland Heights, MO 63043. **Customer Service: 1-800-654-2452 (US and Canada). 314-447-8871 (outside U.S. and Canada). Fax: 314-447-8029. E-mail: journalscustomerservice-usa@elsevier.com** (for print support); **journalsonline support-usa@elsevier.com** (for online support).

Reprints. For copies of 100 or more, of articles in this publication, please contact the Commercial Reprints Department, Elsevier Inc., 360 Park Avenue South, New York, New York 10010-1710. Tel. 212-633-3874; Fax: 212-462-3820; E-mail: reprints@elsevier.com.

Surgical Oncology Clinics of North America is covered in *MEDLINE/PubMed (Index Medicus)* and *EMBASE/ Excerpta Medica, Current Contents/Clinical Medicine,* and *ISI/BIOMED.*

Printed and bound by CPI Group (UK) Ltd, Croydon, CR0 4YY

Transferred to digital print 2013

Contributors

CONSULTING EDITOR

NICHOLAS J. PETRELLI, MD, FACS
Bank of America Endowed Medical Director, Helen F. Graham Cancer Center at
Christiana Care, Newark, Delaware; Professor of Surgery, Thomas Jefferson University,
Philadelphia, Pennsylvania

EDITOR

WILLIAM G. CANCE, MD
Chair, Surgical Oncology and Surgeon-in-Chief, Department of Surgical Oncology,
Roswell Park Cancer Institute, Buffalo, New York

AUTHORS

ARGUN AKCAKANAT, MD, PhD
Assistant Professor, Department of Surgical Oncology, The University of Texas MD
Anderson Cancer Center, Houston, Texas

VINOD P. BALACHANDRAN, MD
Fellow in Surgical Oncology, Department of Surgery, Memorial Sloan-Kettering Cancer
Center, New York, New York

KAREN A. CADOO, MB, BCh, BAO
Breast Cancer Medicine Service, Memorial Sloan-Kettering Cancer Center, Weill Medical
College of Cornell University, New York, New York

WILLIAM G. CANCE, MD
Chair, Surgical Oncology and Surgeon-in-Chief, Department of Surgical Oncology,
Roswell Park Cancer Institute, Buffalo, New York

ALFRED E. CHANG, MD
Hugh Cabot Professor of Surgery, University of Michigan Health System, Ann Arbor,
Michigan

JAMES C. CUSACK Jr, MD
Associate Professor of Surgery, Harvard Medical School; Division of Surgical Oncology,
Massachusetts General Hospital, Boston, Massachusetts

RONALD P. DEMATTEO, MD, FACS
Vice Chairman, Department of Surgery, Memorial Sloan-Kettering Cancer Center,
New York, New York

KELLI BULLARD DUNN, MD, FACS, FASCRS
Professor of Surgery, Associate Director for Clinical Programs, James Graham Brown
Cancer Center, University of Louisville, Louisville, Kentucky

DEREK J. ERSTAD, MD
Department of Surgery, Massachusetts General Hospital, Boston, Massachusetts

JEFFREY M. FARMA, MD
Assistant Clinical Professor of Surgical Oncology, Fox Chase Cancer Center, Philadelphia, Pennsylvania

VITA M. GOLUBOVSKAYA, PhD
Associate Professor of Surgical Oncology, Department of Surgical Oncology, Roswell Park Cancer Institute; Co-Founder, CureFAKtor Pharmaceuticals, Buffalo, New York

BURHAN HASSAN, MD
Postdoctoral Research Fellow, Department of Surgical Oncology, The University of Texas MD Anderson Cancer Center, Houston, Texas

STEVEN N. HOCHWALD, MD
Professor, Department of Surgical Oncology, Roswell Park Cancer Institute, Buffalo, New York

ASHLEY M. HOLDER, MD
Postdoctoral Research Fellow, Department of Surgical Oncology, The University of Texas MD Anderson Cancer Center, Houston, Texas

JAMES R. HOWE, MD
Professor, Department of Surgery, Carver College of Medicine, The University of Iowa, Iowa City, Iowa

CARY HSU, MD
Assistant Professor in Residence, Division of Surgical Oncology, Department of Surgery, David Geffen School of Medicine at the University of California, Los Angeles, Los Angeles, California

FUMITO ITO, MD, PhD
Assistant Professor of Surgery, University of Michigan Health System, Ann Arbor, Michigan

TARI A. KING, MD
Associate Attending Surgeon, Breast Service, Department of Surgery, Jeanne A. Petrek Junior Faculty Chair, Memorial Sloan-Kettering Cancer Center; Associate Professor of Surgery, Weill Medical College of Cornell University, New York, New York

NANCY KLAUBER-DEMORE, MD, FACS
Professor of Surgery, Division of Surgical Oncology, University of North Carolina at Chapel Hill, Chapel Hill, North Carolina

JONATHAN LEWIS, MD, PhD
Boston, Massachusetts

ARI N. MEGUERDITCHIAN, MD, MSc, FRCS, FACS
Assistant Professor of Surgery and Oncology, Department of Surgery, McGill University, Montreal, Quebec, Canada

FUNDA MERIC-BERNSTAM, MD
Chair, Department of Investigational Cancer Therapeutics and Professor, Department of Surgical Oncology, The University of Texas MD Anderson Cancer Center, Houston, Texas

MADHURY RAY, MD
Resident, Division of General Surgery, Department of Surgery, David Geffen School of Medicine at the University of California, Los Angeles, Los Angeles, California

JENNIFER SAMPLES, MD
General Surgical Resident, Division of Surgical Oncology, University of North Carolina at Chapel Hill, Chapel Hill, North Carolina

SARTAJ S. SANGHERA, MD
Department of Surgical Oncology, Roswell Park Cancer Institute, Buffalo, New York

SCOTT K. SHERMAN, MD
Department of Surgery, Carver College of Medicine, The University of Iowa, Iowa City, Iowa

JOSEPH J. SKITZKI, MD, FACS
Assistant Professor, Departments of Surgical Oncology and Immunology, Roswell Park Cancer Institute, Buffalo, New York

TIFFANY A. TRAINA, MD
Breast Cancer Medicine Service, Memorial Sloan-Kettering Cancer Center; Assistant Professor, Department of Medicine, Weill Medical College of Cornell University, New York, New York

MONTE WILLIS, MD, PhD, FAHA, FCAP
Associate Professor of Pathology, Department of Pathology and Laboratory Medicine, McAllister Heart Institute, University of North Carolina at Chapel Hill, Chapel Hill, North Carolina

HAGOP YOUSSOUFIAN, MD
Boston, Massachusetts

JIANLIANG ZHANG, PhD
Associate Professor, Department of Surgical Oncology, Roswell Park Cancer Institute, Buffalo, New York

Contents

> The role of the microenvironment during the initiation and progression of malignancy is appreciated to be of critical importance for improved molecular diagnostics and therapeutics. The tumor microenvironment is the product of a crosstalk between different cells types. Active contribution of tumor-associated stromal cells to cancer progression has been recognized. Stromal elements consist of the extracellular matrix, fibroblasts of various phenotypes, and a scaffold comprised of immune and inflammatory cells, blood and lymph vessels, and nerves. This review focuses on therapeutic targets in the microenvironment related to tumor endothelium, tumor associated fibroblasts, and the extracellular matrix.

> This article presents an overview of the PI3K/Akt/mTOR signaling pathway. As a central regulator of cell growth, protein translation, survival, and metabolism, activation of this signaling pathway contributes to the pathogenesis of many tumor types. Biochemical and genetic aberrations of this pathway observed in various cancer types are explored. Last, pathway inhibitors both in development and already approved by the Food and Drug Administration are discussed.

> The elucidation of the heat shock response (HSR) as a mediator of cellular stress has created a framework for understanding how these processes may promote tumorigenesis. Furthermore, the identification of specific components of the HSR and how they are co-opted by cancer cells has led to the discovery of new therapeutic targets. A wide range of small molecule inhibitors of the HSR are in various stages of development for clinical application in patients with cancer. The introduction of these novel small molecule inhibitors offers the opportunity for synergy with existing therapies and the potential for highly targeted treatments.

Tyrosine kinase (TK) cascades are involved in all stages of tumorigenesis through modulation of transformation and differentiation, cell-cycle progression, and motility. Advances in molecular targeted drug development allow the design and synthesis of inhibitors targeting cancer-associated signal transduction pathways. Potent selective inhibitors with low toxicity can benefit patients with local and metastatic malignancies. This article evaluates information on solid tumor–related TK signaling and inhibitors, including receptor TK signal pathways that lead to successful application in clinical settings, properties of recently approved TK-inhibitor drugs for the treatment of solid tumors, and potential TK pathways for future therapeutic interventions.

Most NF-κB inhibitors target the IKK complex, IκB proteins, or NF-κB transcription factors. The most promising classes of inhibitors include antioxidants, antiinflammatory compounds, natural compounds, statins, proteasome inhibitors, IKKβ inhibitors, biologics, gene therapy, and RNA interference. Targeting NF-κB is limited by intrinsic pathway complexity, cross-talk with other pathways, a lack of biomarkers, poor drug specificity, drug resistance, and difficulty with drug delivery. Future NF-κB targeting will be improved through better understanding of the pathway, more specific inhibitors, and multimodality therapies.

This article summarizes data on translational studies to target the p53 pathway in cancer. It describes the functions of the p53 and Mdm-2 signaling pathways, and discusses current therapeutic approaches to target p53 pathways, including reactivation of p53. In addition, direct interaction and colocalization of the p53 and focal adhesion kinase proteins in cancer cells have been demonstrated, and different approaches to target this interaction are reviewed. This is a broad review of p53 function as it relates to the diagnosis and treatment of a wide range of cancers.

Better understanding of the underlying principles of tumor biology and immunology, enhanced by recent insights into the mechanisms of immune recognition, regulation, and tumor escape has provided new approaches for cancer immunotherapy. This article reviews the current status and future directions of cancer immunotherapy, with a focus on the recent encouraging results from immune-modulating antibodies and adoptive cell therapy.

SURGICAL ONCOLOGY
CLINICS OF NORTH AMERICA

RELATED INTEREST

Surgical Clinics of North America, August 2012 (Vol. 92, Issue 4)
Recent Advances and Future Directions in Trauma Care
LtCOL Jeremy W. Cannon, MD, SM, *Editor*
Available at: http://www.surgical.theclinics.com/

**DOWNLOAD
Free App!**

Review Articles
THE CLINICS

NOW AVAILABLE FOR YOUR iPhone and iPad

Foreword

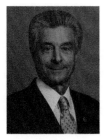

Nicholas J. Petrelli, MD, FACS
Consulting Editor

This issue of the *Surgical Oncology Clinics of North America* is devoted to translational cancer research. The editor is William G. Cance, MD, Chair of the Department of Surgical Oncology and Surgeon-in-Chief at the Roswell Park Cancer Institute. Translational cancer research transforms the latest discoveries in the laboratory into innovative new treatments for cancer patients. In this multidisciplinary environment, basic science benefits from a better understanding of the state of the art in disease management, presentation, and outcomes. In the long run, this results in better research design with the ultimate goal of a successful impact on patient treatment. Translational cancer research saves lives by instituting a rapid development and implementation of thought processes that result from clinician and scientist daily interactions. In 2006, at our own Cancer Center, we created the Center for Translational Cancer Research (CTCR). This center has been a formal alliance with the University of Delaware, the Helen F. Graham Cancer Center at Christiana Care Health System, the Nemours Research Foundation at the A.I. duPont Hospital for Children, and the Delaware Biotechnology Institute at the University of Delaware. The CTCR has created a center without walls to support clinical and basic scientific efforts in basic translational cancer research within the state of Delaware.

Dr Cance has put together an outstanding group of investigators whose careers have been centered around translational cancer research. Uniquely, he has divided this issue of the *Surgical Oncology Clinics of North America* into two sections. The first involves description of the molecular pathways in human cancer, and the second focuses on specific disease sites as applicable to bedside treatment. Surgical oncologists may find that the description of various molecular pathways may not be relevant to their daily practice. However, as aptly put by Dr Cance, the pathways which are described in this issue provide the basis for new therapeutics, and it is important for the surgical oncologists to understand these pathways and also to be part of the evolving process of cancer care.

Surg Oncol Clin N Am 22 (2013) xiii–xiv
http://dx.doi.org/10.1016/j.soc.2013.07.001
1055-3207/13/$ – see front matter © 2013 Published by Elsevier Inc.

surgonc.theclinics.com

I would like to thank Dr Cance and the authors for this outstanding issue of the *Surgical Oncology Clinics of North America*. It is a unique issue that is tremendously educational.

Nicholas J. Petrelli, MD, FACS
Helen F. Graham Cancer Center at Christiana Care
4701 Ogletown-Stanton Road, Suite 1213
Newark, DE 19713, USA

E-mail address:
npetrelli@christianacare.org

Preface

Translational Cancer Research for Surgeons

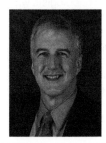

William G. Cance, MD
Editor

Over the last 20 years, we have gained a massive amount of knowledge about the genetic basis of human cancer. Culminating with the sequencing of the human genome, we now have information on a multitude of molecular-based abnormalities that lead to the initiation and progression of cancer. Even with this explosion of knowledge, we are still in the early stages of understanding how cancer cells develop, invade, and metastasize. Nonetheless, as our understanding of the genetic basis of cancer has progressed, a number of novel therapeutic approaches have been developed that target these molecular abnormalities. These discoveries have led to the development of the concept of translational cancer research, in which scientific discoveries are applied to new therapeutics for the patient.

TRANSLATIONAL RESEARCH AND THE SURGICAL ONCOLOGIST

Traditionally, the surgical oncologist has been focused on the operative extirpation of tumors in concert with the multidisciplinary care of the patient. At the same time, the surgeon is typically the "gatekeeper" of the patient with solid tumors, consulted shortly after diagnosis and responsible for directing the overall care of the patient. Thus, the surgical oncologist is first and foremost an oncologist and not simply a surgical specialist. This role has been formally recognized by the creation of a subspecialty certificate in Advanced Surgical Oncology by the American Board of Surgery.

In order for surgical oncologists to maintain their roles as oncologists, it is essential for them to have a broad understanding of the science that underpins the diagnosis and treatment of cancer. This includes the genetic basis of inherited cancer syndromes as well as the various molecular abnormalities that predict cancer behavior and direct targeted therapeutics. Finally, one of the most exciting aspects of the development of

Surg Oncol Clin N Am 22 (2013) xv–xvi
http://dx.doi.org/10.1016/j.soc.2013.06.013
1055-3207/13/$ – see front matter **surgonc.theclinics.com**

these targeted therapeutics is that their high level of specificity can result in fewer toxic side effects. This has already been seen in the area of gastrointestinal stromal tumors where therapy with imatinib is routinely prescribed by surgeons as part of the overall treatment plan for this disease. Every day, new oral-based therapeutics are introduced into the clinical realm, and this heralds an exciting future with many new options for the cancer patient.

In this issue, we have assembled a distinguished group of surgical oncologists who are active translational researchers and who have focused on specific scientific pathways and approaches. The text is organized into two sections. The first section focuses on the various molecular pathways that are operative in human cancer and for which novel therapeutics are actively being developed. The second section focuses on individual disease sites for a more clinical orientation on translational therapeutics that have been taken to early- and late-stage clinical trials, and how this process of translation from the bench to the patient takes place.

It is our hope that this will provide both a broad overview of translational research in cancer and detailed information for specific areas in which the reader wants more information. As we move forward in treating cancer, it is apparent there will be no single "magic bullet" that will cure cancer, but rather a number of therapeutic options that will be tailored for an individual's personalized genetic makeup. The pathways detailed in this monograph will provide the basis for rapidly evolving new therapeutics and it is essential for the surgical oncologist to be a part of this changing process.

William G. Cance, MD
Roswell Park Cancer Institute
Elm and Carlton Streets
Buffalo, NY 14263, USA

E-mail address:
William.Cance@RoswellPark.org

Molecular Pathways and the Development of Targeted Therapeutics

Targeting Angiogenesis and the Tumor Microenvironment

Jennifer Samples, MD[a], Monte Willis, MD, PhD[b],
Nancy Klauber-DeMore, MD[c],*

KEYWORDS

- Angiogenesis • Tumor microenvironment • Tumor associated fibroblast • Integrins
- Growth factors

KEY POINTS

- The role of the microenvironment during the initiation and progression of malignancy is appreciated to be of critical importance for improved molecular diagnostics and therapeutics.
- The tumor microenvironment is the product of a crosstalk between different cells types. Critical elements in the microenvironment include tumor-associated fibroblasts, which provide an essential communication network via secretion of growth factors and chemokines, inducing an altered extracellular matrix, thereby providing additional oncogenic signals that enhance cancer-cell proliferation and invasion.
- Therapeutic targeting of angiogenesis factors, tumor associated fibroblasts, and cell adhesion molecules compose are an active area of clinical trial investigation to determine efficacy of these approaches.
- Some angiogenesis inhibitors are approved by the Food and Drug Administration for cancer, yet further research is needed to improve efficacy in resistant tumors.
- Clinical trials targeting integrins and tumor-activated fibroblasts are being conducted.

TUMOR MICROENVIRONMENT

The role of the microenvironment during the initiation and progression of malignancy is appreciated to be of critical importance for improved molecular diagnostics and

Disclosures: Dr Klauber-DeMore is an inventor on the patent *Discovery of Novel Targets for Angiogenesis Inhibition,* Provisional patent application No. 61/053,397, and is cofounder, shareholder, Chief Scientific Officer, and board member of Enci Therapeutics, Inc, and shareholder and scientific advisory board member of b3bio, Inc.

[a] Division of Surgical Oncology, University of North Carolina at Chapel Hill, 4001 Burnett-Womack Building, CB #7050, Chapel Hill, NC 27599, USA; [b] Department of Pathology & Laboratory Medicine, McAllister Heart Institute, University of North Carolina at Chapel Hill, MBRB 2340b, Chapel Hill, NC 27599, USA; [c] Division of Surgical Oncology, University of North Carolina at Chapel Hill, 170 Manning Drive, Physician's Office Building, CB #7213, Chapel Hill, NC 27599, USA
* Corresponding author.
E-mail address: nancy_demore@med.unc.edu

Surg Oncol Clin N Am 22 (2013) 629–639
http://dx.doi.org/10.1016/j.soc.2013.06.002
1055-3207/13/$ – see front matter © 2013 Elsevier Inc. All rights reserved.

therapeutics.[1] The tumor microenvironment is the product of crosstalk between different cells types. For instance, in epithelial tumors, these cells include the invasive carcinoma and its stromal elements. Critical elements in the microenvironment include tumor-associated fibroblasts, which provide an essential communication network via secretion of growth factors and chemokines, inducing an altered extracellular matrix (ECM), thereby providing additional oncogenic signals that enhance cancer-cell proliferation and invasion. Active contribution of tumor-associated stromal cells to cancer progression has been recognized.[1] Stromal elements consist of the ECM, fibroblasts of various phenotypes, and a scaffold comprised of immune and inflammatory cells, blood and lymph vessels, and nerves. This review focuses on therapeutic targets in the microenvironment related to tumor endothelium, tumor-associated fibroblasts, and the ECM, whereas the immune targets are covered in the immunotherapy article in this issue.

ANGIOGENESIS IS NECESSARY FOR TUMOR GROWTH

The initial evidence that angiogenesis is necessary for tumor growth came from studies transplanting cancer cells into the avascular corneas of rabbits.[2] In these studies, tumors did not grow in rabbit corneas before sprouting vessels were able to grow to connect to the tumor. Additionally, inhibiting blood vessel formation prevented tumor growth beyond 0.4 mm^2. Similar studies found that tumors placed in chicken embryo chorioallantoic membranes shrank during the first 3 days after placement.[3] However, new vessel formation was seen to form from existing vessels after the tumors were placed. When these new vessels connected to the tumor, tumor growth resumed. These studies not only identified a significant role of vessel formation in tumor progression but they also identified that tumors elicited the growth of vessels from existing vessels. This finding suggested that tumors released diffusible factors that initiate angiogenesis to continue and maintain their growth.

There are 4 known strategies by which tumors can augment their blood supply. They can stimulate angiogenesis, use existing vessels directly, induce vasculogenesis, or form vasculogenic networks without vascular cells. The secretion of proangiogenic factors and inhibition of antiangiogenic factors induce vascular sprouting from preexisting capillaries and venules, which constitutes the process of angiogenesis. This mechanism is the most common way tumors gain access to the vasculature. Tumors may also use existing vessels by growing alongside them, as is the case in astrocytomas.[4] The strategy of vasculogenesis involves the formation of blood vessels from bone marrow precursors. This strategy differs markedly from angiogenesis in that the sources of the cells that make up the vessels are from the bone marrow and not from preexisting vessels. However, many of the soluble mediators that initiate vasculogenesis, notably vascular endothelial growth factor (VEGF), parallel those found in angiogenesis.[5] Lastly, tumors themselves can form lumens that can be used to transport blood but lack endothelial cells or other vascular components.[6,7] Multiple strategies may be in play in a particular tumor, depending on their tumor type or stage. In this review, the authors focus on the major pathways of angiogenesis because its contribution has been applicable to therapeutic intervention.

GROWTH FACTORS/RECEPTOR TYROSINE KINASES
VEGF Family

The VEGF family is an essential mediator of angiogenesis, which consists of 5 family members of secreted proteins (VEGFA, VEGFB, VEGFC, VEGFD, VEGFE, and platelet-derived growth factor [PDGF])[8] that bind and activate 3 receptor tyrosine kinases (VEGF receptor [VEGFR]-1, -2 and -3). VEGFA promotes endothelial cell migration, proliferation, vascular permeability, and tube formation. VEGFB was identified as an endothelial cell growth factor expressed in skeletal muscle and heart[9]; however, its role as an angiogenesis factor is not clearly defined. VEGFC and VEGFD play critical roles in lymphangiogenesis, and their expression has been correlated with the development of lymph node metastases.[10] Placental growth factor (PGF) promotes the survival of endothelial cells and regulates the activity of VEGF signaling.[11]

Regulation of VEGF family gene expression is under the control of stresses, such as hypoxia, acidity, and hypoglycemia, which stimulate transcription and increase mRNA stability, resulting in increased protein expression. Under normoxic conditions, prolyl residues in hypoxia inducible factors (HIF) proteins are hydroxylated by prolyl hydroxylase in a reaction that uses molecular oxygen. Hydroxylation of HIF proteins targets them for ubiquitin-mediated proteolysis. Decreased oxygen concentration reduces the efficiency of this process: HIF proteins are stabilized and become available to bind to hypoxia-response elements in the promoters of target genes, thereby activating transcription.[12]

VEGF proteins bind to receptor tyrosine kinases (VEGFR-1, -2 and -3)[13] that mediate cell signaling resulting in their biologic effects. VEGFR-1 (Flt-1) binds 3 of the VEGF family ligands: VEGFA, VEGFB, and PGF. Activation of VEGFR-1 results in hematopoiesis, embryonic vessel development, macrophage chemotaxis, and recruitment of endothelial progenitor cells to tumor blood vessels from the bone marrow.[14] VEGFR-2 (Flk-1/KDR) is the central mediator of VEGF-stimulated tumor angiogenesis and is essential in embryonic vascular development. When VEGF binds to VEGFR-2, the receptor is phosphorylated and activates downstream signaling molecules, including protein kinase C, phospholipase C, mitogen-activated protein kinase (MAPK), Raf, PI3K, and focal adhesion kinase (FAK) pathways, resulting in endothelial cell migration, proliferation, tube formation, and antiapoptosis.[15] VEGFR-3 binds VEGFC and VEGFD and is involved in the formation of lymphatics in tumors and normal tissue.[16]

A humanized version of a monoclonal antibody to VEGFA, bevacizumab, became the first Food and Drug Administration (FDA)–approved antiangiogenic drug in the United States in 2004.[10] It was approved as a first-line treatment agent for metastatic colorectal cancer, in combination with 5-fluorouracil,[17] and was later approved for the treatment of metastatic non–squamous-cell lung cancer, breast cancer, and glioblastoma multiforme.[18]

Additional FDA-approved drugs that block VEGF signaling are sunitinib and sorafenib, both receptor tyrosine kinase inhibitors that are administered orally. In addition to blocking VEGFR signaling, sorafenib also blocks PDGFRB, FLT3, and KIT signaling.[19] Similarly, sunitinib blocks signaling from VEGFR1-3, PDGFRA, PDGFRB, FLT3, and RET.[19] Sorafenib has been approved for unresectable hepatocellular carcinoma, and advanced renal cell carcinoma, whereas sunitinib has been approved for metastatic renal cell carcinoma, gastrointestinal stromal tumors,[10] and neuroendocrine tumors.[20]

Transforming Growth Factor–β

Transforming growth factor–β (TGF-β) is a paracrine polypeptide with 3 homologous forms (TGFβ1, TGFβ2, and TGFβ3). TGF-β is produced in latent form as a zymogen; after secretion, a latency-associated peptide is proteolytically cleaved to release active TGF-β. Active TGF-β binds to constitutively active type 2 receptors (TGFBR2) to activate type 1 receptors (TGFBR1) in a heteromeric complex that controls transcription through the action of a family of SMAD proteins.[21] TGF-β is a proangiogenic agent despite the fact that, in vitro, TGF-β causes apoptosis and growth arrest of endothelial cells. This paradoxic behavior may be explained by the fact that TGF-β activates the secretion of fibroblast growth factor 2, which acts to stimulate the expression of VEGF. VEGF in turn acts in an autocrine manner through its receptor VEGFR2 to activate the MAPK pathway. However, TGF-β will reverse the protective action of VEGF, promoting apoptosis, which occurs in the pruning process, to form the final vascular network.[22] Therapeutic approaches for targeting TGF-β signaling include antagonism of TGF-β ligand binding to the heteromeric receptor complex with isoform-selective antibodies, such as lerdelimumab (TGF-β_2) and metelimumab (TGF-β_1) or the pan-neutralizing antibody GC-1008, and intracellular inhibition of the type I TGF-β receptor kinase with small-molecule inhibitors, such as LY550410, SB-505124, or SD-208.[23]

Fibroblast Growth Factor

Fibroblast growth factors (FGFs) maintain endothelial cell function. FGF1 and FGF2 promote endothelial cell proliferation and migration and stimulate angiogenesis.[24] FGFs produce their biologic effects by binding to transmembrane tyrosine kinase receptors, FGFR1 through FGFR4.[25] FGFR can activate Phospholipase C-gamma (PLC-γ), thereby stimulating the production of diacylglycerol and inositol 1,4,5-tri-sphosphate. This stimulation, in turn, releases intracellular calcium and activates Ca^{2+}-dependent PKCs. The activation of the PI3K-Akt cell survival pathway is one of the important biologic responses induced by FGF2 in endothelial cells.[26]

There are several inhibitors of FGF signaling that are undergoing clinical trials. FP-1039 (FGFR1:Fc) is a soluble fusion protein consisting of the extracellular domain of human FGF receptor 1c (FGFR1) linked to the Fc portion of human IgG1. FP-1039 prevents FGFR1 ligands from binding to any of their related receptors within the family of 7 FGF receptors and may mediate both antitumor and antiangiogenic effects. E-3810 and TKI258 are dual VEGFR and FGFR tyrosine kinase inhibitors in clinical trial.[24]

Notch

The Notch signaling pathway involves gene regulation mechanisms that control multiple cell differentiation processes during embryonic and adult life and is essential for cell-cell communication. This pathway has been directly linked to tumor angiogenesis and to the activation of dormant tumors. VEGFA induces expression of the endothelium-specific Notch ligand deltalike 4 (DLL4): when DLL4 activates the Notch signaling pathway in neighboring cells, it inhibits dorsal sprouting of endothelial tubes. When expressed in tumor cells, DLL4 can activate Notch signaling in host stromal cells, thereby improving vascular function.[27] Inhibition of DLL4-mediated Notch signaling promotes a hyperproliferative response in endothelial cells, a process that leads to an increase in angiogenic sprouting and branching. Despite this increase in vascularity, tumors are poorly perfused, hypoxia increases, and tumor growth is inhibited. Neutralizing anti-DLL4 antibodies have been demonstrated to inhibit tumor growth in vivo.[28] These findings point to the Notch pathway as a potential therapeutic target.

Angiopoietin/Tie Receptors

Angiopoietins belong to a family of endothelial cell-specific molecules that play an important role in endothelial growth, maintenance, and stabilization by binding to Tie receptors.[29] There are 4 types of angiopoietins: Ang-1, -2, -3, and -4. The Tie1 receptor is highly expressed in angioblasts, embryonic vascular endothelium, and endocardium and, in adult tissues, is expressed in lung capillaries.[30] The Tie2 receptor mediates survival signals for endothelial cells resulting in vessel maturation. Ang-2 is an autocrine antagonist that induces vascular destabilization, whereas Ang-1 is an agonist that promotes vessel stabilization in a paracrine fashion. Ang-2 is implicated in tumor-induced angiogenesis and progression and is increased during vascular remodeling.[31] AMG 386 is an investigational peptide-Fc fusion protein that inhibits angiogenesis by preventing the interaction of Ang-1 and Ang-2 with their receptor, Tie2, and is being studied in clinical trials.[32]

Epidermal Growth Factor

The epidermal growth factor (EGF) family consists of 11 members that bind to one of 4 epidermal growth factor receptors (EGFR).[33] All of the receptors, except EGFR3 (HER3), contain an intracellular tyrosine kinase domain.[34] In xenograft models, the activation of EGFR contributes to angiogenesis[35] in addition to cellular proliferation, survival, migration, adhesion, differentiation, and tumor metastasis.[34] The EGFR pathway is more of an indirect regulator of angiogenesis by upregulating the production of proangiogenic factors, such as VEGF. There are 3 FDA-approved EGFR inhibitors: cetuximab and panitumumab, which are monoclonal antibodies, and erlotinib, a tyrosine kinase inhibitor that specifically targets EGFR.[10]

Insulinlike Growth Factor Pathway

The insulinlike growth factor (IGF) pathway plays a major role in cancer cell proliferation, survival, and resistance to anticancer therapies in many human tumors.[36] IGF-1 contributes to the promotion of angiogenesis through increasing VEGF expression via HIF-1a.[37] The 2 main strategies in the development for blocking IGF signaling as an anticancer therapeutic are receptor blockade and tyrosine kinase inhibition.[38] Receptor blockade with the use of monoclonal antibody therapies against the IGF-1R (such as figitumumab)[39] are being investigated. Tyrosine kinase inhibition in general will indiscriminately inhibit the kinase domains of all IGF system receptors. The exception to this is the NVP-AEW541 and NVP-ADW742, which have 15- to 30-fold increased potency for IGF-1R kinase inhibition compared with IR kinase inhibition in cellular assays.[39]

CALCIUM SIGNALING

One of the important intracellular pathways stimulated by a variety of angiogenic growth factors, including VEGF, FGF, and a novel angiogenesis factor secreted frizzled related protein 2 (SFRP2),[40] is activation of calcium signaling. Calcium signaling is mediated through transient increases in cytoplasmic free calcium, which activates the phosphatase calcineurin. Activated calcineurin dephosphorylates nuclear factor of activated T cells (NFAT), which then translocates from the cytoplasm to the nucleus.[41] NFAT plays a critical role of in mediating angiogenic responses.[42,43] NFAT activation was identified as a critical component of SFRP2[40,44] and VEGF-induced angiogenesis and linked to the induction of cyclooxygenase-2.[45] Activation of the Ca^{2+} pathway induces cell proliferation and inhibits apoptosis in cultured endothelial cells, suggesting a proangiogenic activity.[39,40] FK506 is a calcineurin inhibitor that blocks NFAT activation and has been shown to inhibit angiogenesis in vitro and tumor growth in vivo.[40,44] In preclinical models, a monoclonal antibody to SFRP2 reduced tumor growth in vivo and inhibited endothelial and tumor cell NFAT activation in vitro.[46]

ENDOGENOUS ANGIOGENESIS INHIBITORS

The activities of a variety of endogenous angiogenic inhibitors have been described to regulate tumor endothelial growth. These inhibitors include thrombospondin-1,[47] angiostatin,[48] and endostatin.[49] One of the most extraordinary developments in the discovery of endogenous inhibitors came again from the Folkman laboratory[48] via a Lewis Lung Carcinoma mouse model in which lung micrometastases seeded from subcutaneous primary tumors did not develop further when the tumor was intact but grew rapidly after the primary tumor had been surgically removed. It was hypothesized that the primary tumor itself was producing a circulating antiangiogenic agent that inhibited blood vessel growth in the lung micrometastases. After resection of the primary tumor, the source of the endogenous angiogenesis inhibitor was removed and the lung metastases, therefore, grew rapidly. O'Reilly and Folkman isolated a protein they called angiostatin from the urine of mice with intact primary tumors.[48] Angiostatin is a fragment of plasminogen that occurs normally in the circulation, and the cleavage of plasminogen to produce angiostatin occurs in the tumor or itself.[48] Purified angiostatin given daily to mice after resection of the primary tumor completely prevented the development of micrometastases. Angiostatin was subsequently shown to be active against primary tumors established in mice from inoculated human tumor cells, and it also inhibits the proliferation of endothelial cells in culture but had no effect on tumor cell proliferation. Additional proteolytically activated antiangiogenic proteins have been isolated, including endostatin derived from collagen XVIII.[49]

TUMOR ENDOTHELIAL MARKERS

A recent strategy to discovery novel angiogenesis targets is to compare differences in gene expression profiles between tumor and normal endothelium. St Croix and colleagues[50] isolated endothelial cells using magnetic bead selection from a human colon cancer and adjacent normal colon. TEM8 was among the novel genes identified to be overexpressed by tumor endothelium. TEM8 is the anthrax toxin receptor; preclinical targeting of this receptor in tumor models have been successful, making this molecule a candidate for future vascular targeting studies.[51] Subsequent studies have used laser capture microdissection of blood vessels from breast tumors and normal breast tissue,[52] or ovarian cancer and normal ovarian tissue,[53] to identify novel targets that are presently under investigation. One target, SFRP2, has been shown to induce angiogenesis[40]; therapeutic targeting with a monoclonal antibody reduces tumor growth in preclinical models.[46]

CELL ADHESION TO THE ECM

Integrins are heterodimer transmembrane receptors for the ECM comprised of alpha and beta subunits.[54] Integrins bind ligands by recognizing short amino acid stretches on exposed loops, particularly the arginine-glycine-aspartic acid (RGD) sequence. On ligation, integrins mediate signaling events that regulate angiogenesis, cell adhesion, proliferation, survival, and migration. Pathways that are activated include protein kinase B, integrin-linked kinase, MAPK, Rac, or nuclear factor kappa B. In inactive vessels, integrins interact with the basal membrane, thereby maintaining vascular quiescence. During angiogenesis, integrins are essential for endothelial cell migration, proliferation, and survival. In preclinical studies, the inhibition of integrin function suppresses angiogenesis and tumor growth. Of the 24 known integrin heterodimers, $\alpha V\beta 3$[55] and $\alpha V\beta 5$[56] were the first vascular integrins targeted to suppress tumor angiogenesis. Three classes of integrin inhibitors are currently in preclinical and clinical development: synthetic peptides containing an RGD sequence (cilengitide); mono-clonal antibodies targeting the extracellular domain of the heterodimer (Vitaxin); and peptidomimetics (S247), which are orally bioavailable nonpeptidic molecules mimicking the RGD sequence.[57]

FAK is a protein that plays a critical role in intracellular processes of cell spreading, adhesion, motility, survival, and cell-cycle progression and has been shown to play a role in tumor angiogenesis.[58] The pharmacologic blockade of FAK autophosphoryla-tion reduces tumor growth in vivo.[59] The FAK gene encodes a nonreceptor tyrosine kinase that localizes at contact points of cells with ECM and is activated by integrin (cell surface receptor) signaling. Recently, Novartis Inc developed FAK inhibitors down-regulation its kinase activity.[60] TAE-226, a novel FAK inhibitor by Novartis, was recently shown to effectively inhibit FAK signaling in brain cancer by inducing apoptosis.[61] Pfizer-PF-573,228 is another ATP-targeting site inhibitor to be recently described.[62]

TUMOR-ACTIVATED FIBROBLASTS

Fibroblasts in the tumor stroma synthesize fibroblast activation protein (FAP), a type II transmembrane protein that functions as a serine protease. FAP must be assembled into a dimer to become an active protease.[63] More than 90% of human epithelial can-cers overexpress FAP, including colon, breast, lung, and ovarian cancers. The expres-sion of FAP is highly restricted to cancer-associated fibroblasts, but its actual function has yet to be fully identified.[64] This enzyme was reported to cleave gelatin and collagen type I and has, therefore, been implicated in ECM remodeling. It is theorized that FAP has the ability to alter to the tumor microenvironment and partially drive angiogenesis because it is overexpressed in tumors demonstrating increased microvessel density and is overexpressed in human tumor microvessels compared with normal vessels.[52] FAP mRNA is upregulated in endothelial cells that are undergoing capillary morphogen-esis and reorganization. Sibrotuzumab (mAb F19) is a humanized monoclonal antibody to FAP developed for imaging purposes. It is well tolerated and localized to tumor cells but proved to have no effect on metastatic colorectal cancer in a phase II trial.[65] When conjugated to maytansinoid, the antibody did show long-lasting tumor inhibition in mul-tiple xenograft models.[66] Several small molecule inhibitors that block the enzymatic ac-tivity of FAP are under development. However, val-prolineboronic acid (PT-100, talabostat), a selective inhibitor of both FAP and DPPIV, failed to demonstrate any clin-ical benefit in phase II trials of metastatic colorectal cancer, non–small cell lung carci-noma, stage IV melanoma, or chronic lymphocytic leukemia.[67]

SUMMARY

In summary, the tumor microenvironment involves complex biologic signaling path-ways with contributions from endothelial cells, tumor-associated fibroblasts, and the ECM contributing to tumor growth. Antiangiogenic therapy has been shown to increase survival in human tumors, but further research is needed to inhibit tumors that are not responsive to or that become resistant to current antiangiogenic therapy. Further research targeting tumor-associated fibroblasts is needed to validate if this will be a therapeutic approach for treating cancer.

REFERENCES

1. Mbeunkui F, Johann DJ Jr. Cancer and the tumor microenvironment: a review of an essential relationship. Cancer Chemother Pharmacol 2009;63:571–82.

2. Gimbrone MA Jr, Cotran RS, Leapman SB, et al. Tumor growth and neovascularization: an experimental model using the rabbit cornea. J Natl Cancer Inst 1974;52:413–27.

3. Ausprunk DH, Knighton DR, Folkman J. Vascularization of normal and neoplastic tissues grafted to the chick chorioallantois. Role of host and preexisting graft blood vessels. Am J Pathol 1975;79:597–618.

4. Vajkoczy P, Farhadi M, Gaumann A, et al. Microtumor growth initiates angiogenic sprouting with simultaneous expression of VEGF, VEGF receptor-2, and angiopoietin-2. J Clin Invest 2002;109:777–85.

5. Schmidt A, Brixius K, Bloch W. Endothelial precursor cell migration during vasculogenesis. Circ Res 2007;101:125–36.

6. Hillen F, Griffioen AW. Tumour vascularization: sprouting angiogenesis and beyond. Cancer Metastasis Rev 2007;26:489–502.

7. Tang HS, Feng YJ, Yao LQ. Angiogenesis, vasculogenesis, and vasculogenic mimicry in ovarian cancer. Int J Gynecol Cancer 2009;19:605–10.

8. Ferrara N. VEGF and the quest for tumour angiogenesis factors. Nat Rev Cancer 2002;2:795–803.

9. Olofsson B, Pajusola K, Kaipainen A, et al. Vascular endothelial growth factor B, a novel growth factor for endothelial cells. Proc Natl Acad Sci U S A 1996;93:2576–81.

10. Oklu R, Walker TG, Wicky S, et al. Angiogenesis and current antiangiogenic strategies for the treatment of cancer. J Vasc Interv Radiol 2010;21:1791–805.

11. Adini A, Kornaga T, Firoozbakht F, et al. Placental growth factor is a survival factor for tumor endothelial cells and macrophages. Cancer Res 2002;62:2749–52.

12. Mazzone M, Dettori D, Leite de OR, et al. Heterozygous deficiency of PHD2 restores tumor oxygenation and inhibits metastasis via endothelial normalization. Cell 2009;136:839–51.

13. Ferrara N, Gerber HP, LeCouter J. The biology of VEGF and its receptors. Nat Med 2003;9:669–76.

14. Korpanty G, Smyth E, Sullivan LA, et al. Antiangiogenic therapy in lung cancer: focus on vascular endothelial growth factor pathway. Exp Biol Med (Maywood) 2010;235:3–9.

15. Ferrara N. Vascular endothelial growth factor: basic science and clinical progress. Endocr Rev 2004;25:581–611.

16. He Y, Rajantie I, Pajusola K, et al. Vascular endothelial cell growth factor receptor 3-mediated activation of lymphatic endothelium is crucial for tumor cell entry and spread via lymphatic vessels. Cancer Res 2005;65:4739–46.

17. Hurwitz H, Fehrenbacher L, Novotny W, et al. Bevacizumab plus irinotecan, fluorouracil, and leucovorin for metastatic colorectal cancer. N Engl J Med 2004;350:2335–42.

18. Grothey A, Galanis E. Targeting angiogenesis: progress with anti-VEGF treatment with large molecules. Nat Rev Clin Oncol 2009;6:507–18.

19. Wilhelm SM, Adnane L, Newell P, et al. Preclinical overview of sorafenib, a multikinase inhibitor that targets both Raf and VEGF and PDGF receptor tyrosine kinase signaling. Mol Cancer Ther 2008;7:3129–40.

20. Raymond E, Dahan L, Raoul JL, et al. Sunitinib malate for the treatment of pancreatic neuroendocrine tumors. N Engl J Med 2011;364:501–13.

21. Barbara NP, Wrana JL, Letarte M. Endoglin is an accessory protein that interacts with the signaling receptor complex of multiple members of the transforming growth factor-beta superfamily. J Biol Chem 1999;274:584–94.

22. Ferrari G, Cook BD, Terushkin V, et al. Transforming growth factor-beta 1 (TGF-beta1) induces angiogenesis through vascular endothelial growth factor (VEGF)-mediated apoptosis. J Cell Physiol 2009;219:449–58.
23. Yingling JM, Blanchard KL, Sawyer JS. Development of TGF-beta signalling inhibitors for cancer therapy. Nat Rev Drug Discov 2004;3:1011–22.
24. Murakami M, Elfenbein A, Simons M. Non-canonical fibroblast growth factor signalling in angiogenesis. Cardiovasc Res 2008;78:223–31.
25. Eswarakumar VP, Lax I, Schlessinger J. Cellular signaling by fibroblast growth factor receptors. Cytokine Growth Factor Rev 2005;16:139–49.
26. Partovian C, Simons M. Regulation of protein kinase B/Akt activity and Ser473 phosphorylation by protein kinase Calpha in endothelial cells. Cell Signal 2004;16:951–7.
27. Li JL, Sainson RC, Shi W, et al. Delta-like 4 Notch ligand regulates tumor angiogenesis, improves tumor vascular function, and promotes tumor growth in vivo. Cancer Res 2007;67:11244–53.
28. Noguera-Troise I, Daly C, Papadopoulos NJ, et al. Blockade of Dll4 inhibits tumour growth by promoting non-productive angiogenesis. Nature 2006;444:1032–7.
29. Yancopoulos GD, Klagsbrun M, Folkman J. Vasculogenesis, angiogenesis, and growth factors: ephrins enter the fray at the border. Cell 1998;93:661–4.
30. Korhonen J, Polvi A, Partanen J, et al. The mouse tie receptor tyrosine kinase gene: expression during embryonic angiogenesis. Oncogene 1994;9:395–403.
31. Thomas M, Augustin HG. The role of the angiopoietins in vascular morphogenesis. Angiogenesis 2009;12:125–37.
32. Herbst RS, Hong D, Chap L, et al. Safety, pharmacokinetics, and antitumor activity of AMG 386, a selective angiopoietin inhibitor, in adult patients with advanced solid tumors. J Clin Oncol 2009;27:3557–65.
33. Cook KM, Figg WD. Angiogenesis inhibitors: current strategies and future prospects. CA Cancer J Clin 2010;60:222–43.
34. Yarden Y, Sliwkowski MX. Untangling the ErbB signalling network. Nat Rev Mol Cell Biol 2001;2:127–37.
35. Perrotte P, Matsumoto T, Inoue K, et al. Anti-epidermal growth factor receptor antibody C225 inhibits angiogenesis in human transitional cell carcinoma growing orthotopically in nude mice. Clin Cancer Res 1999;5:257–65.
36. Baserga R, Peruzzi F, Reiss K. The IGF-1 receptor in cancer biology. Int J Cancer 2003;107:873–7.
37. Fukuda R, Hirota K, Fan F, et al. Insulin-like growth factor 1 induces hypoxia-inducible factor 1-mediated vascular endothelial growth factor expression, which is dependent on MAP kinase and phosphatidylinositol 3-kinase signaling in colon cancer cells. J Biol Chem 2002;277:38205–11.
38. Weroha SJ, Haluska P. IGF-1 receptor inhibitors in clinical trials–early lessons. J Mammary Gland Biol Neoplasia 2008;13:471–83.
39. Haluska P, Worden F, Olmos D, et al. Safety, tolerability, and pharmacokinetics of the anti-IGF-1R monoclonal antibody figitumumab in patients with refractory adrenocortical carcinoma. Cancer Chemother Pharmacol 2010;65:765–73.
40. Courtwright A, Siamakpour-Reihani S, Arbiser JL, et al. Secreted frizzle-related protein 2 stimulates angiogenesis via a calcineurin/NFAT signaling pathway. Cancer Res 2009;69:4621–8.
41. Nilsson LM, Sun ZW, Nilsson J, et al. Novel blocker of NFAT activation inhibits IL-6 production in human myometrial arteries and reduces vascular smooth muscle cell proliferation. Am J Physiol, Cell Physiol 2007;292:C1167–78.

42. Minami T, Horiuchi K, Miura M, et al. Vascular endothelial growth factor- and thrombin-induced termination factor, Down syndrome critical region-1, attenuates endothelial cell proliferation and angiogenesis. J Biol Chem 2004;279:50537–54.

43. Zaichuk TA, Shroff EH, Emmanuel R, et al. Nuclear factor of activated T cells balances angiogenesis activation and inhibition. J Exp Med 2004;199:1513–22.

44. Siamakpour-Reihani S, Caster J, Bandhu ND, et al. The role of calcineurin/NFAT in SFRP2 induced angiogenesis-a rationale for breast cancer treatment with the calcineurin inhibitor tacrolimus. PLoS One 2011;6:e20412.

45. Armesilla AL, Lorenzo E, Gomez del AP, et al. Vascular endothelial growth factor activates nuclear factor of activated T cells in human endothelial cells: a role for tissue factor gene expression. Mol Cell Biol 1999;19:2032–43.

46. Fontenot E, Rossi E, Mumper R, et al. A novel monoclonal antibody to secreted frizzled related protein 2 inhibits tumor growth. Mol Cancer Ther 2013;12:685–95.

47. Lawler J. Thrombospondin-1 as an endogenous inhibitor of angiogenesis and tumor growth. J Cell Mol Med 2002;6:1–12.

48. O'Reilly MS, Holmgren L, Shing Y, et al. Angiostatin: a novel angiogenesis inhibitor that mediates the suppression of metastases by a Lewis lung carcinoma. Cell 1994;79:315–28.

49. O'Reilly MS, Boehm T, Shing Y, et al. Endostatin: an endogenous inhibitor of angiogenesis and tumor growth. Cell 1997;88:277–85.

50. St Croix B, Rago C, Velculescu V, et al. Genes expressed in human tumor endothelium. Science 2000;289:1197–202.

51. Nanda A, St Croix B. Tumor endothelial markers: new targets for cancer therapy. Curr Opin Oncol 2004;16:44–9.

52. Bhati R, Patterson C, Livasy CA, et al. Molecular characterization of human breast tumor vascular cells. Am J Pathol 2008;172:1381–90.

53. Buckanovich RJ, Sasaroli D, O'brien-Jenkins A, et al. Tumor vascular proteins as biomarkers in ovarian cancer. J Clin Oncol 2007;25:852–61.

54. Stupp R, Ruegg C. Integrin inhibitors reaching the clinic. J Clin Oncol 2007;25:1637–8.

55. Brooks PC, Montgomery AM, Rosenfeld M, et al. Integrin alpha v beta 3 antagonists promote tumor regression by inducing apoptosis of angiogenic blood vessels. Cell 1994;79:1157–64.

56. Friedlander M, Brooks PC, Shaffer RW, et al. Definition of two angiogenic pathways by distinct alpha v integrins. Science 1995;270:1500–2.

57. Alghisi GC, Ruegg C. Vascular integrins in tumor angiogenesis: mediators and therapeutic targets. Endothelium 2006;13:113–35.

58. Golubovskaya VM, Cance W. Focal adhesion kinase and p53 signal transduction pathways in cancer. Front Biosci 2010;15:901–12.

59. Golubovskaya VM, Huang G, Ho B, et al. Pharmacologic blockade of FAK autophosphorylation decreases human glioblastoma tumor growth and synergizes with temozolomide. Mol Cancer Ther 2013;12:162–72.

60. Choi HS, Wang Z, Richmond W, et al. Design and synthesis of 7H-pyrrolo[2,3-d] pyrimidines as focal adhesion kinase inhibitors. Part 2. Bioorg Med Chem Lett 2006;16:2689–92.

61. Shi Q, Hjelmeland AB, Keir ST, et al. A novel low-molecular weight inhibitor of focal adhesion kinase, TAE226, inhibits glioma growth. Mol Carcinog 2007;46:488–96.

62. Slack-Davis JK, Martin KH, Tilghman RW, et al. Cellular characterization of a novel focal adhesion kinase inhibitor. J Biol Chem 2007;282:14845–52.

63. Huang Y, Simms AE, Mazur A, et al. Fibroblast activation protein-alpha promotes tumor growth and invasion of breast cancer cells through non-enzymatic functions. Clin Exp Metastasis 2011;28:567–79.
64. Lai D, Ma L, Wang F. Fibroblast activation protein regulates tumor-associated fibroblasts and epithelial ovarian cancer cells. Int J Oncol 2012;41:541–50.
65. Hofheinz RD, al-Batran SE, Hartmann F, et al. Stromal antigen targeting by a humanised monoclonal antibody: an early phase II trial of sibrotuzumab in patients with metastatic colorectal cancer. Onkologie 2003;26:44–8.
66. Liu R, Li H, Liu L, et al. Fibroblast activation protein: a potential therapeutic target in cancer. Cancer Biol Ther 2012;13:123–9.
67. Brennen WN, Isaacs JT, Denmeade SR. Rationale behind targeting fibroblast activation protein-expressing carcinoma-associated fibroblasts as a novel chemotherapeutic strategy. Mol Cancer Ther 2012;11:257–66.

Targeting the PI3-Kinase/Akt/ mTOR Signaling Pathway

Burhan Hassan, MD[a], Argun Akcakanat, MD, PhD[a],
Ashley M. Holder, MD[a], Funda Meric-Bernstam, MD[b],*

KEYWORDS

- PI3K/Akt/mTOR signaling pathway • PTEN • Cell signaling
- Molecular targeted therapy

KEY POINTS

- PI3K/Akt/mTOR pathway:
  - Essential role in cell growth, protein translation, survival, and metabolism.
  - Activation contributes to pathogenesis of many cancers.
  - Second most frequently activated pathway in cancer.
- Preclinical studies and clinical trials ongoing with inhibitors targeting PI3K, PDK-1, Akt, and mTOR.
- Rational combination therapies likely key to targeting this pathway effectively.

Cells communicate with each other and respond to environmental conditions through signal transduction pathways. In cancer, deregulation of these pathways results in altered responses, such as increased cell survival and proliferation under conditions that would usually promote cell death or cell cycle arrest. The phosphatidylinositol 3-kinase (PI3K)/Akt/mammalian Target of Rapamycin (mTOR) signaling pathway assimilates both intracellular and extracellular signals to control cell metabolism, growth, proliferation, and survival.[1] Activation of PI3K/Akt/mTOR signaling contributes to the

Funding Sources: This work was supported in part by the National Cancer Institute T32 CA009599-23 (A.M.H, F.M.B), Susan G. Komen for the Cure SAC10006 (F.M.B), Stand Up to Cancer Dream Team Translational Research Grant, a Program of the Entertainment Industry Foundation (SU2C-AACR-DT0209) (F.M.B, A.A), National Cancer Institute 5R21 CA159270, the Kleberg Center for Molecular Markers at The University of Texas MD Anderson Cancer Center, the National Center for Research Resources Grants 3UL1RR024148 and UL1TR000371 (F.M.B and A.A).
Conflict of Interest: Funda Meric-Bernstam has research funding from AstraZeneca and Celgene.
[a] Department of Surgical Oncology, The University of Texas MD Anderson Cancer Center, 6767 Bertner Avenue, Unit 0107, Houston, TX 77030, USA; [b] Department of Surgical Oncology, The University of Texas MD Anderson Cancer Center, 1400 Holcombe Boulevard, Unit 455, Houston, TX 77030, USA
* Corresponding author.
E-mail address: fmeric@mdanderson.org

Surg Oncol Clin N Am 22 (2013) 641–664
http://dx.doi.org/10.1016/j.soc.2013.06.008
1055-3207/13/$ – see front matter © 2013 Elsevier Inc. All rights reserved.

pathogenesis of many tumor types, suggesting that targeted inhibition of individual players in this pathway, including PI3K, phosphoinositide-dependent kinase-1 (PDK-1), Akt, and mTOR, is a potential strategy for cancer therapy.[1-3] This article offers an overview of the pathway, a review of the biochemical and genetic aberrations of the pathway observed in cancer, and a description of pathway inhibitors that are approved and in clinical development.

PI3K/AKT/mTOR SIGNALING PATHWAY

Initiation of signaling through the PI3K/Akt/mTOR pathway occurs through several mechanisms, all of which result in increased activation of the pathway, as commonly seen in many cancer subtypes. Once PI3K signaling is activated, it can act on a diverse array of substrates including mTOR, a master regulator of protein translation.[4] The PI3K/Akt/mTOR pathway is an attractive therapeutic target in cancer not only because it is the second most frequently altered pathway after p53,[5,6] but also because it serves as a convergence point for many stimuli. Through its downstream substrates, this pathway controls key cellular processes, such as transcription, apoptosis, cell cycle progression, and translation (**Fig. 1**).

PI3 Kinase

PI3K signaling can be activated by multiple stimuli: activated tyrosine kinase growth factor receptors; cell adhesion molecules, such as integrins and G-protein-coupled receptors (GPCR); and oncogenes, such as *Ras*. PI3K is a member of the lipid kinase family that is divided into 3 classes, each differentially activated by stimuli. Class IA isoforms are activated by tyrosine kinase receptors or *Ras*; class IB are activated by heterotrimeric G proteins or *Ras*; class II PI3K isoforms are activated through insulin receptors, growth factor receptors, and integrins; and class III kinases are thought to be constitutively active.[7] Despite all isoforms having unique lipid substrate specificity, all initiate downstream signaling by phosphorylating the D3 position of phosphatidylinositol rings at the cell membrane.

The class IA PI3K enzymes are the most relevant to activation of the PI3K/Akt/mTOR pathway, because they catalyze the generation of phosphatidylinositol-3, 4, 5-trisphosphate (PIP3) from phosphatidylinositol-4, 5-bisphosphate (PIP2). PI3K activation occurs through engagement of Src homology 2 (SH2) domains with phosphotyrosine residues on activated growth factor receptors or through direct interaction with activated *Ras*.[8,9]

PDK-1 and Akt are the crucial downstream kinases, and their activation depends on the generation of PIP3 and PIP2. These 3-phosphoinositides bind to the pleckstrin homology (PH) domains of PDK-1 and Akt to cause translocation of each kinase to the plasma membrane, where both are subsequently activated.

Akt

The phosphatase and tensin homolog deleted from chromosome 10 (PTEN), a tumor suppressor that dephosphorylates membrane phosphatidylinositols, is a key negative regulator of the effects of PI3K.[10,11] Once PDK-1 is activated by PIP3, it propagates the signal to the serine/threonine kinase Akt by phosphorylating its catalytic domain. Akt has 3 isoforms (Akt1, 2, and 3), which are structurally similar and are expressed in most tissues.[12] PDK-1 phosphorylates Akt1 in its activation loop on threonine 308 (T308), an event that alone stimulates partial activation of Akt.[13,14] Full activation of Akt1 also requires phosphorylation at serine 473 (S473) in its regulatory domain. Phosphorylation of homologous residues in Akt2 and Akt3 occurs by the same mechanism.

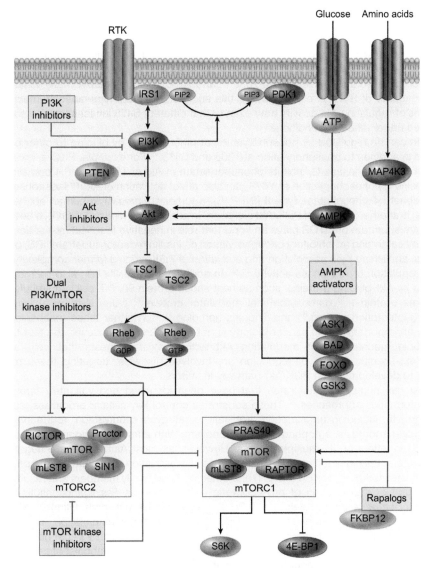

Fig. 1. Growth factors, insulin, nutrients, and energy status regulate the activation of the PI3K/Akt/mTOR signaling network. Protein synthesis, cell growth and proliferation, and metabolic functions are regulated by downstream effectors of the pathway, such as 4E-BP1 and S6K. *Boxes* indicate therapies targeting the pathway. *Arrows* represent activation and *bars* represent inhibition. 4E-BP1, eukaryotic translation initiation factor 4E-binding protein 1; AMPK, adenosine monophosphate-activated protein kinase; ASK1, apoptosis signal-regulating kinase 1; ATP, adenosine-5′-triphosphate; BAD, BCL2-associated agonist of cell death; FKBP-12, FK506-binding protein, 12 kD; FoxO, forkhead box O; GDP, guanosine diphosphate; GSK3, glycogen synthase kinase 3; GTP, guanosine-5′-triphosphate; IRS1, insulin receptor substrate 1; MAP4K3, mitogen-activated protein kinase kinase kinase kinase 3; mLST8, mTOR associated protein, LST8 homolog; mTOR, mammalian target of rapamycin; mTORC1, mTOR complex 1; mTORC2, mTOR complex 2; PDK-1, phosphoinositide-dependent kinase 1; PI3K, phosphatidylinositol 3-kinase; PIP2, phosphatidylinositol-4, 5-biphosphate; PIP3, phosphatidylinositol-3, 4, 5-triphosphate; PRAS40, proline-rich Akt1 substrate 40; PTEN, phosphatase and tensin homolog deleted from chromosome 10; Rheb, Ras homolog enriched in brain; RTK, receptor tyrosine kinase; S6K, ribosomal protein S6 kinase; SIN1, stress-activated mitogen-activated protein kinase associated protein 1; TSC1, tuberous sclerosis complex 1; TSC2, tuberous sclerosis complex 2.

Several kinases are capable of phosphorylating Akt at S473, including PDK-1,[15] integrin-linked kinase (ILK), an ILK-associated kinase,[16,17] Akt itself,[18] DNA-dependent protein kinase (DNA-PK),[19,20] and mTORC2.[21] Because many kinases are capable of S473 phosphorylation, this suggests that cell type–specific mechanisms of regulating Akt activity may exist or that different S473 kinases may be stimulated under different conditions.

Akt can be regulated by phosphorylation at other sites or by binding to other proteins in addition to phosphorylation at T308 and S473.[22] For example, PKC-z, an isoform of protein kinase C, inhibits phosphorylation of Akt at T34 in the PH domain.[23] Tyrosine (Y) phosphorylation at Y474 can also affect activation of Akt.[24] Inositol polyphosphate 4-phosphatase type II (INPP4B), a tumor suppressor in human epithelial cells, is another inhibitor of PI3K/Akt signaling. In addition, S6 kinase 1 (S6K1), a downstream substrate of mTOR plays an important role in negative feedback regulation of Akt by catalyzing an inhibitory phosphorylation on insulin receptor substrate (IRS) proteins, abolishing their association and activation of PI3K, adding further complexity to the regulation of Akt kinase activity.[25–27] In addition, Akt activity can also be modulated by Akt-binding proteins, such as heat shock protein 90,[28] T-cell leukemia/lymphoma protein-1,[29] carboxyterminal modulator protein,[30] c-Jun N-terminal kinase (JNK)-interaction protein,[31] and Tribbles homolog 3.[32] Whether these mechanisms play an important role in cancer biology is not clearly known; however, the fact that multiple mechanisms of modulating Akt activity exist suggests that cell- and context-specific modes of regulation are involved; likewise, targeting these may lead to developments in PI3K/Akt pathway inhibitors.

Akt has numerous substrates that have been identified and validated through bioinformatics approaches.[33] These substrates control key cellular processes, such as growth, including transcription, translation, cell cycle progression, and survival, including apoptosis, autophagy, and metabolism. With a few exceptions, Akt has an inhibitory effect on its multiple targets. However, as most Akt targets are negative regulators, the net result of Akt activation is cellular activation. For example, Akt phosphorylates forkhead box O1 (FoxO1) and other forkhead family members and results in inhibition of transcription of pro-apoptotic genes, such as *Fas* ligand, insulin-like growth factor binding protein 1 (*IGFBP1*), and bisindolyl maleimide (*Bim*).[34,35]Conversely, the inflammatory kinases (IKK), following Akt phosphorylation, increase NF-*k*B activity and the transcription of prosurvival genes.[36,37] Akt, by phosphorylating and inactivating proapoptotic proteins, such as BCL2-associated agonist of cell death (Bad), directly regulates apoptotic machinery through Bad's regulation and control of cytochrome c release from mitochondria. Akt is also involved in the regulation of apoptosis signal-regulating kinase-1 (ASK-1) and mitogen-activated protein kinase (MAPK) kinase, both of which are involved in stress and cytokine-induced cell death.[38–40] Akt regulates cell cycle progression through the cyclin-dependent kinase inhibitors, p21WAF1/CIP1 and p27KIP1.[36–39,41] Inhibition of glycogen synthase kinase-3beta (GSK-3beta) by Akt also stimulates cell cycle progression by stabilizing cyclin D1 expression.[40] Akt also plays an important role in protein translation by phosphorylating tuberous sclerosis complex 2 (TSC2, also called tuberin) and mTOR. Thus, Akt inhibition can result in numerous effects on cancer cells that could contribute to an antitumor response.

mTOR

mTOR is an atypical serine/threonine protein kinase that belongs to the PI3K-related kinase family. mTOR exists in 2 multiprotein complexes: mTOR complex 1 and 2 (mTORC1 and mTORC2). mTORC1 is a complex of the mTOR protein, mammalian

LST8, proline-rich Akt1 substrate 40 (PRAS40), and raptor,[42,43] whereas mTORC2 consists of a complex of mTOR, mLST8, mSIN1, protor, and rictor.[44–49] Akt activates mTOR through at least 2 mechanisms: either directly by phosphorylating mTORC1 at S2448[50] or indirectly through TSC2. TSC2 inactivation through phosphorylation by Akt results in upregulation of mTORC1 activity through a cascade of signaling molecules.[51–53] A GTPase-activating domain of TSC2 catalyzes the conversion of the Ras-like protein, Ras homolog enriched in brain (Rheb)-GTP to Rheb-GDP leading to inactivation of mTOR function.[54,55] Thus, Akt by decreasing TSC2 activity, increases levels of Rheb-GTP, which then leads to activation of mTORC1. mTORC1 plays a pivotal role in protein translation through its substrate: eukaryotic initiation factor 4E-binding protein 1 (4E-BP1) and S6 kinase 1 (S6K1). Hyperphosphorylation of 4E-BP1 by mTORC1, inhibits its binding to eukaryotic initiation factor 4E (eIF4E), thereby activating cap-dependent translation.[54] In addition to protein translation, mTORC1 regulates cell proliferation, survival, and angiogenesis by regulating eIF4E-mediated translation of Bcl-2, Bcl-xL, and vascular endothelial growth factor (VEGF).[56–58] mTORC1 also phosphorylates S6K1, which in turn leads to phosphorylation of S6 ribosomal protein, and other targets, including insulin receptor substrate 1 (IRS-1), eukaryotic initiation factor 4B (eIF4B), programmed cell death 4 (PDCD4), eukaryotic elongation factor-2 kinase (eEF2K), mTOR, and glycogen synthase kinase-3, which are implicated in cellular transformation.[56,59,60] In addition, mTORC1 regulates the transition from G1 to S phase through downregulation of cyclin D1 and c-Myc, which are required for progression through this phase of the cell cycle.[61]

In comparison with mTORC1, little is known about mTORC2 signaling. mTORC2 responds to growth factors, such as insulin, through a poorly defined mechanism that requires PI3K and ribosomes, as ribosomes are needed for mTORC2 activation and mTORC2 binds them in a PI3K-dependent fashion.[62] mTORC2 controls several members of the AGC subfamily of kinases, including Akt, serum-induced and glucocorticoid-induced protein kinase 1 (SGK1), and protein kinase C-α (PKC-α). Akt is phosphorylated by mTORC2 at its hydrophobic motif (S473), a site required for its maximal activation.[21] mTORC2 deletion, associated with defective Akt-Ser473 phosphorylation, impairs the phosphorylation of some Akt targets, including forkhead box O1/3a (FoxO1/3a), whereas other Akt targets, such as TSC2 and GSK-3beta, remain unaffected.[44,63] mTORC2 also directly activates SGK1, a kinase controlling ion transport and growth.[64] In contrast to Akt, mTORC2 deletion results in complete loss of SGK-1 activity. As SGK1 phosphorylates FoxO1/3a residues that are also phosphorylated by Akt, loss of SGK1 activity is probably responsible for the reduction in FoxO1/3a phosphorylation in mTORC2-depleted cells. PKC-α is another AGC kinase regulated by mTORC2. Along with other effectors, such as paxillin and Rho GTPases, mTORC2 plays a role in cell migration by regulating phosphorylation of PKC-α and control of the actin cytoskeleton in cell-type-specific fashion.[49,65,66]

PATHOGENESIS OF CANCER BY ABERRATIONS IN THE PI3K/AKT/mTOR PATHWAY

Aberrations in the PI3K/Akt/mTOR pathway can occur through multiple mechanisms, resulting in pathway activation and contributing to the development of many human cancer types. Genomic aberrations affecting the PI3K pathway include germline and somatic mutations, amplifications, rearrangements, methylation, overexpression, and aberrant splicing, resulting in decreased expression or function of PTEN, amplification or mutation of *PIK3CA*, or amplification of *Akt*.[67–70] The pathway is also triggered by activation of growth factor receptors, including human epidermal growth factor receptor 2 (HER2) and insulin-like growth factor receptor (IGFR), through autocrine growth loops, through mutations or overexpression of the growth factor receptors themselves, or by additional intracellular signaling molecules (**Table 1**).[10,71,72]

Loss of PTEN Function

PTEN is targeted by a number of regulatory events, many of which are aberrant in cancer, suggesting that PTEN is a critical regulator of pathway function. PTEN functions both as a protein and lipid phosphatase. Its tumor suppressive function is attributed to lipid phosphatases, as loss of lipid phosphatase function of PTEN results in increased PI3k/Akt/mTOR pathway activation. Loss of PTEN function and its activity in cancer occurs through multiple mechanisms, which include mutations, loss of heterozygosity, methylation, aberrant expression of regulatory microRNA, protein instability, and protein phosphorylation.[54] PTEN is the second most frequently mutated tumor

Table 1
Pathogenesis of cancer by aberrations in the PI3K/Akt/mTOR pathway

Genetic Aberration	Tumor Type	Frequency, %
PTEN loss	Glioblastoma	54–74
	Endometrial	32–83
	Gastric	47
	Prostate	29
	Breast	39
	Melanoma	44–57
PTEN mutation	Glioblastoma	17–44
	Endometrial	36–50
	Gastric	7
	Prostate	12
	Breast	0–4
	Melanoma	7
PIK3CA amplification	Cervix	69
	Gastric	36
	Lung (squamous)	60
	Head and neck	37
	Ovary	25
PIK3CA mutation	Breast	21–40
	Colorectal	13–32
	Glioblastoma	5–8
	Endometrial	24–32
	Hepatocellular	6–36
	Ovarian	10
	Gastric	7
Akt amplification	Head and neck	30
	Gastric	20
	Pancreas	20
	Ovary	12
Akt1 mutation	Thyroid	5
	Endometrial	4
	Breast	4
Akt2 mutation	Breast	0.8–1
Akt3 mutation	Breast	1

Abbreviations: mTOR, mammalian Target of Rapamycin; PI3K, phosphatidylinositol 3-kinase; PTEN, phosphatase and tensin homolog deleted from chromosome 10.
 Data from Refs.[74–80,85,94,95,99,102,104,105,175–211]

suppressor gene[73] and, as shown in multiple studies, it is mutated or deleted in many human cancer types, including brain, bladder, breast, prostate, and endometrial cancers.[74–85] Epigenetic silencing is seen in some tumor types, in which *PTEN* mutations are rare[86–88]; methylation of *PTEN* has been observed in 69% of non–small-cell lung cancer.[89] Methylation of the promoter region in *PTEN* is also seen in endometrial and gastric cancer.[90–92]

PIK3CA Amplification or Mutation

PI3K can be activated as a result of overexpression of structurally normal protein or from mutations in the catalytic p110 or regulatory p85 subunits. *PIK3CA* is the gene that encodes the p110a catalytic subunit and is overexpressed in 40% of ovarian[93] and 50% of cervical cancers.[94] In several cancer types, somatic mutations of this gene have been detected that result in increased kinase activity. Nonsynonymous mutations that encode the helical and kinase domains of the protein have been seen in 32% of colorectal cancers. In breast cancer, *PIK3CA* mutations have been observed in 21.4% of tumors.[10] *PIK3CA* mutations have also been detected in 27% of glioblastomas and 25% of gastric cancers.[95] Mutations in the regulatory subunit p85 have also been detected. For example, p65, a truncated version of p85, was isolated from a tumor cell line that has shown to cause constitutive activation of PI3K and cellular transformation.[96] Moreover, a constitutively active p85 mutant, as a result of SH2 domain deletion, has been detected in colon and ovarian cancers.[97] Notably, mutations, particularly in exons 9 and 20 of *PIK3CA*, encoding the helical and kinase domains respectively, activate Akt signaling in some models.[98–100] However, *PIK3CA* mutations are not always associated with PI3K/Akt/mTOR pathway activation in vitro and were not associated with PI3K/Akt/mTOR pathway activation in breast cancers in The Cancer Genome Atlas.[101] This suggests that the effect of *PIK3CA* mutations may also be cell context–dependent, and in certain cancer types, such as in breast cancer, other major regulators of the pathway may need to be considered.

Amplification of Akt

Amplification of Akt isoforms has been observed in some cancer subtypes. *Akt1* amplification has been detected in gastric carcinomas,[102] and amplification of *Akt2* has been observed in 12% of ovarian cancers, 10% to 20% of pancreatic carcinomas,[103,104] and a subset of pancreatic cancers.[93,104,105] In breast cancer, amplification of either *Akt1* or *Akt2* has been reported. *Akt3* amplification has been observed in prostate cancer and hormone-independent breast cancer cell lines.[106] E17K mutation in the Pleckstrin homology (PH) protein domain of Akt has been identified.[5,107] This mutation allows Akt1 recruitment to the cellular membrane independent of PI3K, conferring transforming activity. Sequencing based on mass spectroscopy showed mutations in *Akt1-E17K* in fewer than 2% of the breast tumors evaluated, and in none of the cell lines evaluated.[10]

Activation of Growth Factor Receptors

The PI3K/Akt/mTOR pathway is also activated by cell surface growth factor receptors. Increased activation of growth factor receptors in cancer can occur via amplification, activating mutations, or the release of growth factors that stimulate their receptors in an autocrine fashion. The ERBB family of receptor tyrosine kinases is the most important family of growth factor receptors that is frequently activated in cancer cells. ERBB includes ERBB1/epidermal growth factor receptor (EGFR), HER2, HER3, and HER4. These receptors dimerize to activate the PI3K/Akt/mTOR pathway. HER2/HER3 heterodimers are especially considered to be strong activators of the PI3K/Akt pathway,[108] whereas tumor cells with HER2 overexpression exhibit constitutive activation of the pathway.[71] HER2 receptor mutations can also lead to constitutive activation of the pathway. EGFRvIII, a truncated version of EGFR, lacks the extracellular ligand-binding domain and is constitutively active, resulting in activation of the PI3K/Akt pathway.[109] Mutations in the kinase domains of EGFR and *HER2*, but not in *HER3* or *HER4*, result in pathway activation and have also been described in lung cancer.[110–113] Aberrant autocrine growth loops can also result in increased pathway activation via activation of ERBB family members. For example, overexpression of 2 ligands of EGFR, transforming growth factor-a (TGF-a) and amphiregulin, is associated with activation of EGFR and the PI3K/Akt pathway.[114,115]

Pathway Activation in Human Dysplastic Lesions

PI3K/Akt/mTOR pathway activation is an early event in the tumorigenesis of multiple cancers, as activation of the pathway has been described in multiple preneoplastic lesions. Hamartoma syndromes such as Cowden syndrome (*PTEN* mutations), Peutz-Jeghers syndrome (*LKB1* mutations), tuberous sclerosis (*TSC1/2* mutations), neurofibromatosis (*NF1* mutations), and probably Birt-Hogg-Dubé (*BHD*/*Folliculin* mutations)[116–120] have increased activation of PI3K/Akt/mTOR pathway. Compared with a normal nevus, a dysplastic nevus has increased Akt activation,[121] whereas in case of breast tissue, phosphorylation of Akt, mTOR, and 4E-BP1 increases progressively from normal breast epithelium to hyperplasia and from abnormal hyperplasia to tumor invasion.[122]

PI3K/AKT/mTOR PATHWAY TARGETED THERAPY

The PI3K/Akt/mTOR pathway holds multiple putative therapeutic targets. Because homeostasis of the pathway is tightly regulated, it is necessary to identify mechanistic feedback loops and cross-talk with other signaling cascades to anticipate mechanisms of adaptive response and acquired resistance and thereby to develop rational combination therapies. The PI3K/Akt/mTOR pathway can be targeted by a variety of approaches, including (1) targeting kinases that lead to activation of Akt, PI3K, and PDK-1; (2) directly targeting PI3K; (3) directly inhibiting Akt; (4) targeting downstream effectors of Akt, such as mTOR; or (5) combination approaches (**Table 2**).

PI3K Kinase Inhibitors

Wortmannin, an irreversible pan-isoform PI3K inhibitor, and LY294002, a reversible inhibitor of mTOR and PI3K, are first-generation PI3K inhibitors. Although these commercially available inhibitors were effective in treating cancer xenografts by inhibiting PI3K, poor solubility and high toxicity limited their clinical application. Both Wortmannin and LY294002 failed to enter clinical trials in humans. Meanwhile, derivatives of both drugs, as well as inhibitors of the p110 catalytic subunit of PI3K and isoform specific inhibitors, are in development and even in clinical trials.

Most of the PI3K inhibitors under development target all 3 isoforms of the p110 catalytic subunit of class IA PI3K. Most of them have been effective in cancer cell lines in in vitro settings, particularly in those harboring *PIK3CA* mutations. Severe adverse effects, which were the limiting factor in cases of the Wortmannin and LY294002 drug, were not observed in newer drugs. In BKM120, mood disorders have been reported as the dose-limiting toxicity, when used in combination with endocrine therapy.[123] Prolonged stable disease has been observed even in heavily pretreated patients. The inhibitors currently in development include NVP-BKM120, BAY80-6946, PX866, XL147, and GDC-0941. Some of these inhibitors are currently

Table 2
Selected PI3K/Akt/mTOR pathway targeted agents

Molecular Targets	Agent	Company	Phase
PI3K inhibitors	BAY80-6946	Bayer (Pitssburg, PA)	I/II
	BKM120	Novartis (New York, NY)	II/III
	GDC-0941	Genentech (San Francisco, CA)	II
	PX866	Oncothyreon (Seattle, WA)	I/II
	XL147	Exelixis (San Francisco, CA)	I/II
PIK3Cd	CAL-101	Calistoga/Gilead (Seattle, WA)	III
PI3Kα	BYL719	Novartis	I/II
	MLN1117	Millennium (Cambridge, MA)	I
PDK-1 inhibitors	OSU-03012 (AR-12)	Arno (Flemington, MA)	I
	UCN-01	Keryx (New York, NY)	I/II
Dual PI3K/mTOR inhibitors	BEZ235	Novartis	I/II
	GDC-0980	Genentech	I/II
	PF-04691502	Pfizer (New York, NY)	I/II
	PF-05212384	Pfizer	I/II
	XL765	Exelixis	I/II
Multimodal inhibitor (PI3K, mTOR, DNA-PK, HIF-1α)	SF1126	Semafore (Westfield, IN)	I
Akt inhibitors	AZD5363	AstraZeneca (Wilmington, DE)	I
	MK-2206	Merck (Whitehouse Station, NJ)	I/II
	GSK2110183	GlaxoSmithKline (Philadelphia, PA)	I
	Perifosine	Keryx	III
mTOR kinase inhibitors	AZD2014	AstraZeneca	I/II
	AZD8055	AstraZeneca	I
	MLN0128	Millennium	I
	OSI-027	OSI Oncology/Astellas (Long Island, NY)	I
Rapalogs	Everolimus (RAD001)	Novartis	IV/FDA approved for breast cancer, RCC, PNET, subependymal giant cell astrocytoma (in TSC)
	Ridaforolimus (MK8669)	ARIAD (Cambridge, MA)/ MERCK	II
	Sirolimus	Wyeth/Pfizer (New York, NY)	III
	Temsirolimus (CCI779)	Wyeth/Pfizer	III/FDA approved for RCC

Abbreviations: FDA, Food and Drug Administration; mTOR, mammalian Target of Rapamycin; PI3K, phosphatidylinositol 3-kinase; PNET, pancreatic neuroendocrine tumor; RCC, renal cell carcinoma; TSC, tuberous sclerosis.

Data from National Institutes of Health. Available at: http://clinicaltrials.gov/. Accessed March 13, 2013.

tested in association with chemotherapy (PX866 and docetaxel; XL147 or GDC-0941 and carboplatin/paclitaxel), with RTK inhibitors (XL147 and erlotinib; NVP-BKM120 and trastuzumab), and with other new agents (GDC-0941 and GDC-0973, an oral MAPK inhibitor).[124]

PI3K Isoform-Specific Inhibitors

To limit unintended off-target effects, isoform-specific inhibitors of PI3K have also been developed. CAL-101, BYL719, and MLN1117 (formerly INK1117) are a few examples of such inhibitors. They have been shown to be more effective in cancer cells with PI3K activation than in PTEN-deficient tumors. CAL-101 is an isoform-specific inhibitor with high selectivity for the PI3Kδ isoform and low nanomolar half maximal inhibitory concentration (IC50). It is available in oral formulation and has displayed an acceptable safety profile and promising clinical activity in patients with advanced chronic lymphocytic leukemia,[125] mantle cell lymphoma, and indolent non-Hodgkin lymphoma (NHL). In B-cell malignancies, CAL-101, in association with anti-CD20 monoclonal antibodies and/or bendamustine, has shown promising results and acceptable toxicity in phase I clinical trials.[126] MLN1117 is a potent and orally efficacious PI3Kα-selective kinase inhibitor currently in clinical development. BYL719, another PI3Kα-selective kinase inhibitor, has shown promising preliminary clinical activity as a single agent in patients with *PIK3CA* mutant ER+ metastatic breast cancer.[127]

PDK-1 Inhibitors

To be completely active, Akt requires phosphorylation at 2 sites: one in its catalytic domain (T308) and one in its regulatory domain (S473). PDK-1, once activated by the products of PI3K, PIP2, and PIP3, phosphorylates Akt at its T308 residue.[34,128] Because PDK-1 has a central role in the activation of the pathway, it is possible that PDK-1 inhibitors could be an effective therapeutic option in cancer types that rely on this pathway. PDK-1 has been shown to be inhibited by 2 groups of drugs: staurosporine and its analogs and celecoxib and its analogs.

Staurosporine, a broad-spectrum kinase inhibitor, was isolated from *Streptomyces staurosporeus* in an attempt to identify inhibitors of PKC. Derivatives of staurosporine were developed, as its activity was limited to in vitro settings. 7-Hydroxystaurosporine (UCN-01) is a PKC inhibitor that inhibits a variety of kinases, including cdc2/CDK1,[129] PDK-1,[130] and PKC.[131] UCN-01 has shown antiproliferative effects in head and neck cancer cells.[132] Clinical trials have shown promising results for UCN-01, with preliminary evidence of antitumor activity in melanoma and large-cell lymphoma.[133] Despite limited promising results in clinical trials, the nonspecific nature of UCN-01 and its insufficient efficacy as a single agent[134] make it less attractive as a targeted, single-agent therapy.

Celecoxib derivatives, OSU-03012 and OSU-0301, are another group of drugs that are PDK-1 inhibitors, with IC50s in the millimolar range in 60 different human cancer cell lines. Their biologic efficacy stems from their ability to delay G2/M cell cycle progression and induce apoptosis independently of PDK-1 inhibition.[135] Although celecoxib derivatives may be very effective in growth inhibition and apoptosis, their cyclooxygenase-independent mechanism of action likely involves the inhibition of other pathways in addition to PDK-1 inhibition.

Akt Inhibitors

Inhibition of Akt by biochemical and genetic means induces apoptosis and increases a cancer's responsiveness to chemotherapy or radiation in both in vitro and in vivo settings. Thus, the rationale to target Akt in cancer is strong. Lipid-based Akt inhibitors, small molecules that target the ATP-binding domain of Akt or the PH domain of Akt, or peptides that inhibit Akt function, are a few of the approaches used in the development of Akt inhibitors.

Lipid-Based Akt Inhibitors

The alkylphospholipid (ALK) perifosine bears structural similarity to ceramide: a sphingomyelin derivative that has been shown to inhibit the Akt pathway.[136] Perifosine inhibits Akt translocation and activity.[137] Perifosine has shown a broad spectrum of activity in melanoma, lung, prostate, colon, and breast cancer cells in vitro.[138] In a phase I clinical trial, gastrointestinal toxicity proved to be dose-limiting.[138] In another clinical trial, a loading dose/maintenance dose schedule was used that limited the side effects observed earlier. Perifosine is currently in Phase II/III clinical trials. Other lipid-based Akt inhibitors, such as Phosphatidylinositol Ether Lipid Analogs (PIAs) and d-3-deoxy-phosphatidyl-myoinositol-1-[(R)-2-methoxy-3-octadecyloxyropyl   hydrogen phosphate] (PX-316), are in the early phases of development.

MK-2206 is a novel, selective allosteric inhibitor of Akt. MK-2206 inhibits Akt signaling and cell cycle progression and increases apoptosis in a dose-dependent manner. MK-2206 sensitivity was significantly greater in cell lines with *PTEN* or *PIK3CA* mutation; however, not all cell lines with PI3K pathway aberrations were sensitive. MK-2206 had a growth-inhibitory effect in vivo and enhanced the antitumor activity of paclitaxel.[98] Phase II clinical trials of MK-2206 have begun for the treatment of a variety of tumor types, including endometrial cancer, breast cancer, and colon cancer.

AZD5363 is a potent inhibitor of all isoforms of Akt. Cell lines with *PIK3CA* mutation, *PTEN* mutation, or *HER2* amplification, without coincident *RAS* mutation, showed the highest frequency of response to AZD5363 in vitro.[139] This drug is currently in phase I clinical trials for advanced metastatic breast cancer, prostate cancer, and solid tumors.

Isoform-Specific Akt Inhibitors

High-throughput kinase activity screen has helped to identify isoform-specific Akt inhibitors. Akti1 inhibits Akt1; Akti2 inhibits Akt2; and Akti1,2 inhibits both Akt1 and Akt2 in vitro with IC50s in the micromolar range.[140,141] These inhibitors act through a PH domain-dependent mechanism that prevents phosphorylation of the enzyme. Treatment with either Akti1 or Akti2 sensitizes cancer cells to chemotherapy-induced cell death, but inhibition of both isoforms by Akti1,2 was necessary for maximum sensitization.[142]

Allosteric mTOR Inhibitors

mTOR inhibitors are the best-characterized PI3K/Akt/mTOR pathway inhibitors, as they target the most distal actor. In 1975, rapamycin, the prototypic mTOR inhibitor, was discovered as a potent antifungicide.[143,144] Originally, it was approved by the Food and Drug Administration (FDA) to prevent allograft rejection, but later, its potential as an antiproliferative drug in cancer cell lines was discovered.[145–147]

Temsirolimus, everolimus, and ridaforolimus are rapamycin analogs that have been explicitly designed as cancer drugs. These inhibitors bind to the FK506-binding protein, FKBP-12, which then binds to and inhibits mTOR, resulting in activation of mTOR signaling. Rapamycin, temsirolimus, ridaforolimus, and everolimus have potent activity as single agents and in combination with cytotoxic chemotherapy in vitro. Rapalogs promote cell cycle arrest in some cell lines, whereas it promotes apoptosis in others by sensitizing tumor cells to DNA damage–induced apoptosis through inhibition of p21 translation. They also sensitize cancer cells to chemotherapeutic agents, including cisplatin, paclitaxel, and camptothecin.[147–150] Rapamycin analogs have been FDA-approved for the treatment of pancreatic neuroendocrine tumors, renal cell carcinoma, breast cancer (in combination with exemestane) and subependymal giant cell astrocytoma associated with tuberous sclerosis; they have also shown promise in clinical trials in other tumor types, such as mesothelioma and endometrial cancer.[54,151]

Several trials have examined the efficacy of rapamycin analogs in combination with other anticancer agents in addition to being investigated as single agents. For example, a recent phase I/II trial examined the effect of everolimus administration in combination with imatinib mesylate in patients with gastrointestinal stromal tumors. Patients whose tumors were refractory to imatinib alone were responsive to combination therapy.[152] This result provides evidence that, in cancer types that exhibit chemotherapeutic resistance, the use of signal transduction inhibitors in combination may be an effective treatment strategy. There are other clinical trials going on that are looking at the therapeutic benefit of combining temsirolimus with other signal transduction inhibitors in solid tumors. Because the PI3K/Akt/mTOR pathway is one of the most frequently activated pathways in cancer cells, targeting it seems natural. However, the possibility of feedback activation of Akt due to mTOR inhibition suggests that combination therapy or a newer class of drugs, such as mTOR kinase inhibitors, might be more effective than rapalogs alone.

mTOR Kinase Inhibitors

mTOR kinase inhibitors are ATP-competitive inhibitors of mTOR, including Torin1, PP242, PP30, Ku-0063794, AZD8055, AZD2014, and MLN0128. These drugs share remarkable selectivity toward mTOR with IC50 values in the low nanomolar range.[153–156] mTOR kinase inhibitors are potent inhibitors of both mTORC1 and mTORC2. They effectively inhibit both protein translation and S473 Akt phosphorylation via direct inhibition of mTORC2. PP242 has been observed to cause cell death in models of acute leukemia harboring the Philadelphia chromosome (Ph) translocation and to delay leukemia onset in vivo.[157] mTOR kinase inhibitors induce cell death in several hematologic malignancies, such as acute myeloid leukemia[158,159] and T-lineage acute lymphoblastic leukemia,[160] and in a broad range of in vitro cancer settings.[154,161] Some of these second-generation mTOR inhibitors are currently in phase I/II trials (OSI-027, MLN0128, and AZD2014). The mTOR kinase inhibitors strongly inhibit phosphorylation of Akt at S473 residue but with, however, a biphasic regulation of Akt, characterized by a rapid but only transient dephosphorylation of Akt T308.[162] Moreover, the loss of mTORC1-mediated feedback on PI3K might activate PIP3-dependant PI3K effectors other than Akt. These potential mechanisms of resistance have encouraged the development of dual PI3K/mTOR kinase inhibitors.

PI3K/mTOR Dual Inhibitors

The PI3K/mTOR dual inhibitors hypothetically have the potential to be more effective than rapamycin, yet may have more toxicity. The dual pathway inhibitors are more efficient in blocking Akt activity than pure ATP-competitive mTOR inhibitors. Akt is more active when it is phosphorylated at both T308 and S473 residues. PP242 (pure mTOR inhibitor) has no effect on Akt T308 phosphorylation, Akt1 activity, or phosphorylation of the Akt substrate GSK-3beta in human platelets.[163] PI-103 and NVP-BEZ235 are 2 dual PI3K/mTOR inhibitors that have been tested in a wide range of tumors in preclinical studies.[164–169] They efficiently inhibit Akt phosphorylation and both T308 and S473 residues. NVP-BEZ235 and other dual inhibitors (GDC-0980, XL675) have demonstrated biologic activity in clinical trials. Side effects included nausea, vomiting, diarrhea, hyperglycemia, and loss of appetite. Furthermore, the concomitant use of rapalogs and dual PI3K/mTOR inhibitors at low concentrations has demonstrated decreased toxicity along with synergistic treatment effects in vitro and in xenograft models.[170–172]

SF116, a multimodal inhibitor (PI3K, mTOR, DNA-PK, PIM1, and HIF-1α) has been developed as an RGDS-conjugated LY294002 prodrug with site selectivity. SF116, a multimodal inhibitor (PI3K, mTOR, DNA-PK, PIM1, and HIF-1α) has been developed as a peptide-coated LY294002 prodrug with site selectivity, which binds to specific integrins.[173] SF1126 has shown significant disease stabilization in phase I study[174] and is now being tested in B-cell malignancies.

SUMMARY

The PI3K/Akt/mTOR pathway plays a central role in cell growth, protein translation, survival, and metabolism. Activation of PI3K/Akt/mTOR signaling contributes to the pathogenesis of many tumor types. Because it is the second most frequently activated signaling pathway, there is intense interest in targeting this pathway for cancer therapy. Numerous preclinical studies and clinical trials are ongoing with inhibitors targeting PI3K, PDK-1, Akt, and mTOR. Although the results of these trials are eagerly anticipated, it is likely that the optimal activity of PI3K/Akt/mTOR pathway inhibitors will be manifested only through the development, evaluation, and implementation of rational combination therapies based on biomarkers of response.

REFERENCES

1. Meric-Bernstam F, Akcakanat A, Chen HQ, et al. PIK3CA/PTEN mutations and Akt activation as markers of sensitivity to allosteric mTOR inhibitors. Clin Cancer Res 2012;18:1777–89.
2. Vivanco I, Sawyers CL. The phosphatidylinositol 3-kinase-AKT pathway in human cancer. Nat Rev Cancer 2002;2:489–501.
3. Guertin DA, Sabatini DM. Defining the role of mTOR in cancer. Cancer Cell 2007;12:9–22.
4. Laplante M, Sabatini DM. mTOR signaling in growth control and disease. Cell 2012;149:274–93.
5. Brugge J, Hung MC, Mills GB. A new mutational aktivation in the PI3K pathway. Cancer Cell 2007;12:104–7.
6. Agarwal R, Carey M, Hennessy B, et al. PI3K pathway-directed therapeutic strategies in cancer. Curr Opin Investig Drugs 2010;11:615–28.
7. Vanhaesebroeck B, Leevers SJ, Panayotou G, et al. Phosphoinositide 3-kinases: a conserved family of signal transducers. Trends Biochem Sci 1997;22:267–72.
8. Vanhaesebroeck B, Alessi DR. The PI3K-PDK1 connection: more than just a road to PKB. Biochem J 2000;346:561–76.
9. Vanhaesebroeck B, Waterfield MD. Signaling by distinct classes of phosphoinositide 3-kinases. Exp Cell Res 1999;253:239–54.
10. Stemke-Hale K, Gonzalez-Angulo AM, Lluch A, et al. Integrative genomic and proteomic analysis of PIK3CA, PTEN, and AKT mutations in breast cancer. Cancer Res 2008;68:6084–91.
11. Stocker H, Andjelkovic M, Oldham S, et al. Living with lethal PIP3 levels: viability of flies lacking PTEN restored by a PH domain mutation in Akt/PKB. Science 2002;295:2088–91.

12. Zinda MJ, Johnson MA, Paul JD, et al. AKT-1, -2, and-3 are expressed in both normal and tumor tissues of the lung, breast, prostate, and colon. Clin Cancer Res 2001;7:2475–9.
13. Alessi DR, Saito Y, Campbell DG, et al. Identification of the sites in MAP kinase kinase-1 phosphorylated by p74(raf-1). EMBO J 1994;13:1610–9.
14. Andjelkovic M, Alessi DR, Meier R, et al. Role of translocation in the activation and function of protein kinase B. J Biol Chem 1997;272:31515–24.
15. Balendran A, Currie R, Armstrong CG, et al. Evidence that 3-phosphoinositide-dependent protein kinase-1 mediates phosphorylation of p70 56 kinase in vivo at Thr-412 as well as Thr-252. J Biol Chem 1999;274:37400–6.
16. Lynch DK, Ellis CA, Edwards PA, et al. Integrin-linked kinase regulates phosphorylation of serine 473 of protein kinase B by an indirect mechanism. Oncogene 1999;18:8024–32.
17. Delcommenne M, Tan C, Gray V, et al. Phosphoinositide-3-OH kinase-dependent regulation of glycogen synthase kinase 3 and protein kinase B/AKT by the integrin-linked kinase. Proc Natl Acad Sci U S A 1998;95:11211–6.
18. Toker A, Newton AC. Akt/protein kinase B is regulated by autophosphorylation at the hypothetical PDK-2 site. J Biol Chem 2000;275:8271–4.
19. Hill MM, Feng JH, Hemmings BA. Identification of a plasma membrane raft-associated PKB Ser473 kinase activity that is distinct from ILK and PDK1. Curr Biol 2002;12:1251–5.
20. Feng JH, Park J, Cron P, et al. Identification of a PKB/Akt hydrophobic motif Ser-473 kinase as DNA-dependent protein kinase. J Biol Chem 2004;279:41189–96.
21. Sarbassov DD, Guertin DA, Ali SM, et al. Phosphorylation and regulation of Akt/PKB by the rictor-mTOR complex. Science 2005;307:1098–101.
22. Brazil DP, Park J, Hemmings BA. PKB binding proteins: getting in on the Akt. Cell 2002;111:293–303.
23. Powell DJ, Hajduch E, Kular G, et al. Ceramide disables 3-phosphoinositide binding to the pleckstrin homology domain of protein kinase B (PKB)/Akt by a PKCzeta-dependent mechanism. Mol Cell Biol 2003;23:7794–808.
24. Conus NM, Hannan KM, Cristiano BE, et al. Direct identification of tyrosine 474 as a regulatory phosphorylation site for the Akt protein kinase. J Biol Chem 2002;277:38021–8.
25. Harrington LS, Findlay GM, Gray A, et al. The TSC1-2 tumor suppressor controls insulin-PI3K signaling via regulation of IRS proteins. J Cell Biol 2004;166:213–23.
26. Shah OJ, Wang ZY, Hunter T. Inappropriate activation of the TSC/Rheb/mTOR/S6K cassette induces IRS1/2 depletion, insulin resistance, and cell survival deficiencies. Curr Biol 2004;14:1650–6.
27. Tremblay F, Brule S, Um SH, et al. Identification of IRS-1 Ser-1101 as a target of S6K1 in nutrient- and obesity-induced insulin resistance. Proc Natl Acad Sci U S A 2007;104:14056–61.
28. Basso AD, Solit DB, Chiosis G, et al. Akt forms an intracellular complex with heat shock protein 90 (Hsp90) and Cdc37 and is destabilized by inhibitors of Hsp90 function. J Biol Chem 2002;277:39858–66.
29. Pekarsky Y, Koval A, Hallas C, et al. Tcl1 enhances Akt kinase activity and mediates its nuclear translocation. Proc Natl Acad Sci U S A 2000;97:3028–33.
30. Maira SM, Galetic I, Brazil DP, et al. Carboxyl-terminal modulator protein (CTMP), a negative regulator of PKB/Akt and v-Akt at the plasma membrane. Science 2001;294:374–80.

31. Kim AH, Sasaki T, Chao MV. JNK-interacting protein 1 promotes Akt1 activation. J Biol Chem 2003;278:29830–6.
32. Du KY, Herzig S, Kulkarni RN, et al. TRB3: a tribbles homolog that inhibits Akt/PKB activation by insulin in liver. Science 2003;300:1574–7.
33. Obenauer JC, Cantley LC, Yaffe MB. Scansite 2.0: proteome-wide prediction of cell signaling interactions using short sequence motifs. Nucleic Acids Res 2003; 31:3635–41.
34. Datta SR, Brunet A, Greenberg ME. Cellular survival: a play in three Akts. Genes Dev 1999;13:2905–27.
35. Nicholson KM, Anderson NG. The protein kinase B/Akt signalling pathway in human malignancy. Cell Signal 2002;14:381–95.
36. Ozes ON, Mayo LD, Gustin JA, et al. NF-kappa B activation by tumour necrosis factor requires the Akt serine-threonine kinase. Nature 1999;401:82–5.
37. Romashkova JA, Makarov SS. NF-kappaB is a target of AKT in anti-apoptotic PDGF signalling. Nature 1999;401:86–90.
38. Shin I, Yakes FM, Rojo F, et al. PKB/Akt mediates cell-cycle progression by phosphorylation of p27(Kip1) at threonine 157 and modulation of its cellular localization. Nat Med 2002;8:1145–52.
39. Zhou BP. Cytoplasmic localization of p21(Cip1/WAF1) by Akt-induced phosphorylation in HER-2/neu-overexpressing cells. Nat Cell Biol 2001;3: 245–52.
40. Diehl JA, Cheng MG, Roussel MF, et al. Glycogen synthase kinase 3 beta regulates cyclin D1 proteolysis and subcellular localization. Genes Dev 1998;12: 3499–511.
41. Liang J, Zubovitz J, Petrocelli T, et al. PKB/Akt phosphorylates p27, impairs nuclear import of p27 and opposes p27-mediated G1 arrest. Nat Med 2002;8: 1153–60.
42. Wullschleger S, Loewith R, Hall MN. TOR signaling in growth and metabolism. Cell 2006;124:471–84.
43. Wang L, Harris TE, Lawrence JC. Regulation of proline-rich Akt substrate of 40 kDa (PRAS40) function by mammalian target of rapamycin complex 1 (mTORC1)-mediated phosphorylation. J Biol Chem 2008;283:15619–27.
44. Jacinto E, Facchinetti V, Liu D, et al. SIN1/MIP1 maintains rictor-mTOR complex integrity and regulates Akt phosphorylation and substrate specificity. Cell 2006; 127:125–37.
45. Yang Q, Inoki K, Ikenoue T, et al. Identification of Sin1 as an essential TORC2 component required for complex formation and kinase activity. Genes Dev 2006;20:2820–32.
46. Pearce LR, Huang X, Boudeau J, et al. Identification of Protor as a novel Rictor-binding component of mTOR complex-2. Biochem J 2007;405:513–22.
47. Frias MA, Thoreen CC, Jaffe JD, et al. mSin1 is necessary for Akt/PKB phosphorylation, and its isoforms define three distinct mTORC2s. Curr Biol 2006; 16:1865–70.
48. Martin J, Masri J, Bernath A, et al. Hsp70 associates with Rictor and is required for mTORC2 formation and activity. Biochem Biophys Res Commun 2008;372: 578–83.
49. Sarbassov DD, Ali SM, Kim DH, et al. Rictor, a novel binding partner of mTOR, defines a rapamycin-insensitive and raptor-independent pathway that regulates the cytoskeleton. Curr Biol 2004;14:1296–302.
50. Nave BT, Ouwens DM, Withers DJ, et al. Mammalian target of rapamycin is a direct target for protein kinase B: identification of a convergence point for

opposing effects of insulin and amino-acid deficiency on protein translation. Biochem J 1999;344:427–31.

51. Inoki K, Li Y, Zhu TQ, et al. TSC2 is phosphorylated and inhibited by Akt and suppresses mTOR signalling. Nat Cell Biol 2002;4:648–57.

52. Manning BD, Tee AR, Logsdon MN, et al. Identification of the tuberous sclerosis complex-2 tumor suppressor gene product tuberin as a target of the phosphoinositide 3-Kinase/Akt pathway. Mol Cell 2002;10:151–62.

53. Potter CJ, Pedraza LG, Xu T. Akt regulates growth by directly phosphorylating Tsc2. Nat Cell Biol 2002;4:658–65.

54. Meric-Bernstam F, Gonzalez-Angulo AM. Targeting the mTOR signaling network for cancer therapy. J Clin Oncol 2009;27:2278–87.

55. Garami A, Zwartkruis FJ, Nobukuni T, et al. Insulin activation of Rheb, a mediator of mTOR/S6K/4E-BP signaling, is inhibited by TSC1 and 2. Mol Cell 2003;11: 1457–66.

56. De Benedetti A, Graff JR. eIF-4E expression and its role in malignancies and metastases. Oncogene 2004;23:3189–99.

57. Soni A, Akcakanat A, Singh G, et al. eIF4E knockdown decreases breast cancer cell growth without activating Akt signaling. Mol Cancer Ther 2008;7:1782–8.

58. Culjkovic B, Tan K, Orolicki S, et al. The eIF4E RNA regulon promotes the Akt signaling pathway. J Cell Biol 2008;181:51–63.

59. Jastrzebski K, Hannan KM, Tchoubrieva EB, et al. Coordinate regulation of ribosome biogenesis and function by the ribosomal protein S6 kinase, a key mediator of mTOR function. Growth Factors 2007;25:209–26.

60. Barlund M, Forozan F, Kononen J, et al. Detecting activation of ribosomal protein S6 kinase by complementary DNA and tissue microarray analysis. J Natl Cancer Inst 2000;92:1252–9.

61. Sawyers CL. Will mTOR inhibitors make it as cancer drugs? Cancer Cell 2003;4: 343–8.

62. Zinzalla V, Stracka D, Oppliger W, et al. Activation of mTORC2 by association with the ribosome. Cell 2011;144:757–68.

63. Guertin DA, Stevens DM, Thoreen CC, et al. Ablation in mice of the mTORC components raptor, rictor, or mLST8 reveals that mTORC2 is required for signaling to Akt-FOXO and PKC alpha but not S6K1. Dev Cell 2006;11:859–71.

64. Garcia-Martinez JM, Alessi DR. mTOR complex 2 (mTORC2) controls hydrophobic motif phosphorylation and activation of serum- and glucocorticoid-induced protein kinase 1 (SGK1). Biochem J 2008;416:375–85.

65. Jacinto E, Loewith R, Schmidt A, et al. Mammalian TOR complex 2 controls the actin cytoskeleton and is rapamycin insensitive. Nat Cell Biol 2004;6:1122–8.

66. Hernandez-Negrete I, Carretero-Ortega J, Rosenfeldt H, et al. P-Rex1 links mammalian target of rapamycin signaling to Rac activation and cell migration. J Biol Chem 2007;282:23708–15.

67. Hennessy BT, Smith DL, Ram PT, et al. Exploiting the PI3K/AKT pathway for cancer drug discovery. Nat Rev Drug Discov 2005;4:988–1004.

68. Karni R, de Stanchina E, Lowe SW, et al. The gene encoding the splicing factor SF2/ASF is a proto-oncogene. Nat Struct Mol Biol 2007;14:185–93.

69. Kumar R, Hung NC. Signaling intricacies take center stage in cancer cells. Cancer Res 2005;65:2511–5.

70. Manning BD, Cantley LC. AKT/PKB signaling: navigating downstream. Cell 2007;129:1261–74.

71. Zhou BP, Hu MC, Miller SA, et al. HER-2/neu blocks tumor necrosis factor-induced apoptosis via the Akt/NF-kappa B pathway. J Biol Chem 2000;275:8027–31.

72. Cui XJ, Zhang P, Deng WL, et al. Insulin-like growth factor-I inhibits progesterone receptor expression in breast cancer cells via the phosphatidylinositol 3-kinase/akt/mammalian target of rapamycin pathway: progesterone receptor as a potential indicator of growth factor activity in breast cancer. Mol Endocrinol 2003;17:575–88.
73. Stokoe D. PTEN. Curr Biol 2001;11:R502.
74. Wang SI, Puc J, Li J, et al. Somatic mutations of PTEN in glioblastoma multiforme. Cancer Res 1997;57:4183–6.
75. Chiariello E, Roz L, Albarosa R, et al. PTEN/MMAC1 mutations in primary glioblastomas and short-term cultures of malignant gliomas. Oncogene 1998;16: 541–5.
76. Feilotter HE, Coulon V, McVeigh JL, et al. Analysis of the 10q23 chromosomal region and the PTEN gene in human sporadic breast carcinoma. Br J Cancer 1999;79:718–23.
77. Freihoff D, Kempe A, Beste B, et al. Exclusion of a major role for the PTEN tumour-suppressor gene in breast carcinomas. Br J Cancer 1999;79:754–8.
78. Smith JS, Tachibana I, Passe SM, et al. PTEN mutation, EGFR amplification, and outcome in patients with anaplastic astrocytoma and glioblastoma multiforme. J Natl Cancer Inst 2001;93:1246–56.
79. McMenamin ME, Soung P, Perera S, et al. Loss of PTEN expression in paraffin-embedded primary prostate cancer correlates with high Gleason score and advanced stage. Cancer Res 1999;59:4291–6.
80. Rasheed BK, Stenzel TT, McLendon RE, et al. PTEN gene mutations are seen in high-grade but not in low-grade gliomas. Cancer Res 1997;57:4187–90.
81. Ali IU, Schriml LM, Dean M. Mutational spectra of PTEN/MMAC1 gene: a tumor suppressor with lipid phosphatase activity. J Natl Cancer Inst 1999;91: 1922–32.
82. Aveyard JS, Skilleter A, Habuchi T, et al. Somatic mutation of PTEN in bladder carcinoma. Br J Cancer 1999;80:904–8.
83. Dahia PL. PTEN, a unique tumor suppressor gene. Endocr Relat Cancer 2000;7: 115–29.
84. Dreher T, Zentgraf H, Abel U, et al. Reduction of PTEN and p27(kip1) expression correlates with tumor grade in prostate cancer. Analysis in radical prostatectomy specimens and needle biopsies. Virchows Arch 2004;444:509–17.
85. Li J, Yen C, Liaw D, et al. PTEN, a putative protein tyrosine phosphatase gene mutated in human brain, breast, and prostate cancer. Science 1997;275: 1943–7.
86. Yokomizo A, Tindall DJ, Drabkin H, et al. PTEN/MMAC1 mutations identified in small cell, but not in non-small cell lung cancers. Oncogene 1998;17:475–9.
87. Forgacs E, Biesterveld EJ, Sekido Y, et al. Mutation analysis of the PTEN/ MMAC1 gene in lung cancer. Oncogene 1998;17:1557–65.
88. Kohno T, Takahashi M, Manda R, et al. Inactivation of the PTEN/MMACI/TEPI gene in human lung cancers. Genes Chromosomes Cancer 1998;22:152–6.
89. Soria JC, Lee HY, Lee JI, et al. Lack of PTEN expression in non-small cell lung cancer could be related to promoter methylation. Clin Cancer Res 2002;8: 1178–84.
90. Salvesen HB, MacDonald N, Ryan A, et al. PTEN methylation is associated with advanced stage and microsatellite instability in endometrial carcinoma. Int J Cancer 2001;91:22–6.
91. Kang YH, Lee HS, Kim WH. Promoter methylation and silencing of PTEN in gastric carcinoma. Lab Invest 2002;82:285–91.

92. Tamura G. Promoter methylation status of tumor suppressor and tumor-related genes in neoplastic and non-neoplastic gastric epithelia. Histol Histopathol 2004;19:221–8.
93. Shayesteh L, Lu YL, Kuo WL, et al. PIK3CA is implicated as an oncogene in ovarian cancer. Nat Genet 1999;21:99–102.
94. Ma YY, Wei SJ, Lin YC, et al. PIK3CA as an oncogene in cervical cancer. Oncogene 2000;19:2739–44.
95. Samuels Y, Wang ZH, Bardelli A, et al. High frequency of mutations of the PIK3CA gene in human cancers. Science 2004;304:554.
96. Jimenez C, Jones DR, Rodriguez-Viciana P, et al. Identification and characterization of a new oncogene derived from the regulatory subunit of phosphoinositide 3-kinase. EMBO J 1998;17:743–53.
97. Philp AJ, Campbell IG, Leet C, et al. The phosphatidylinositol 3 '-kinase p85 alpha gene is an oncogene in human ovarian and colon tumors. Cancer Res 2001;61:7426–9.
98. Sangai T, Akcakanat A, Chen HQ, et al. Biomarkers of response to Akt inhibitor MK-2206 in breast cancer. Clin Cancer Res 2012;18:5816–28.
99. Bachman KE, Argani P, Samuels Y, et al. The PIK3CA gene is mutated with high frequency in human breast cancers. Cancer Biol Ther 2004;3:772–5.
100. Kang SY, Bader AG, Vogt PK. Phosphatidylinositol 3-kinase mutations identified in human cancer are oncogenic. Proc Natl Acad Sci U S A 2005;102:802–7.
101. Koboldt DC, Fulton RS, McLellan MD, et al. Comprehensive molecular portraits of human breast tumours. Nature 2012;490:61–70.
102. Staal SP. Molecular-cloning of the Akt oncogene and its human homologs Akt1 and Akt2-amplification of Akt1 in a primary human gastric adenocarcinoma. Proc Natl Acad Sci U S A 1987;84:5034–7.
103. Cheng JQ, Ruggeri B, Klein WM, et al. Amplification of AKT2 in human pancreatic cancer cells and inhibition of ATK2 expression and tumorigenicity by antisense RNA. Proc Natl Acad Sci U S A 1996;93:3636–41.
104. Ruggeri BA, Huang LY, Wood M, et al. Amplification and overexpression of the AKT2 oncogene in a subset of human pancreatic ductal adenocarcinomas. Mol Carcinog 1998;21:81–6.
105. Bellacosa A, Defeo D, Godwin AK, et al. Molecular alterations of the Akt2 oncogene in ovarian and breast carcinomas. Int J Cancer 1995;64:280–5.
106. Nakatani K, Thompson DA, Barthel A, et al. Up-regulation of Akt3 in estrogen receptor-deficient breast cancers and androgen-independent prostate cancer lines. J Biol Chem 1999;274:21528–32.
107. Carpten JD, Faber AL, Horn C, et al. A transforming mutation in the pleckstrin homology domain of AKT1 in cancer. Nature 2007;448:439–44.
108. Prigent SA, Gullick WJ. Identification of c-erbB-3 binding-sites for phosphatidylinositol 3'-kinase and SHC using an EGF receptor c-erbB-3 chimera. EMBO J 1994;13:2831–41.
109. Moscatello DK, Holgado-Madruga M, Emlet DR, et al. Constitutive activation of phosphatidylinositol 3-kinase by a naturally occurring mutant epidermal growth factor receptor. J Biol Chem 1998;273:200–6.
110. Shigematsu H, Takahashi T, Nomura M, et al. Somatic mutations of the HER2 kinase domain in lung adenocarcinomas. Cancer Res 2005;65:1642–6.
111. Pao W, Miller V, Zakowski M, et al. EGF receptor gene mutations are common in lung cancers from "never smokers" and are associated with sensitivity of tumors to gefitinib and erlotinib. Proc Natl Acad Sci U S A 2004;101:13306–11.

112. Paez JG, Janne PA, Lee JC, et al. EGFR mutations in lung cancer: correlation with clinical response to gefitinib therapy. Science 2004;304:1497–500.
113. Lynch TJ, Bell DW, Sordella R, et al. Activating mutations in the epidermal growth factor receptor underlying responsiveness of non-small-cell lung cancer to gefitinib. N Engl J Med 2004;350:2129–39.
114. Rusch V, Baselga J, Cordoncardo C, et al. Differential expression of the epidermal growth-factor receptor and its ligands in primary nonsmall cell lung cancers and adjacent benign lung. Cancer Res 1993;53:2379–85.
115. Tateishi M, Ishida T, Mitsudomi T, et al. Immunohistochemical evidence of autocrine growth-factors in adenocarcinoma of the human lung. Cancer Res 1990;50:7077–80.
116. Liaw D, Marsh DJ, Li J, et al. Germline mutations of the PTEN gene in Cowden disease, an inherited breast and thyroid cancer syndrome. Nat Genet 1997;16:64–7.
117. Johannessen CM, Reczek EE, James MF, et al. The NF1 tumor suppressor critically regulates TSC2 and mTOR. Proc Natl Acad Sci U S A 2005;102:8573–8.
118. Kamm MA. The small intestine and colon: scintigraphic quantitation of motility in health and disease. Eur J Nucl Med 1992;19:902–12.
119. Shackelford DB, Shaw RJ. The LKB1-AMPK pathway: metabolism and growth control in tumour suppression. Nat Rev Cancer 2009;9:563–75.
120. Hartman TR, Nicolas E, Klein-Szanto A, et al. The role of the Birt-Hogg-Dube protein in mTOR activation and renal tumorigenesis. Oncogene 2009;28:1594–604.
121. Dai DL, Martinka M, Li G. Prognostic significance of activated Akt expression in melanoma: a clinicopathologic study of 292 cases. J Clin Oncol 2005;23:1473–82.
122. Zhou XY, Tan M, Hawthorne VS, et al. Activation of the Akt/mammalian target of rapamycin/4E-BP1 pathway by ErbB2 overexpression predicts tumor progression in breast cancers. Clin Cancer Res 2004;10:6779–88.
123. Mayer IA, Abramson VG, Balko JM, et al. SU2C phase Ib study of pan-PI3K inhibitor BKM120 with letrozole in ER1/HER2- metastatic breast cancer (MBC). J Clin Oncol 2012;30(Suppl) (abstract 510).
124. Bowles DW, Jimeno A. New phosphatidylinositol 3-kinase inhibitors for cancer. Expert Opin Investig Drugs 2011;20:507–18.
125. Sharman J, de Vos S, Leonard JP, et al. A phase 1 study of the selective phosphatidylinositol 3-kinase-delta (PI3K delta) inhibitor, CAL-101 (GS-1101), in combination with rituximab and/or bendamustine in patients with relapsed or refractory chronic lymphocytic leukemia (CLL). Blood 2011;118:779–80.
126. Leonard J, Schreeder M, Coutre S, et al. A phase 1 study of Cal-101, an isoform-selective inhibitor of phosphatidylinositol 3-kinase P110d, in combination with anti-Cd20 monoclonal antibody therapy and/or bendamustine in patients with previously treated B-cell malignancies. Ann Oncol 2011;22:137.
127. Juric D, Argiles G, Burris H, et al. Phase I study of BYL719, an alpha-specific PI3K inhibitor, in patients with PIK3CA mutant advanced solid tumors: preliminary efficacy and safety in patients with PIK3CA mutant ER-positive (ER+) metastatic breast cancer (MBC). Cancer Res 2012;72(24 Supplement):P6–10–07.
128. Kandel ES, Hay N. The regulation and activities of the multifunctional serine/threonine kinase Akt/PKB. Exp Cell Res 1999;253:210–29.
129. Graves PR, Yu LJ, Schwarz JK, et al. The Chk1 protein kinase and the Cdc25C regulatory pathways are targets of the anticancer agent UCN-01. J Biol Chem 2000;275:5600–5.

130. Sato S, Fujita N, Tsuruo T. Interference with PDK1-Akt survival signaling pathway by UCN-01 (7-hydroxystaurosporine). Oncogene 2002;21:1727–38.
131. Mizuno K, Noda K, Ueda Y, et al. Ucn-01, an antitumor drug, is a selective inhibitor of the conventional Pkc subfamily. FEBS Lett 1995;359:259–61.
132. Patel V, Lahusen T, Leethanakul C, et al. Antitumor activity of UCN-01 in carcinomas of the head and neck is associated with altered expression of cyclin D3 and p27(KIP1). Clin Cancer Res 2002;8:3549–60.
133. Sausville EA, Arbuck SG, Messmann R, et al. Phase I trial of 72-hour continuous infusion UCN-01 in patients with refractory neoplasms. J Clin Oncol 2001;19: 2319–33.
134. Li TH, Christensen SD, Frankel PH, et al. A phase II study of cell cycle inhibitor UCN-01 in patients with metastatic melanoma: a California Cancer Consortium trial. Invest New Drugs 2012;30:741–8.
135. Ding HM, Han CH, Zhu JX, et al. Celecoxib derivatives induce apoptosis via the disruption of mitochondrial membrane potential and activation of caspase 9. Int J Cancer 2005;113:803–10.
136. Summers SA, Garza LA, Zhou HL, et al. Regulation of insulin-stimulated glucose transporter GLUT4 translocation and Akt kinase activity by ceramide. Mol Cell Biol 1998;18:5457–64.
137. Kondapaka SB, Singh SS, Dasmahapatra GP, et al. Perifosine, a novel alkylphospholipid, inhibits protein kinase B activation. Mol Cancer Ther 2003;2: 1093–103.
138. Crul M, Rosing H, de Klerk GJ, et al. Phase I and pharmacological study of daily oral administration of perifosine (D-21266) in patients with advanced solid tumours. Eur J Cancer 2002;38:1615–21.
139. Davies BR, Greenwood H, Dudley P, et al. Preclinical pharmacology of AZD5363, an inhibitor of AKT: pharmacodynamics, antitumor activity, and correlation of monotherapy activity with genetic background. Mol Cancer Ther 2012; 11:873–87.
140. Lindsley CW, Zhao ZJ, Leister WH, et al. Allosteric Akt (PKB) inhibitors: discovery and SAR of isozyme selective inhibitors. Bioorg Med Chem Lett 2005;15: 761–4.
141. Barnett SF, Defeo-Jones D, Fu S, et al. Identification and characterization of pleckstrin-homology-domain-dependent and isoenzyme-specific Akt inhibitors. Biochem J 2005;385:399–408.
142. DeFeo-Jones D, Barnett SF, Fu S, et al. Tumor cell sensitization to apoptotic stimuli by selective inhibition of specific Akt/PKB family members. Mol Cancer Ther 2005;4:271–9.
143. Sehgal SN, Baker H, Vezina C. Rapamycin (Ay-22,989), a new antifungal antibiotic. 2. fermentation, isolation and characterization. J Antibiot (Tokyo) 1975;28: 727–32.
144. Vezina C, Kudelski A, Sehgal SN. Rapamycin (Ay-22,989), a new antifungal antibiotic. 1. taxonomy of producing streptomycete and isolation of active principle. J Antibiot (Tokyo) 1975;28:721–6.
145. Douros J, Suffness M. New anti-tumor substances of natural origin. Cancer Treat Rev 1981;8:63–87.
146. Houchens DP, Ovejera AA, Riblet SM, et al. Human-brain tumor xenografts in nude-mice as a chemotherapy model. Eur J Cancer Clin Oncol 1983;19: 799–805.
147. Geoerger B, Kerr K, Tang CB, et al. Antitumor activity of the rapamycin analog CCI-779 in human primitive neuroectodermal tumor/medulloblastoma models

as single agent and in combination chemotherapy. Cancer Res 2001;61: 1527–32.

148. Shi YF, Frankel A, Radvanyi LG, et al. Rapamycin enhances apoptosis and increases sensitivity to cisplatin in-vitro. Cancer Res 1995;55:1982–8.

149. Wan XL, Helman LJ. Effect of insulin-like growth factor II on protecting myoblast cells against cisplatin-induced apoptosis through p70 s6 kinase pathway. Neoplasia 2002;4:400–8.

150. Mondesire WH, Jian W, Zhang H, et al. Targeting mammalian target of rapamycin synergistically enhances chemotherapy-induced cytotoxicity in breast cancer cells. Clin Cancer Res 2004;10:7031–42.

151. Chan S, Scheulen ME, Johnston S, et al. Phase II study of temsirolimus (CCI-779), a novel inhibitor of mTOR, in heavily pretreated patients with locally advanced or metastatic breast cancer. J Clin Oncol 2005;23:5314–22.

152. Van Oosterom AT, Dumez H, Desai J, et al. Combination signal transduction inhibition: a phase I/II trial of the oral mTOR-inhibitor everolimus (E, RAD001) and imatinib mesylate (IM) in patients (pts) with gastrointestinal stromal tumor (GIST) refractory to IM. J Clin Oncol 2004;22(15 Supplement):3002.

153. Garcia-Martinez JM, Moran J, Clarke RG, et al. Ku-0063794 is a specific inhibitor of the mammalian target of rapamycin (mTOR). Biochem J 2009;421: 29–42.

154. Chresta CM, Davies BR, Hickson I, et al. AZD8055 Is a potent, selective, and orally bioavailable atp-competitive mammalian target of rapamycin kinase inhibitor with in vitro and in vivo antitumor activity. Cancer Res 2010;70:288–98.

155. Feldman ME, Apsel B, Uotila A, et al. Active-site inhibitors of mTOR target rapamycin-resistant outputs of mTORC1 and mTORC2. PLoS Biol 2009;7: 371–83.

156. Hsieh AC, Liu Y, Enlind MP, et al. The translational landscape of mTOR signalling steers cancer initiation and metastasis. Nature 2012;485:55–61.

157. Janes MR, Limon JJ, So LM, et al. Effective and selective targeting of leukemia cells using a TORC1/2 kinase inhibitor. Nat Med 2010;16:205–13.

158. Altman JK, Sassano A, Kaur S, et al. Dual mTORC2/mTORC1 targeting results in potent suppressive effects on acute myeloid leukemia (AML) progenitors. Clin Cancer Res 2011;17:4378–88.

159. Willems L, Chapuis N, Puissant A, et al. The dual mTORC1 and mTORC2 inhibitor AZD8055 has anti-tumor activity in acute myeloid leukemia. Leukemia 2012; 26:1195–202.

160. Evangelisti C, Ricci F, Tazzari P, et al. Targeted inhibition of mTORC1 and mTORC2 by active-site mTOR inhibitors has cytotoxic effects in T-cell acute lymphoblastic leukemia. Leukemia 2011;25:781–91.

161. Bhagwat SV, Gokhale PC, Crew AP, et al. Preclinical characterization of OSI-027, a potent and selective inhibitor of mTORC1 and mTORC2: distinct from rapamycin. Mol Cancer Ther 2011;10:1394–406.

162. Rodrik-Outmezguine VS, Chandarlapaty S, Pagano NC, et al. mTOR kinase inhibition causes feedback-dependent biphasic regulation of AKT signaling. Cancer Discov 2011;1:248–59.

163. Moore SF, Hunter RW, Hers I. mTORC2 protein complex-mediated Akt (protein kinase B) serine 473 phosphorylation is not required for Akt1 activity in human platelets [corrected]. J Biol Chem 2011;286:24553–60.

164. Raynaud FI, Eccles S, Clarke PA, et al. Pharmacologic characterization of a potent inhibitor of class I phosphatidylinositide 3-kinases. Cancer Res 2007; 67:5840–50.

165. Park S, Chapuis N, Bardet V, et al. PI-103, a dual inhibitor of Class IA phosphatidylinositide 3-kinase and mTOR, has antileukemic activity in AML. Leukemia 2008;22:1698–706.

166. Chiarini F, Fala F, Tazzari PL, et al. Dual inhibition of class IA phosphatidylinositol 3-kinase and mammalian target of rapamycin as a new therapeutic option for T-cell acute lymphoblastic leukemia. Cancer Res 2009;69:3520–8.

167. Maira SM, Stauffer F, Brueggen J, et al. Identification and characterization of NVP-BEZ235, a new orally available dual phosphatidylinositol 3-kinase/mammalian target of rapamycin inhibitor with potent in vivo antitumor activity. Mol Cancer Ther 2008;7:1851–63.

168. Serra V, Markman B, Scaltriti M, et al. NVP-BEZ235, a dual PI3K/mTOR inhibitor, prevents PI3K signaling and inhibits the growth of cancer cells with activating PI3K mutations. Cancer Res 2008;68:8022–30.

169. Chapuis N, Tamburini J, Green AS, et al. Dual inhibition of PI3K and mTORC1/2 signaling by NVP-BEZ235 as a new therapeutic strategy for acute myeloid leukemia. Clin Cancer Res 2010;16:5424–35.

170. Xu CX, Li YK, Yue P, et al. The combination of RAD001 and NVP-BEZ235 exerts synergistic anticancer activity against non-small cell lung cancer in vitro and in vivo. PLoS One 2011;6:e20899.

171. Mazzoletti M, Bortolin F, Brunelli L, et al. Combination of PI3K/mTOR inhibitors: antitumor activity and molecular correlates. Cancer Res 2011;71: 4573–84.

172. Werzowa J, Koehrer S, Strommer S, et al. Vertical inhibition of the mTORC1/mTORC2/PI3K pathway shows synergistic effects against melanoma in vitro and in vivo. J Invest Dermatol 2011;131:495–503.

173. Garlich JR, De P, Dey N, et al. A vascular targeted pan phosphoinositide 3-kinase inhibitor prodrug, SF1126, with antitumor and antiangiogenic activity. Cancer Res 2008;68:206–15.

174. Garlich JR, Becker MD, Shelton CF, et al. Phase I study of novel prodrug dual PI3K/mTOR inhibitor SF1126 in B-cell malignancies. Blood 2010;116:744.

175. Tashiro H, Blazes MS, Wu R, et al. Mutations in PTEN are frequent in endometrial carcinoma but rare in other common gynecological malignancies. Cancer Res 1997;57:3935–40.

176. Risinger JI, Hayes K, Maxwell GL, et al. PTEN mutation in endometrial cancers is associated with favorable clinical and pathologic characteristics. Clin Cancer Res 1998;4:3005–10.

177. Bilbao C, Rodriguez G, Ramirez R, et al. The relationship between microsatellite instability and PTEN gene mutations in endometrial cancer. Int J Cancer 2006; 119:563–70.

178. Byun DS, Cho K, Ryu BK, et al. Frequent monoallelic deletion of PTEN and its reciprocal association with PIK3CA amplification in gastric carcinoma. Int J Cancer 2003;104:318–27.

179. Gray IC, Stewart LM, Phillips SM, et al. Mutation and expression analysis of the putative prostate tumour-suppressor gene PTEN. Br J Cancer 1998;78:1296–300.

180. Cairns P, Okami K, Halachmi S, et al. Frequent inactivation of PTEN/MMAC1 in primary prostate cancer. Cancer Res 1997;57:4997–5000.

181. Pesche S, Latil A, Muzeau F, et al. PTEN/MMAC1/TEP1 involvement in primary prostate cancers. Oncogene 1998;16:2879–83.

182. Reifenberger J, Wolter M, Bostrom J, et al. Allelic losses on chromosome arm 10q and mutation of the PTEN (MMAC1) tumour suppressor gene in primary and metastatic malignant melanomas. Virchows Arch 2000;436:487–93.

183. Birck A, Ahrenkiel V, Zeuthen J, et al. Mutation and allelic loss of the PTEN/MMAC1 gene in primary and metastatic melanoma biopsies. J Invest Dermatol 2000;114:277–80.

184. Celebi JT, Shendrik I, Silvers DN, et al. Identification of PTEN mutations in metastatic melanoma specimens. J Med Genet 2000;37:653–7.

185. Pollock PM, Walker GJ, Glendening JM, et al. PTEN inactivation is rare in melanoma tumours but occurs frequently in melanoma cell lines. Melanoma Res 2002;12:565–75.

186. Duerr EM, Rollbrocker B, Hayashi Y, et al. PTEN mutations in gliomas and glioneuronal tumors. Oncogene 1998;16:2259–64.

187. Liu W, James CD, Frederick L, et al. PTEN/MMAC1 mutations and EGFR amplification in glioblastomas. Cancer Res 1997;57:5254–7.

188. Bedolla R, Prihoda TJ, Kreisberg JI, et al. Determining risk of biochemical recurrence in prostate cancer by immunohistochemical detection of PTEN expression and Akt activation. Clin Cancer Res 2007;13:3860–7.

189. Depowski PL, Rosenthal SI, Ross JS. Loss of expression of the PTEN gene protein product is associated with poor outcome in breast cancer. Mod Pathol 2001; 14:672–6.

190. Rhei E, Kang L, Bogomolniy F, et al. Mutation analysis of the putative tumor suppressor gene PTEN/MMAC1 in primary breast carcinomas. Cancer Res 1997; 57:3657–9.

191. Tsao H, Zhang X, Benoit E, et al. Identification of PTEN/MMAC1 alterations in uncultured melanomas and melanoma cell lines. Oncogene 1998;16:3397–402.

192. Guldberg P, thor Straten P, Birck A, et al. Disruption of the MMAC1/PTEN gene by deletion or mutation is a frequent event in malignant melanoma. Cancer Res 1997;57:3660–3.

193. Massion PP, Kuo WL, Stokoe D, et al. Genomic copy number analysis of non-small cell lung cancer using array comparative genomic hybridization: implications of the phosphatidylinositol 3-kinase pathway. Cancer Res 2002;62: 3636–40.

194. Bjorkqvist AM, Husgafvel-Pursiainen K, Anttila S, et al. DNA gains in 3q occur frequently in squamous cell carcinoma of the lung, but not in adenocarcinoma. Genes Chromosomes Cancer 1998;22:79–82.

195. Pedrero JM, Carracedo DG, Pinto CM, et al. Frequent genetic and biochemical alterations of the PI 3-K/AKT/PTEN pathway in head and neck squamous cell carcinoma. Int J Cancer 2005;114:242–8.

196. Campbell IG, Russell SE, Choong DY, et al. Mutation of the PIK3CA gene in ovarian and breast cancer. Cancer Res 2004;64:7678–81.

197. Wu G, Xing M, Mambo E, et al. Somatic mutation and gain of copy number of PIK3CA in human breast cancer. Breast Cancer Res 2005;7:R609–16.

198. Lee JW, Soung YH, Kim SY, et al. PIK3CA gene is frequently mutated in breast carcinomas and hepatocellular carcinomas. Oncogene 2005;24:1477–80.

199. Saal LH, Holm K, Maurer M, et al. PIK3CA mutations correlate with hormone receptors, node metastasis, and ERBB2, and are mutually exclusive with PTEN loss in human breast carcinoma. Cancer Res 2005;65:2554–9.

200. Levine DA, Bogomolniy F, Yee CJ, et al. Frequent mutation of the PIK3CA gene in ovarian and breast cancers. Clin Cancer Res 2005;11:2875–8.

201. Samuels Y, Velculescu VE. Oncogenic mutations of PIK3CA in human cancers. Cell Cycle 2004;3:1221–4.

202. Velho S, Oliveira C, Ferreira A, et al. The prevalence of PIK3CA mutations in gastric and colon cancer. Eur J Cancer 2005;41:1649–54.

203. Ikenoue T, Kanai F, Hikiba Y, et al. Functional analysis of PIK3CA gene mutations in human colorectal cancer. Cancer Res 2005;65:4562–7.
204. Knobbe CB, Trampe-Kieslich A, Reifenberger G. Genetic alteration and expression of the phosphoinositol-3-kinase/Akt pathway genes PIK3CA and PIKE in human glioblastomas. Neuropathol Appl Neurobiol 2005;31:486–90.
205. Kang S, Seo SS, Chang HJ, et al. Mutual exclusiveness between PIK3CA and KRAS mutations in endometrial carcinoma. Int J Gynecol Cancer 2008;18:1339–43.
206. Cheng JQ, Godwin AK, Bellacosa A, et al. AKT2, a putative oncogene encoding a member of a subfamily of protein-serine/threonine kinases, is amplified in human ovarian carcinomas. Proc Natl Acad Sci U S A 1992;89:9267–71.
207. Ricarte-Filho JC, Ryder M, Chitale DA, et al. Mutational profile of advanced primary and metastatic radioactive iodine-refractory thyroid cancers reveals distinct pathogenetic roles for BRAF, PIK3CA, and AKT1. Cancer Res 2009;69:4885–93.
208. Cohen Y, Shalmon B, Korach J, et al. AKT1 pleckstrin homology domain E17K activating mutation in endometrial carcinoma. Gynecol Oncol 2010;116:88–91.
209. Stephens PJ, Tarpey PS, Davies H, et al. The landscape of cancer genes and mutational processes in breast cancer. Nature 2012;486:400–4.
210. Gonzalez-Angulo AM, Blumenschein GR Jr. Defining biomarkers to predict sensitivity to PI3K/Akt/mTOR pathway inhibitors in breast cancer. Cancer Treat Rev 2013;39:313–20.
211. Banerji S, Cibulskis K, Rangel-Escareno C, et al. Sequence analysis of mutations and translocations across breast cancer subtypes. Nature 2012;486:405–9.

Targeting the Heat Shock Response in Cancer
Tipping the Balance in Transformed Cells

Sartaj S. Sanghera, MD[a], Joseph J. Skitzki, MD[a,b],*

KEYWORDS

- Heat shock response • HSF-1 • Curaxins • Small molecule inhibitors

KEY POINTS

- Components of the heat shock response (HSR) have become increasingly well defined.
- The HSR is active in all phases of tumorigenesis.
- Targeting the substrates of the HSR is an attractive and novel means of cancer therapy.
- Agents that target the HSR are in various stages of development for clinical use in a variety of cancer types.
- The ability of these new agents to synergize with current therapies may be significant.

INTRODUCTION

The heat shock response (HSR) is a highly conserved, precisely orchestrated, and internally regulated series of genetic and biochemical events that is triggered by the exposure of eukaryotic cells to various forms of stress.[1,2] The response was first reported in 1962 by Ritossa,[3] who observed the appearance of a new pattern of chromatin puffs on the salivary gland chromosomes of the fruit fly, *Drosophila bucksii*, in response to exposure to increased temperatures. Subsequent studies revealed that this response could be induced by a variety of other stresses such as exposure to heavy metals and oxidative stress. In 1973, Tissières and colleagues[4] further defined this response at a molecular level, describing a brisk and dramatic increase in the synthesis of a small, interrelated family of proteins that came to be known as the heat shock proteins (HSPs). This transcriptional response to stress was then discovered to be mediated by a family of heat shock transcription factors (HSFs) that are negatively regulated and activated by the initiation of specific cellular events.

Disclosures: The authors have nothing to disclose.
[a] Department of Surgical Oncology, Roswell Park Cancer Institute, Elm and Carlton Streets, Buffalo, NY 14263, USA; [b] Department of Immunology, Roswell Park Cancer Institute, Elm and Carlton Streets, Buffalo, NY 14263, USA
* Corresponding author. Department of Surgical Oncology, Roswell Park Cancer Institute, Elm and Carlton Streets, Buffalo, NY 14263.
E-mail address: joseph.skitzki@roswellpark.org

Cell stress is a defining event and efficient use of the stress response can be the difference between cell survival and extinction. The HSR serves a primarily cytoprotective function and is autoregulated so that it is just as promptly switched off, either when the stress has been overcome and homeostasis restored or when the cell has been overwhelmed and cell death ensues.[5] The seamless coordination of these complex interactions involves multilevel crosstalk between the HSR and multiple, diverse, proliferative, antiapoptotic, and death receptor pathways.[6] If these environmental or physiologic stresses are prolonged, then aberrations of the HSR can result in defective development and the establishment of a wide variety of disorders associated with a broad spectrum of disease states ranging from neurodegenerative diseases to ischemia-reperfusion injury.[7]

Given their role in proteostasis, and therefore cytoprotection, increased expression of molecular chaperones is noted in several pathologic disease states that are characterized by increased synthesis and accumulation of aberrant proteins, notable among which is cancer. Demonstration of the increased expression of HSPs in cancer has led to the hypothesis that transformed cells co-opt the HSR to perpetuate the malignant phenotype.[8] This increased expression has been noted in several different cancers: solid organ, gastrointestinal, and hematopoietic. Further, increased expression correlates with aggressiveness and resistance to therapy,[9] which has resulted in extensive research in the past decade to elucidate mechanisms whereby transformed cells might exploit the stress machinery. Increased understanding of these interactions has sparked an interest in developing modulators of the HSR as a means of treatment.[10]

In this article, the various components and mechanisms driving the HSR are detailed with special emphasis on its importance in fostering and maintaining the malignant phenotype. Current research, clinical applications, and future directions in the area of pharmacotherapy targeting this ubiquitous cellular response to stress are discussed.

THE HSR

The rapid and prolific transcriptional activation of the HSP genes is under the control of HSFs. Four HSFs are known to exist, of which HSF-1, HSF-2 and HSF-4 are found in humans. HSF-1 is the primary activator of the inducible stress response in human tissues.[11] At baseline conditions of homeostasis, HSF-1 exists in a repressed state in the cytoplasm where it is bound to the complex of HSP40/HSP70 and HSP90 as an inert monomer.[12] On activation, it undergoes hyperphosphorylation at serine residues, forms homotrimers that have DNA-binding capacity, and translocates to the nucleus. There it binds to promoter regions on the 5′ end of the HSP genes, located at variable distances upstream from the site of transcription initiation. These promoter regions contain specific DNA sequence motifs that constitute the stress-responsive heat shock elements (HSEs). It is widely thought that the appearance of many nonnative and/or nascent polypeptides within the cell as a result of environmental or physiologic stress is the primary activator of HSF-1.[13] HSF-1 activity is turned off via internally regulated and autoregulated mechanisms. Acting as a feedback loop, HSP70, which is elaborated from HSF-1 activity, binds to the transactivation domain of HSF-1 and represses further transcription of heat shock genes.

HSPS

At a molecular level, the hallmark of the HSR is the increased synthesis of the HSP family of proteins.[2] HSPs constitute subsets within at least 2 larger, well-characterized families of proteins, namely molecular chaperones and proteases. Their presumed primary function is to combat the proteotoxic state induced by various forms of cell stress.[14] By virtue of their structure and function, proteins are particularly susceptible to physiologic stress. Increased temperatures, oxidative agents, heavy metals, and low pH can all lead to unfolding of proteins, thus exposing their hydrophobic core motifs and making them prone to misfolding. Misfolding may promote the aggregation and precipitation of unstable intermediaries, which eventually threatens cell survival. Molecular chaperones perform the task of protein assembly, folding, refolding of intermediates, membrane translocation, and sequestration in subcellular compartments. In situations in which the exposure is of a lethal intensity, irreversibly damaged proteins are processed by a related family of proteins, the proteases, to ensure prompt degradation and removal.[15]

HSPs were initially classified into 6 major families, based on approximate molecular weight: HSP100, HSP90, HSP70, HSP60, HSP50, and small HSPs.[16] More recently, the nomenclature was revised by Kampinga and colleagues[17] to align with that of the Human Genome Organisation (HUGO) Gene Nomenclature Committee and thereby promote consistent reporting. The new nomenclature classifies the HSPs into the following groups: HSPH (HSP110), HSPC (HSP90), HSPA (HSP70), DNAJ (HSP40), and HSPB (small HSPs). This article discuss in further detail 2 of the most widely studied and targeted families of HSPs.

HSPA

Members of this subclass of HSPs are major molecular chaperones and cytokine chaperokines found in the cytoplasm, nucleus, mitochondria, and endoplasmic reticulum. There are at least 13 homologous proteins in the human HSPA chaperone family and they seem to be highly conserved in eukaryotes.[17] These proteins can be either stress-inducible (HSPA1) or constitutively expressed (HSPA8). They have the ability to interact with newly synthesized polypeptides as they emerge from ribosomes or to bind to nonnative or damaged proteins that result from exposure to stress. In addition, they assist in trafficking proteins into cell organelles, and they also seem to play a role in dissociation of aggregated proteins. These multiple, diverse functions underline the significance of HSPA to the maintenance of protein homeostasis during normal biochemical cellular processes as well as in the stressed state.[18]

All HSPA family members have a multidomain organization that consists of an N-terminal nucleotide-binding domain ($\sim$40 kDa) with ATPase activity and a C-terminal peptide-binding domain ($\sim$25 kDa) with a short linker. The interaction of HSPA with protein substrates depends on ATP hydrolysis. In the ATP-bound state, HSPA has low binding affinity for substrates. Functional activation requires assembly into large, complex chaperone machines constituted through association with cochaperones including the DNAJ family of HSPs. DNAJ causes stimulation of ATP hydrolysis, and the resulting ADP-bound HSPA has high substrate-binding affinity. All cellular functions performed by the HSPA family depend on ATP-dependent association with, and dissociation from, substrate proteins. By regulating the configuration and affinity of HSPA within the chaperone machines, DNAJ, and other cochaperones, can modulate its substrate selectivity and therefore recruit it for a multitude of intracellular functions.[19]

HSPC

HSPC is another example of an evolutionarily highly conserved molecular chaperone, existing from bacteria to mammals. Another ATP-dependent chaperone, it is essential in the cellular response to stress. The proteostatic functions of HSPC are even more diverse, playing an integral role in constitutive cell signaling in the nonstressed state. More than 200 client proteins are stabilized and/or activated via interaction with HSPC.[20] Similar to HSPA, this task is accomplished through the construction, together with HSPA, DNAJ, and other cochaperones, of a dynamic, interactive complex called the HSPC chaperone machine. HSPC is abundant even in nonstressed cells, and a multitude of client proteins rely on interactions with the chaperone machinery to acquire their active conformations.[21]

The molecular mechanisms underlying the function of HSPCs remain less well understood compared with other chaperone proteins. The reasons for this are multifactorial. The complexes formed between HSPC and its client proteins are dynamic and short lived, complicated further by the abundant and variable participation of cochaperones.[22] HSPC interacts with more than 20 cochaperones, and each of them plays a part in modulating substrate affinity, specificity, and activity. Via abundant expression and numerous interactions with a variety of proteins, HSPC creates a dynamic reservoir that serves to buffer proteotoxic stress. However, under extreme conditions this reservoir is prone to rapid depletion, leaving the cell susceptible to the altered structure and function of a plethora of HSPC client proteins.[23]

A broad classification of the functions of molecular chaperones has traditionally been entertained, defined as protein holding and protein folding. Both HSPA and HSPC are involved mainly in protein holding. HSPA primarily interacts with nascent polypeptides, safeguarding their refolding potential and preventing the formation of misfolded, insoluble intermediates, and then guides them back to productive, on-pathway folding.[24] Protein folding takes place once the substrate has been released and is regulated primarily by HSPD. However, these distinctions are not absolute and there is overlap and redundancy. For example, HSPA can cooperate with other ATP-dependent chaperones (including HSPC) and chaperonins to mediate folding of certain substrates.[18] In deciding the fate of damaged proteins, HSPA and HSPC seem to have divergent functions: HSPA promotes substrate ubiquitination leading to elimination, whereas HSPC favors protein preservation.[8,25]

THE HSR AND TUMORIGENESIS
Essential Steps in Tumorigenesis

Hanahan and Weinberg[26] examined the molecular, biochemical, and cellular traits displayed by most human cancers. In a landmark review, they set forth the principles that govern the transformation of normal cells to malignant tumors. There is now almost universal agreement that the evolution of the malignant phenotype requires these key alterations in cell physiology: self-sufficiency in growth signals, insensitivity to growth-inhibitory (antigrowth) signals, evasion of programmed cell death (apoptosis), limitless replicative potential, sustained angiogenesis, and tissue invasion and metastasis. Via their ability to hold a large pool of proteins in their active conformations, HSPs modulate the function of several important signaling proteins and are therefore involved in many of these steps on the pathway to tumor progression,[8,27] as summarized in **Table 1**.

Levels of HSPs are increased in a wide variety of cancers. Despite various hypotheses, the mechanism by which this increased expression is effected remains elusive. A general hypothesis proposes that stress stimuli encountered within the tumor microenvironment (hypoglycemia, hypoxia, and low pH) cause canonical induction of the HSR.[2] However, Tang and colleagues[38] showed that although overexpression of HSPs was preserved from tumor samples to cells grown in culture, expression was

Table 1
Influence of HSPs in the key steps of tumorigenesis

Hallmarks of Cancer	HSPs Implicated	Molecules	References, Year
Self-sufficiency in growth signals	HSP70 HSP90	Cyclin D1 HER-2, c-Src, c-*Raf*, ERK1, Akt, Bcr-Abl, EGFR, BRAF, HCK, Cdk4, and eIF-2α	Diehl et al,[28] 2003 Taipale et al,[29] 2010
Insensitivity to growth inhibition	HSP90	CDK4, CDK6	Bishop et al,[30] 2007
Evasion of programmed cell death	HSP27 HSP70 HSP90	Bid, cytochrome C Caspases, Bax, AIF, APAF-1, JNK, Akt Caspases, APAF-1, RIP1, AKT	Beere et al,[47] 2001 Calderwood et al,[8] 2006
Limitless replicative potential	HSP72 HSP70 HSP90	Hdm2, p53 and Cdc2 p53 Telomerase (h-TERT)	Yaglom et al,[31] 2007 Sherman et al,[32] 2007 Holt et al,[33] 1999
Sustained angiogenesis	HSP27 HSP70 HSP90	VEGF HIF1α HIF1α, VEGF, NOS	Keezer et al,[34] 2003 Zhou et al,[35] 2004 Garcia-Cardena et al,[36] 1998
Tissue invasion and metastasis	HSP90	MMP2	Eustace et al,[37] 2004

Abbreviations: EGFR, epidermal growth factor receptor; HER-2, human epidermal growth factor 2; HIF1α, hypoxia inducible factor 1; MMP2, matrix metalloproteinase 2; NOS, nitric oxide synthase; VEGF, vascular endothelial growth factor.
Data from Refs.[6,8,28-37]

subsequently downregulated on the establishment of tumor xenografts in vivo using the cultured cells. The mechanisms for HSP overexpression are likely to be complex and multifactorial. Multiple alterations in protein homeostasis occur during the stepwise progression to carcinogenesis that could lead to induction, or derepression, of HSP genes. This process includes the early stages such as infection by oncogenic viruses or exposure to environmental carcinogens; progressive expression of mutated proteins; changes in the immune and endocrine systems; and also cell exposure to a multitude of stresses including hypoxia, starvation, and other proteotoxic stressors.[39]

Coupling of HSF-1 Activation to Malignant Cell Signal Transduction

The activation of HSF-1 during stress has evolved to be a brisk response. Therefore, it does not rely on an increase in transcription or translation, but relies solely on the posttranslational modification of existing levels of HSF-1. However, activation of HSF-1 in cancers is associated with an increase in the detected overall level of the protein. Although the mechanism for this increase is unclear, it has been theorized to involve an increase in transcription/translation or certain epigenetic changes.[40]

Addiction to Chaperones

Genetic mutations and increased protein expression are key events in tumor progression. Transformation is therefore accompanied by an exponential increase in protein load, with many of those proteins being mutated and therefore being inherently unstable. Maintenance of proteostasis within this mutated phenotype causes an enhanced dependence on the chaperoning function of HSPs. Chaperones stabilize oncoproteins and permit, or even enhance, their tumorigenic potential. Therefore, tumor cells show an addiction to chaperones and this may be the cause of their increased HSP expression.[41]

The ability of HSPs to hold large amounts of altered proteins, including protein kinases and transcription factors, may significantly affect vital biologic processes such as signal transduction, chromatin remodeling and epigenetic regulation, development, and morphologic evolution has earned them the nickname capacitors of evolution.[42] Cancer cells co-opt this capacitance machinery to protect an array of mutated and overexpressed oncoproteins from misfolding and therefore from proteasomal degradation. These oncoproteins have a host of different functions that affect each of the physiologic changes that must occur in the pathway to transformation.[8]

Growth Signaling and Anti-apoptosis

HSPs are vital for maintaining signaling proteins in active conformations so as to enable an expeditious response to growth signals. HSPC, along with HSPA and HSPB, organized within high-molecular-weight chaperone machinery, is required for the stability and activity of various significant growth-promoting oncoproteins.[43] Prominent among these is HER-2 and its downstream effectors including Akt, c-Src, and Raf-1.[44] In addition, it has also been shown that HSP90 association is essential for the function and stability of the androgen receptor in prostate cancer cells.

Activation of several oncogenes, notably c-Myc and Ras, also induces pathways of programmed cell death or apoptosis.[26] Therefore, several of the apoptotic pathways must be subverted during the progression to transformation and attainment of the malignant phenotype. HSPA and HSPB, unlike HSPC, do not influence cellular proliferation. However, they do play a role in the inhibition of programmed cell death and, thereby, in the creation of a profoundly resilient state. Some of the high-profile targets of HSPA and HSPB include members of the caspase-dependent apoptotic pathways such as c-Jun kinase, Apaf-1, and caspase 8.[6,45] In addition, HSPA also plays a role in the inhibition of an alternative death pathway involving digestion of cellular contents by lysosome-derived cathepsins.[46] Inactivation or knockdown of HSPA and/or HSPB in tumor cells leads to spontaneous activation of apoptosis.[47]

Inhibition of Replicative Senescence

All somatic cells have a built-in, preset limit on the number of cell divisions. This limit is regulated by the length of end-chromosomal telomeres, which undergo shortening with every successive cell division. At the preprogrammed point of crisis, the cell enters the pathway of senescence.[48] In some cells, expression of p53-sensitive telomerase is sufficient to bypass crisis and escape senescence.[49] HSPC is essential for telomerase stability. Recent data indicate that specific members of the HSPC and HSPA family are overexpressed in tumors and inhibit senescence via both a p53-dependent and p53-independent manner.[50]

Angiogenesis

To meet increasing tissue demands for oxygen delivery, growing tumor cells use angiogenic growth factor signaling to create neocirculatory pathways at the microscopic level. The primary signal for angiogenesis is hypoxia and the most important sensor for hypoxia in tumor tissues is the hypoxia-inducible factor 1α (HIF1α).[51] HIF1α is regulated primarily at the level of protein stability and both HSPA and HSPC are necessary for its stabilization and accumulation.[52] Several key downstream signaling molecules such as vascular endothelial growth factor (VEGF) and nitric oxide synthase (NOS) require HSPC for their induction and stable functionality.[53]

Invasion and Metastasis

There is evidence to support the involvement of HSPs in this final stage of tumor dissemination. For example, tumor cells that overexpress HSF-1 and HSPs show a higher propensity and capability for invasion and metastases.[9] However, the mechanisms involved in these processes are poorly understood at this time. Existing data show that the induction in some tumor cells of an anchorage-independent state, mediated by heregulin, requires the HFS-1 gene.[40] Other recent studies have also suggested a role for extracellular HSPC. HSPC expressed on the surface of tumor cells can bind to matrix metalloproteinase 2 (MMP2), a key protein in the development of invasion.[37]

Implications of HSP Overexpression

The involvement of HSPs in various stages of oncogenesis, and their aberrant overexpression in a wide variety of tumor specimens, has generated interest in their role as biomarkers, both diagnostic and predictive. There is a potential for the use of circulating levels of HSPs and anti-HSP antibodies for diagnostic purposes, although this potential remains unrealized. However, there is increasing evidence that the overexpression of HSPs in tissue samples is a biomarker of carcinogenesis and the level of expression has been correlated with the degree of differentiation, response to therapy, and outcome prognostication.[9,27]

Increased levels of HSP27 have been detected in breast and endometrial cancer as well as in leukemia. Moreover, there is variability of the phosphorylation patterns of HSP27 in tumor samples compared with corresponding normal tissue. The expression of this protein confers a poor prognosis in patients with gastric, liver, and prostate cancer. Likewise, expression of the HSP70 protein correlates with unfavorable outcomes in breast, endometrial, uterine cervical, and bladder carcinomas. In addition, increased expression of HSP90 has been linked with disease progression in melanoma and correlated with poor survival outcomes in cancers of the breast and lung as well as in gastrointestinal stromal tumors (GIST).[9]

The HSP27 gene also contains an estrogen-responsive element that might significantly alter expression in hormone receptor–positive tumors. However, this has not been shown to reliably predict response to hormonal therapy. In contrast, both HSP27 and HSP70 seem to confer resistance to chemotherapy in breast cancer. Although HSP27 correlates with poor response to chemotherapy in patients with leukemia, HSP70 predicts a favorable response to chemotherapy in osteosarcomas.[9]

Targeting the HSR in Cancer

Via their function as molecular chaperones, HSPs aid the accumulation of mutated proteins within the cancer phenotype, thus conferring cytoprotection against otherwise lethal levels of cellular stress. In addition, via crosstalk with interconnected signal transduction pathways, HSPs influence several key steps in tumorigenesis, which makes HSPs and their protective mechanisms an attractive target for antitumor therapy.

The abundance and ubiquitous expression of HSPs in normal cells seem to render them unlikely targets for meaningful drug development secondary to a lack of selectivity. However, the addiction to chaperones prevalent in transformed cells renders them particularly vulnerable to inhibition of the activity of HSPs. Because the heat shock machinery is already being driven and used at maximal levels in the cancer cell, any decrease in the activity of HSR mechanisms can cause a dangerous imbalance favoring cell death. In addition, not only are cancer cells enriched in HSPs but studies show that there is preferential expression of a certain cancer phenotype of HSPs in tumors compared with normal cells. In the case of HSP90, the altered conformation of the proteins in tumor cells leads to a 20-fold to 200-fold higher specificity for small molecule inhibitors compared with normal cells.[8]

Another perceived obstacle for drug development has been that HSPs interact with substrates in a stoichiometric manner and lack catalytic activity. Therefore, researchers have used high-throughput models that provide a reliable readout of the transcriptional response to cell stress to successfully screen millions of small molecules. An ever-increasing number of molecules are currently in preclinical or clinical evaluation with some promising results.

Modulation of HSF-1

Given the central role of HSF-1 in the regulation of HSP expression in the stressed cell, it has attracted attention as a target for drug development. Drugs have been developed to both positively as well as negatively modulate HSF-1. Induction of the HSR is a useful therapeutic strategy, mainly in diseases in which the aggregation of misfolded proteins is the key underlying pathogenic defect, exemplified by neurodegenerative disorders (**Table 2**).

Examples of drugs that induce the HSR include proteasome inhibitors such as MG-132 and lactacystin, which activate HSF-1 via an increase in the intracellular concentration of misfolded proteins. This process is hypothesized to cause the dissociation of HSF-1 from its complex, which then undergoes hyperphosphorylation and translocation to the nucleus, triggering the HSR.[54] Bortezomib, another proteasome inhibitor, is clinically approved for the treatment of multiple myeloma.[55] Several other molecules also activate the HSR via an indirect activation of HSF-1. These molecules include agents that cause oxidative stress, such as terrecyclic acid as well as several specific chaperone inhibitors.[56] In addition, inflammatory mediators such as phospholipase A_2, arachidonic acid, cyclopentanone, and prostaglandins promote the DNA-binding activity of HSF-1.[57] Other compounds, although unable to induce the HSR independently, are known to function synergistically to enhance the HSR in response to low levels of stress. For example, nonsteroidal antiinflammatory drugs facilitate the trimerization of HSF-1 and allow maximal activation of the HSR at reduced levels of thermal stress.[58] The hydroxylamine derivatives bimoclomol and arimoclomol prolong the duration of HSF-1 binding to DNA.[59] The induction of the HSR is also relevant to other clinically important scenarios ranging from ischemia-reperfusion to radiation toxicity.[60]

Inhibition of the HSR via the negative modulation of HSF-1 offers the prospect of blocking a wide spectrum of pathways that cancer cells rely on to spur autonomous cell growth and escape apoptosis. The potential benefit of this approach has been shown by proof-of-principle studies that used siRNAs to target HSF-1. Targeting HSF-1 in this manner increased the sensitivity of tumor cells to heat shock, proteasome inhibition, and hyperthermic chemotherapy as a result of the decreased HSF-1 expression.[61] One of the first discovered inhibitory agents of HSF-1 was the naturally occurring flavonoid, quercetin. By downregulating the activity of HSF-1 at several steps (hyperphosphorylation, DNA binding, and transcriptional activity), quercetin inhibited tumor cell growth both in vitro and in vivo. Treatment with quercetin also rendered the cells more susceptible to apoptosis resulting from exposure to hyperthermia and chemotherapy. Moreover, the drug seemed to show tumor cell selectivity compared with normal cells.[62] However, the molecular actions of quercetin were

Table 2
Summary of HSR-targeted therapeutics

HSF-1 inhibitors	—	Quercetin KNK-437 NZ28 Emunin
HSP70 inhibitors	ABD	Dihydropyrimidines • NSC630668 • MAL3-101 VER-155008 MKT-077
	PBD	PES
	Aptamers	ADD70
HSP90 inhibitors	Natural	Geldanamycin • 17-AAG (tanespimycin) • 17-DMAG (alvespimycin) • IPI-504 (retaspimycin) Radicicol derivatives • VER-52296 • KF58333 Novobiocin • Coumermycin A1
	Synthetic	PU series • PU-H71 • CNF-2024 Pyrazole/isoxazole compounds • CCT-018159 • VER-52296 Shepherdin
	Isoform specific	NECA (GRP-94)
	Posttranslational	HDAC inhibitors • LAQ824 • FK228
Inhibitors of cochaperones	HSP40	MAL2-11B
	DNAJ	D-peptide
	Hop	Pyrimidotriazinediones
Multitargeted agents	HSF-1, NF-kB and AP-1	Triptolide
	HSR, p53 and NF-kB	Curaxins

Abbreviations: ABD, ATPase-binding domain; HDAC, histone deacetylase; NECA, 5'-N-ethylcarbox-amidoadenosine; PBD, peptide-binding domain; PES, 2-phenylethynesulfonamide.

nonspecific because several protein kinases were downregulated on treatment.[63] Subsequent interest focused on a benzylidene lactam, KNK 437, which was found to be more specific and less toxic. However, both quercetin and KNK 437 did not show enough potency to enable clinical application.[60] In an attempt to provide clinical efficacy, the Chinese herbal medicine triptolide, derived from diterpene triepoxide, was found to potently inhibit the transcriptional activity of the C-terminal transactivation domain of HSF-1, but specificity was an issue, because this compound targeted other transcription factors including NF-kB and AP-1.[64] A recent development in HSF-1 inhibitors was the discovery of 2 novel compounds, NZ28 and emunin, whose predominant mechanism involves the posttranscriptional phase of the induced stress response.[61] In addition, a novel class of agents, termed curaxins, seems to inhibit HSF-1 and are discussed in more detail later.[65]

Inhibition of Chaperones

Given the problems encountered during the development of drugs that modulate the HSR, focus has shifted toward targeting the function of individual HSPs. Given their role in maintaining the malignant phenotype, the HSP90 and HSP70 families have been at the center of concerted efforts for drug development in the past decade.[66,67]

HSP90

This most abundant member of the HSP family constitutes approximately 2% of the cellular protein content of eukaryotic cells. It displays interaction with more than 200 client proteins that carry out diverse, pivotal functions in the cell cycle, including cell cycle regulators (eg, CDK4, h-TERT), mediators of apoptosis (eg, Bcl-2, APAF), tumor suppressor genes (eg, p53), signaling molecules (eg, SRC, AKT), transcription factors (eg, HSF-1, HIF1α), steroid hormone receptors (eg, androgen and progesterone receptors), and mutant fusion kinases (eg, Bcr-Abl). As discussed earlier, many tumor types overexpress this chaperone protein. Considerable research in the past decade has focused on the elucidation of the effector mechanisms of this chaperone as well as strategies to effectively target its functions for cancer therapy.[29]

Natural Inhibitors of HSP90

This high-molecular-weight chaperone functions in an ATP-dependent manner and several of the naturally occurring inhibitors of HSP90 bind to its ATP-binding and hydrolyzing pocket with an affinity higher than natural nucleotides. This action interferes with the client protein folding functions that are regulated by the N-terminal domain. Radicicol (Monorden) is an antifungal compound that, although effective in blocking HSP90 activity in vitro, failed to prove efficacious in vivo because of chemical instability.[68] However, some oxime derivatives of radicicol have been developed that show therapeutic efficacy in human tumor xenograft models (eg, KF58333).[69]

The benzoquinone ansamycins are a second class of naturally occurring antibiotics that inhibit HSP90 activity via competitive inhibition of ATP binding at the N-terminal nucleotide-binding site.[70] Geldanamycin was the lead compound investigated within this class of drugs but, despite its activity in vitro and in vivo, preclinical trials advised caution because of evidence of compound instability and hepatotoxicity.[71] Further efforts to widen the therapeutic window of these agents led to the discovery of the 17-allylamino-17-desmethoxygeldanamycin (17-AAG) analogue, which went on to become the first drug in its class to enter clinical trials. However, progress in the clinic was again thwarted by its poor solubility and lack of oral bioavailability. These issues were overcome by its successor, the N,N-dimethylethylamino analogue 17-DMAG, which exhibited superior potency and water solubility.[68] In phase I trials, 17-DMAG has been tested in a variety of leukemias and solid tumors, with an acceptable toxicity profile. Other 17-AAG analogues such as IPI-504 (retaspimycin) are currently in various phases of clinical testing against a variety of tumor types including lung cancer, GIST, and breast cancer.[72]

The antibiotic novobiocin is another natural inhibitor of HSP90 activity. The mechanism of action of this antibiotic and its analogues, such as coumermycin A1, is distinct from the other natural inhibitors. These compounds bind to the C-terminal domain, which directs the homodimerization of HSP90 and leads to destabilization of several HSP90 client proteins including Her-2, mutant p53, and Bcr-Abl. These agents have growth-inhibitory effects on various cancer cell lines in vitro.[73]

Synthetic Inhibitors of HSP90

Purine (PU)-based compounds that mimic the scaffolds targeting the ATPase activity of HSP90 were the earliest agents tested. The first among these were the PU series, derived from data based on the crystallographic study interactions of ADP and geldanamycin inside the ATP-binding domain. PU-H71 selectively suppresses the BCL-6–dependent growth of lymphoma cells, BCL-6 being a client protein of HSP90.[74] Another purine scaffold compound, CNF-2024, induces death of Hodgkin lymphoma cells via inhibition of the NF-kB pathway.[75] Both these compounds are active against tumor cells in circumstances in which 17-AAG derivatives have failed to show therapeutic efficacy either as a result of tumor cell expression of resistant proteins (P-gp, MRP-1) or because of the lack of overexpression of steroid receptors (eg, ER/PR and Her-2 in breast cancer).[76,77]

High-throughput screening assays designed to investigate the binding affinity of small molecules to the N-terminal domain of HSP90 yielded another novel class of compounds with anti-HSP90 activity, the pyrazole/isoxazole resorcinols, of which 3,4-diarylpyrazole (CCT-018159) has been the lead compound. Exposure of cancer cells to this drug leads to decreased expression of c-raf and cdk4, and an increase in the expression of HSP70, with the result being cytostasis and apoptosis. In the search for structural analogues with enhanced potency, the amide derivatives were discovered, of which the most advanced compound currently being tested is VER-52296.[78]

Another approach that allows more selectivity is the use of peptide mimetics to exclusively disrupt the interaction of HSP90 with specific client proteins. Shepherdin is one such agent, and binds to the N-terminal end of HSP90 through a scaffold that mimics the I74-L87 sequence on survivin, a client protein of HSP90 with key antiapoptotic and proliferative functions. Exposure to shepherdin dramatically increases cell death in acute myeloid leukemia cells both in cell culture and in tumor xenograft models.[79] Selective inhibition has also been targeted against the different isoforms of HSP90. An example is 5′-N-ethylcarboxamidoadenosine (NECA), which has a high binding affinity for the GRP-94 isoform found in mitochondria.[80] The lack of binding to the other HSP90 isoforms holds promise for targeted therapy because the different isoforms display tumor-specific expression. However, it remains to be seen whether these strategies afford better therapeutic efficacy and/or selectivity.

HSP90 activity can also be modulated via its posttranscriptional modification. HSP90 undergoes acetylation, ubiquitination, and S-nitrosylation. Histone deacetylase (HDAC) inhibitors, such as LAQ824 and FK228, effect an epigenetic modulation of HSP90 gene expression by causing the hyperacetylation of HSP90,[81] which inhibits the ATP-binding activity of HSP90 and leads to client protein degradation.

HSP70

Many human cancer cells express increased levels of HSP70, and transformed cells are preferentially enriched with the inducible form of this chaperone protein as opposed to the constitutively expressed form that is widely prevalent in nontransformed cells.[9,82] Moreover, increased expression of HSP70 is encountered in many tumor cells as a result of exposure to chemotherapeutic agents. This phenomenon is widely thought to provide enhanced cytoprotection, and is possibly one of the mechanisms underlying the development of drug resistance. The broad-based antiapoptotic functions of HSP70, which include the inhibition of both caspase-dependent and caspase-independent cell death, therefore make an attractive target for the development of novel cancer therapeutics.[83]

Targeting the Amino-terminal ATPase-binding Domain

Analogous to the HSP90 inhibitors, compounds that disrupt ATP-HSP70 interactions should display therapeutic benefit against tumor cell proliferation and resistance to apoptosis. 15-Deoxyspergualin (15-DSG) was the first compound described to have the ability to stimulate the ATPase activity of HSP70.[82] Subsequent endeavors were designed to discover drugs with enhanced potency and the National Cancer Institute identified the structurally analogous dihydropyrimidine, NSC 630668, which blocked protein translocation mediated by yeast HSC70 in vitro. Next generation dihydropyr-imidines showed even more promise, with MAL3-101 blocking proliferation of breast cancer cells in vitro and showing antimyeloma effects in vivo. Further screening has yielded a variety of small molecules that display divergent pharmacologic activity based on their ability to modulate the ATPase activity of HSP70, but their meaningful clinical application awaits accurate delineation of their mechanistic properties.

VER-155008 is an adenosine derivative with affinity for the ADP-binding site of various HSP70 isoforms, but not for HSP90 chaperones. As a single agent, this compound can induce caspase-dependent and caspase-independent apoptotic cell death in breast and colon cancer cells respectively. This compound sets a precedent for formulating drugs targeting specific isoforms of HSP70, but has not yet been tested in vivo.[84]

MKT, a cationic rhodacyanine dye, also acts via binding to the amino-terminal ATPase-binding domain (ABD) of HSP70. In vitro studies showed that this molecule has a 100-fold higher potency against tumor cells compared with normal healthy cell lines. This finding led to its evaluation in phase I clinical trials against a variety of solid tumors. However, severe nephrotoxicity was encountered at clinically relevant dosages, limiting its usefulness. Researchers are pursuing modifications based on the allosteric association of this compound with HSP70, to evaluate agents with similar binding affinity but without the associated renal toxicity.[85]

Targeting the C-terminal Peptide-binding Domain

Only a few molecules have been developed that target the peptide-binding domain of HSP70. A recently described agent is the small molecule inhibitor called 2-phenylethy-nesulfonamide (PES). Although it has proved to be a potent anticancer agent, debate continues as to the role of HSP in mediating cell death triggered by exposure to this compound. Although some studies show that it directly activates an independent apoptotic, caspase-dependent cell death, others indicate that it may not be specific for HSP70 but may have a role in additionally modulating HSP90.[86]

Given the paucity of small molecules that directly inhibit the function of HSP70, the focus of drug development has shifted toward the formulation of peptide aptamers (molecules that inhibit HSP70 function indirectly by mimicking the binding domains of substrate proteins). One class of such rationally designed decoy targets derives from the amino acid sequence 150 to 228 of apoptosis-inducing factor (AIF). They are referred to as ADD70 (AIF-derived decoy for HSP70), and they bind to and inhibit the activity of HSP70. Treatment with ADD70 produces cytostasis and tumor regres-sion in animal models of colon cancer and melanoma. In addition, in a mechanism that depends on HSP70 neutralization, ADD70 also sensitizes rat colon cancer cells and mouse melanoma cells to treatment with cisplatin.[87] Other peptide aptamers are in various stages of preclinical discovery.

Inhibition of Cochaperones

Because HSP90 and HSP70 function as a part of a larger, macromolecular chaperone machine in association with several other cochaperones, there is the opportunity to indirectly inhibit their activity via inhibition of the cochaperones. One such cochaper-one for HSP90 is AHA1 (activator of HSP90 ATPase), a stress-regulated protein that activates the intrinsic ATPase activity of HSP90. Decreased expression of AHA1 using a variety of methods reduced the activities of HSP90 client proteins such as v-Src and glucocorticoid receptors, as well as reducing HSP90-dependent signaling via the RAS-RAF-MEK-ERK1/2 and PI3K-AKT/PKB pathways.[88] Treatment with HDAC inhibitors also leads to a substantial decrease in the association of HSP90 with some of its cochaperones.[81]

HSP40 is an important cochaperone of HSP70. There is significant heterogeneity of HSP40 homologues, and interaction of each subtype with HSP70 is hypothesized to have distinct effects on cell proteostasis.[89] MAL2-11B is one compound known to negatively modulate the ability of HSP40 to stimulate HSP70 ATPase activity. A high-throughput alpha screen approach used by one group has led to the discovery of pyrimidotriazinediones, compounds that disrupt the interaction of Hop (HSP70/90 organizing protein) with HSP70. Hop is a modular protein that is essential for the transfer of client proteins between the HSP70 and HSP90 chaperone machines. These compounds were found to be toxic to tumor cells in vitro.[90] Whether this approach will realize the promise of higher selectivity and improved therapeutic efficacy remains to be seen.

Combination Strategies

Combination use of selective inhibitors of different aspects of the HSR may improve the therapeutic potential of targeting this pathway (see **Table 2**). A well-known consequence of the treatment of tumor cells with HSP90 inhibitors is the induction of other HSPs, especially HSP70 and HSP27, both cochaperones with significant anti-apoptotic properties.[45] Therefore, combining HSP90 inhibitors with either specific modulators of HSP70/HSP27 or with HSF-1 inhibitors capable of preventing their induction would result in synergy, enhancing the anticancer properties of those compounds. Combination therapy has shown efficacy in vitro as well as in vivo. Pretreatment of human leukemic cells with the HSF-1 inhibitor KNK-437 rendered them more susceptible to treatment with the HSP90 inhibitor 17-AAG.[83] Treatment of colon cancer cell lines with the HSP70 inhibitors VER-155008 and ADD70 similarly caused a significant increase in the anticancer activity of 17-AAG.[84,87] Because resistance to therapy has been attributed to overexpression of certain HSPs, combined modulation of more than one HSP, or the use of HSP modulation in combination with standard chemotherapeutics, has the potential to overcome drug resistance.

CURAXINS: A NOVEL GROUP OF MULTITARGETED THERAPEUTICS

A novel class of anticancer therapeutics has recently been discovered by Gurova and colleagues,[91] and consist of a new family of multitargeted, nongenotoxic drugs named curaxins. In their initial efforts to target the HSR to augment the efficacy of drugs such as bortezomib and geldanamycin, their group analyzed known antimalarial agents with the hypothesis that, like cancer cells, the malarial parasite must survive by using adaptive mechanisms to combat proteotoxic stress. Both quinacrine (QC) and emetine abolished the HSR in treated cancer cells. Although emetine inhibited general translation, QC had a more specific mechanism of action, via suppression of the inducible HSF-1-dependent transcription of the HSP70 gene. It was therefore able to block the induction of HSR in cells exposed to geldanamycin or to heat. Combination treatments with QC and proteotoxic stressors led to tumor cell apoptosis in vitro and regression of tumors in vivo.[92]

It had been shown previously by the same group that QC is a powerful inducer of p53 and inhibitor of NF-kB. Because of its multitargeted efficacy, lack of genotoxicity, and established safety profile, the profound antitumor potential of QC initiated research into the development of analogous compounds with enhanced potency and optimized pharmacologic characteristics. A structure-activity relationship study was used to evaluate libraries of structural analogues of QC in cell-based p53 and NF-kB reporter assays, which gave rise to the curaxins.[91] The mechanism of action of these compounds has been further elucidated and involves the chromatin trapping of FACT (facilitates chromatin transcription), a target protein that is selectively overexpressed in tumor cells.[65] Further research will likely establish a role for the use of these drugs as effective ways to modulate several critical pathways involved in carcinogenesis without invoking the inherent risks of traditional genotoxic chemotherapeutics.

SYNERGY WITH HYPERTHERMIA

As a primary initiator of the HSR, hyperthermia for the treatment of a variety of disease states, including cancer, has been appreciated for centuries. There are accounts from ancient India, Egypt, and Greece describing the use of heat to treat breast cancer. Parmenides is thought to have said "Give me a chance to create fever and I will cure any disease." In the second half of the nineteenth century, reports emerged from Europe describing the regression of a small number of tumors after patients experienced a high fever. In 1893, Coley introduced the use of toxins that induced prolonged high-grade fevers as a means to treat tumors. Around this same time, Westermark used intracavitary circulating heated water to palliate uterine cervical cancer. In 1909, Keating-Hart was the first to use electrical current to produce local hyperthermia in the treatment of tumors: an example of electrocoagulation, which continues to be an efficient ablative strategy to this day. The use of hyperthermia (local, regional, or whole body) in combination with chemotherapy or radiotherapy for the treatment of a wide variety of tumors has subsequently evolved.[93]

There is a clear scientific rationale for the use of hyperthermia in cancer therapy. By virtue of a tumor microenvironment that is typically hypoxic and acidic, tumor cells are especially sensitive to levels of thermal stress that are nonlethal in normal tissues ($40–44°C$).[94] This hostile tumor core is also the region that is least sensitive to radiation therapy and has the lowest delivered concentration of systemically administered cytotoxic agents, owing to poor perfusion. The benefits of hyperthermia in this setting can be attributed to a multitude of factors, including the direct cytotoxic effect of heat, induced alterations in the tumor microenvironment, synergy with chemotherapy or radiotherapy, as well effects at the cellular level, including the induction of the HSR.[95] Studies have shown the generation of enhanced antitumor immune responses with the use of mild hyperthermia. Besides the activation of antigen-presenting cells and altered patterns of lymphocyte trafficking, this is also, at least in part, caused by the increased production of HSPs.[96] Current clinical applications involve local hyperthermia using external or internal sources of energy; regional hyperthermia via perfusion of limbs, organs, or body cavities; and whole-body hyperthermia.

Direct intratumoral placement of a probe that emits an alternating electrical current (radiofrequency ablation) or microwaves (microwave ablation) is the prototypical application of tumor ablative strategies that use hyperthermia. These modalities have allowed the treatment of otherwise unresectable liver lesions, both primary and metastatic, with curative intent, enabling a meaningful prolongation of disease-free and overall survival.[93] Depending on the modality used and the intensity of treatment delivered, there is the creation of a core of intratumoral coagulative necrosis, a middle zone of apoptotic cell death, and an outer zone of hyperemia/hyperthermia without cell death. Clinicians strive to achieve a margin of normal tissue ablation surrounding the tumor edges to achieve the equivalence of an R0 resection.[97] With the addition of inhibitors of the HSR, the potential zone of tumor cell destruction may be improved with minimal damage to surrounding normal structures. Blockade of HSPs in tumor cells that already maximize their HSR may tip the balance in favor of apoptosis, whereas normal tissues have a greater threshold for undergoing cell death.

The application of hyperthermia is not limited to local therapies and is routinely used in the treatment of a variety of cancers in the form of regional therapies. Regional therapies include isolated limb perfusion for extremity melanoma or sarcoma, and heated intraperitoneal chemoperfusion following cytoreduction for the treatment of peritoneal carcinomatosis. Temperatures of 42°C are typically reached and are associated with the HSR. The introduction of agents capable of blocking the HSR in these scenarios is expected to increase tumor cell kill while simultaneously allowing a dose reduction in toxic chemotherapeutics.

SUMMARY

The discovery of the importance of the HSR in cancer development and progression has created a promising avenue in oncologic translational research. Novel techniques of screening large libraries of small molecule inhibitors have provided a potential new generation of targeted and specific chemotherapeutics. Ongoing translational research and clinical trials in modulating the HSR in cancer are gaining momentum and offer the opportunity for synergy with existing therapies.

REFERENCES

1. Lindquist S. The heat-shock response. Annu Rev Biochem 1986;55:1151–91.
2. Lindquist S, Craig E. The heat-shock proteins. Annu Rev Genet 1988;22(1): 631–77.
3. Ritossa F. A new puffing pattern induced by temperature shock and DNP in *Drosophila*. Cell Mol Life Sci 1962;18(12):571–3.
4. Tissières A, Mitchell HK, Tracy UM. Protein synthesis in salivary glands of *Drosophila melanogaster*: relation to chromosome puffs. J Mol Biol 1974; 84(3):389–98.
5. Hightower LE. Heat shock, stress proteins, chaperones, and proteotoxicity. Cell 1991;66(2):191–7.
6. Beere HM. "The stress of dying": the role of heat shock proteins in the regulation of apoptosis. J Cell Sci 2004;117(13):2641–51.
7. Thomas PJ, Qu B, Pedersen PL. Defective protein folding as a basis of human disease. Trends Biochem Sci 1995;20(11):456–9.
8. Calderwood SK, Khaleque MA, Sawyer DB, et al. Heat shock proteins in cancer: chaperones of tumorigenesis. Trends Biochem Sci 2006;31(3):164–72.
9. Ciocca DR, Calderwood SK. Heat shock proteins in cancer: diagnostic, prognostic, predictive, and treatment implications. Cell Stress Chaperones 2005; 10(2):86.
10. Morimoto RI, Santoro MG. Stress-inducible responses and heat shock proteins: new pharmacologic targets for cytoprotection. Nat Biotechnol 1998;16(9): 833–8.
11. Sarge KD, Murphy SP, Morimoto RI. Activation of heat shock gene transcription by heat shock factor 1 involves oligomerization, acquisition of DNA-binding activity, and nuclear localization and can occur in the absence of stress. Mol Cell Biol 1993;13(3):1392–407.

12. Zou J, Guo Y, Guettouche T, et al. Repression of heat shock transcription factor HSF1 activation by HSP90 (HSP90 complex) that forms a stress-sensitive complex with HSF1. Cell 1998;94(4):471–80.
13. Ananthan J, Goldberg AL, Voellmy R. Abnormal proteins serve as eukaryotic stress signals and trigger the activation of heat shock genes. Science 1986; 232(4749):522.
14. Morimoto RI, Tissières A, Georgopoulos C. The biology of heat shock proteins and molecular chaperones. New York: Cold Spring Harbor Laboratory Press; 1994.
15. Spiess C, Beil A, Ehrmann M. A temperature-dependent switch from chaperone to protease in a widely conserved heat shock protein. Cell 1999;97(3):339–47.
16. Buchberger A, Bakau B, Gething M. Guidebook to molecular chaperones and protein-folding catalysts. Oxford (UK): Oxford University Press; 1997.
17. Kampinga HH, Hageman J, Vos MJ, et al. Guidelines for the nomenclature of the human heat shock proteins. Cell Stress Chaperones 2009;14(1):105–11.
18. Mayer M, Bukau B. Hsp70 chaperones: cellular functions and molecular mechanism. Cell Mol Life Sci 2005;62(6):670–84.
19. Laufen T, Mayer MP, Beisel C, et al. Mechanism of regulation of Hsp70 chaperones by DnaJ cochaperones. Proc Natl Acad Sci U S A 1999;96(10):5452–7.
20. Panaretou B, Prodromou C, Roe SM, et al. ATP binding and hydrolysis are essential to the function of the Hsp90 molecular chaperone in vivo. EMBO J 1998;17(16):4829–36.
21. Pratt WB, Toft DO. Regulation of signaling protein function and trafficking by the hsp90/hsp70-based chaperone machinery. Exp Biol Med 2003;228(2):111–33.
22. Pearl LH, Prodromou C. Structure and mechanism of the Hsp90 molecular chaperone machinery. Annu Rev Biochem 2006;75:271–94.
23. Queitsch C, Sangster TA, Lindquist S. Hsp90 as a capacitor of phenotypic variation. Nature 2002;417(6889):618–24.
24. Wegele H, Müller L, Buchner J. Hsp70 and Hsp90—a relay team for protein folding. Ergeb Physiol 2004;151(1):1–44.
25. Young JC, Agashe VR, Siegers K, et al. Pathways of chaperone-mediated protein folding in the cytosol. Nat Rev Mol Cell Biol 2004;5(10):781–91.
26. Hanahan D, Weinberg RA. The hallmarks of cancer. Cell 2000;100(1):57–70.
27. Ciocca DR, Arrigo AP, Calderwood SK. Heat shock proteins and heat shock factor 1 in carcinogenesis and tumor development: an update. Arch Toxicol 2013;87(1):19–48.
28. Diehl JA, Yang W, Rimerman RA, et al. Hsc70 regulates accumulation of cyclin D1 and cyclin D1-dependent protein kinase. Mol Cell Biol 2003;23(5):1764–74.
29. Taipale M, Jarosz DF, Lindquist S. HSP90 at the hub of protein homeostasis: emerging mechanistic insights. Nat Rev Mol Cell Biol 2010;11(7):515–28.
30. Bishop SC, Burlison JA, Blagg J, et al. Hsp90: a novel target for the disruption of multiple signaling cascades. Curr Cancer Drug Targets 2007;7(4):369–88.
31. Yaglom JA, Gabai VL, Sherman MY. High levels of heat shock protein Hsp72 in cancer cells suppress default senescence pathways. Cancer Res 2007;67(5): 2373–81.
32. Sherman M, Gabai V, O'Callaghan C, et al. Molecular chaperones regulate p53 and suppress senescence programs. FEBS Lett 2007;581(19):3711–5.
33. Holt SE, Aisner DL, Baur J, et al. Functional requirement of p23 and Hsp90 in telomerase complexes. Genes Dev 1999;13(7):817–26.
34. Keezer SM, Ivie SE, Krutzsch HC, et al. Angiogenesis inhibitors target the endothelial cell cytoskeleton through altered regulation of heat shock protein 27 and cofilin. Cancer Res 2003;63(19):6405–12.

35. Zhou J, Schmid T, Frank R, et al. PI3K/Akt is required for heat shock proteins to protect hypoxia-inducible factor 1α from pVHL-independent degradation. J Biol Chem 2004;279(14):13506–13.

36. Garcia-Cardena G, Fan R, Shah V, et al. Dynamic activation of endothelial nitric oxide synthase by Hsp90. Nature 1998;392(6678):821–4.

37. Eustace BK, Sakurai T, Stewart JK, et al. Functional proteomic screens reveal an essential extracellular role for hsp90α in cancer cell invasiveness. Nat Cell Biol 2004;6(6):507–14.

38. Tang D, Khaleque MA, Jones EL, et al. Expression of heat shock proteins and heat shock protein messenger ribonucleic acid in human prostate carcinoma in vitro and in tumors in vivo. Cell Stress Chaperones 2005;10(1):46.

39. Ciocca DR, Fanelli MA, Cuello-Carrion FD, et al. Heat shock proteins in prostate cancer: from tumorigenesis to the clinic. Int J Hyperthermia 2010;26(8): 737–47.

40. Hoang AT, Huang J, Rudra-Ganguly N, et al. A novel association between the human heat shock transcription factor 1 (HSF1) and prostate adenocarcinoma. Am J Pathol 2000;156(3):857–64.

41. Luo J, Solimini NL, Elledge SJ. Principles of cancer therapy: oncogene and non-oncogene addiction. Cell 2009;136(5):823–37.

42. Rutherford SL, Lindquist S. Hsp90 as a capacitor for morphological evolution. Nature 1998;396(6709):336–42.

43. Jolly C, Morimoto RI. Role of the heat shock response and molecular chaperones in oncogenesis and cell death. J Natl Cancer Inst 2000;92(19): 1564–72.

44. Zhang H, Burrows F. Targeting multiple signal transduction pathways through inhibition of Hsp90. J Mol Med (Berl) 2004;82(8):488–99.

45. Lanneau D, Brunet M, Frisan E, et al. Heat shock proteins: essential proteins for apoptosis regulation. J Cell Mol Med 2008;12(3):743–61.

46. Nylandsted J, Gyrd-Hansen M, Danielewicz A, et al. Heat shock protein 70 promotes cell survival by inhibiting lysosomal membrane permeabilization. J Exp Med 2004;200(4):425–35.

47. Beere HM. Stressed to death: regulation of apoptotic signaling pathways by the heat shock proteins. Sci STKE 2001;93:1–6.

48. Campisi J. Senescent cells, tumor suppression, and organismal aging: good citizens, bad neighbors. Cell 2005;120(4):513–22.

49. Bodnar AG, Ouellette M, Frolkis M, et al. Extension of life-span by introduction of telomerase into normal human cells. Science 1998;279(5349):349–52.

50. Rohde M, Daugaard M, Jensen MH, et al. Members of the heat-shock protein 70 family promote cancer cell growth by distinct mechanisms. Genes Dev 2005; 19(5):570–82.

51. Semenza GL. Targeting HIF-1 for cancer therapy. Nat Rev Cancer 2003;3(10): 721–32.

52. Zhang D, Li J, Costa M, et al. JNK1 mediates degradation HIF-1α by a VHL-independent mechanism that involves the chaperones Hsp90/Hsp70. Cancer Res 2010;70(2):813–23.

53. Fleming I, Busse R. Molecular mechanisms involved in the regulation of the endothelial nitric oxide synthase. Am J Physiol Regul Integr Comp Physiol 2003;284(1):R1–12.

54. Kim D, Kim S, Li GC. Proteasome inhibitors MG132 and lactacystin hyperphosphorylate HSF1 and induce hsp70 and hsp27 expression. Biochem Biophys Res Commun 1999;254(1):264–8.

55. Richardson PG, Sonneveld P, Schuster MW, et al. Bortezomib or high-dose dexamethasone for relapsed multiple myeloma. N Engl J Med 2005;352(24): 2487–98.

56. Turbyville TJ, Wijeratne EK, Whitesell L, et al. The anticancer activity of the fungal metabolite terrecyclic acid A is associated with modulation of multiple cellular stress response pathways. Mol Cancer Ther 2005;4(10):1569–76.

57. Whitesell L, Bagatell R, Falsey R. The stress response: implications for the clinical development of hsp90 inhibitors. Curr Cancer Drug Targets 2003;3(5):349–58.

58. Jurivich DA, Pangas S, Qiu L, et al. Phospholipase A2 triggers the first phase of the thermal stress response and exhibits cell-type specificity. J Immunol 1996; 157(4):1669–77.

59. Hargitai J, Lewis H, Boros I, et al. Bimoclomol, a heat shock protein co-inducer, acts by the prolonged activation of heat shock factor-1. Biochem Biophys Res Commun 2003;307(3):689–95.

60. Powers MV, Workman P. Inhibitors of the heat shock response: biology and pharmacology. FEBS Lett 2007;581(19):3758–69.

61. Zaarur N, Gabai VL, Porco JA, et al. Targeting heat shock response to sensitize cancer cells to proteasome and Hsp90 inhibitors. Cancer Res 2006;66(3): 1783–91.

62. Jakubowicz-Gil J, Rzymowska J, Gawron A. Quercetin, apoptosis, heat shock. Biochem Pharmacol 2002;64(11):1591–5.

63. Ferry DR, Smith A, Malkhandi J, et al. Phase I clinical trial of the flavonoid quercetin: pharmacokinetics and evidence for in vivo tyrosine kinase inhibition. Clin Cancer Res 1996;2(4):659–68.

64. Jiang X, Wong BC, Lin MC, et al. Functional p53 is required for triptolide-induced apoptosis and AP-1 and nuclear factor-kB activation in gastric cancer cells. Oncogene 2001;20(55):8009–18.

65. Gasparian AV, Burkhart CA, Purmal AA, et al. Curaxins: anticancer compounds that simultaneously suppress NF-kB and activate p53 by targeting FACT. Sci Transl Med 2011;3(95):95ra74.

66. Neckers L. Hsp90 inhibitors as novel cancer chemotherapeutic agents. Trends Mol Med 2002;8(4):S55–61.

67. Galluzzi L, Giordanetto F, Kroemer G. Targeting HSP70 for cancer therapy. Mol Cell 2009;36(2):176–7.

68. Sharp S, Workman P. Inhibitors of the HSP90 molecular chaperone: current status. Adv Cancer Res 2006;95:323–48.

69. Soga S, Shiotsu Y, Akinaga S, et al. Development of radicicol analogues. Curr Cancer Drug Targets 2003;3(5):359–69.

70. Stebbins CE, Russo AA, Schneider C, et al. Crystal structure of an Hsp90-geldanamycin complex: targeting of a protein chaperone by an antitumor agent. Cell 1997;89(2):239.

71. Supko JG, Hickman RL, Grever MR, et al. Preclinical pharmacologic evaluation of geldanamycin as an antitumor agent. Cancer Chemother Pharmacol 1995; 36(4):305–15.

72. Kim Y, Alarcon S, Lee S, et al. Update on Hsp90 inhibitors in clinical trial. Curr Top Med Chem 2009;9(15):1479–92.

73. Trepel J, Mollapour M, Giaccone G, et al. Targeting the dynamic HSP90 complex in cancer. Nat Rev Cancer 2010;10(8):537–49.

74. Cerchietti LC, Lopes EC, Yang SN, et al. A purine scaffold Hsp90 inhibitor destabilizes BCL-6 and has specific antitumor activity in BCL-6–dependent B cell lymphomas. Nat Med 2009;15(12):1369–76.

75. Böll B, Eltaib F, Reiners KS, et al. Heat shock protein 90 inhibitor BIIB021 (CNF2024) depletes NF-κB and sensitizes Hodgkin's lymphoma cells for natural killer cell–mediated cytotoxicity. Clin Cancer Res 2009;15(16):5108–16.
76. Zhang H, Neely L, Lundgren K, et al. BIIB021, a synthetic Hsp90 inhibitor, has broad application against tumors with acquired multidrug resistance. Int J Cancer 2010;126(5):1226–34.
77. Caldas-Lopes E, Cerchietti L, Ahn JH, et al. Hsp90 inhibitor PU-H71, a multimodal inhibitor of malignancy, induces complete responses in triple-negative breast cancer models. Proc Natl Acad Sci U S A 2009;106(20):8368–73.
78. Sharp SY, Prodromou C, Boxall K, et al. Inhibition of the heat shock protein 90 molecular chaperone in vitro and in vivo by novel, synthetic, potent resorcinylic pyrazole/isoxazole amide analogues. Mol Cancer Ther 2007;6(4):1198–211.
79. Plescia J, Salz W, Xia F, et al. Rational design of shepherdin, a novel anticancer agent. Cancer Cell 2005;7(5):457–68.
80. Rosser MF, Nicchitta CV. Ligand interactions in the adenosine nucleotide-binding domain of the Hsp90 chaperone, GRP94 I. evidence for allosteric regulation of ligand binding. J Biol Chem 2000;275(30):22798–805.
81. Glaser KB. HDAC inhibitors: clinical update and mechanism-based potential. Biochem Pharmacol 2007;74(5):659–71.
82. Powers MV, Jones K, Barillari C, et al. Targeting HSP70: the second potentially druggable heat shock protein and molecular chaperone? Cell Cycle 2010;9(8):1542–50.
83. Guo F, Rocha K, Bali P, et al. Abrogation of heat shock protein 70 induction as a strategy to increase antileukemia activity of heat shock protein 90 inhibitor 17-allylamino-demethoxy geldanamycin. Cancer Res 2005;65(22):10536–44.
84. Massey AJ, Williamson DS, Browne H, et al. A novel, small molecule inhibitor of Hsc70/Hsp70 potentiates Hsp90 inhibitor induced apoptosis in HCT116 colon carcinoma cells. Cancer Chemother Pharmacol 2010;66(3):535–45.
85. Rousaki A, Miyata Y, Jinwal UK, et al. Allosteric drugs: the interaction of anti-tumor compound MKT-077 with human Hsp70 chaperones. J Mol Biol 2011;411(3):614–32.
86. Leu J, Pimkina J, Pandey P, et al. HSP70 inhibition by the small-molecule 2-phenylethynesulfonamide impairs protein clearance pathways in tumor cells. Mol Cancer Res 2011;9(7):936–47.
87. Schmitt E, Maingret L, Puig P, et al. Heat shock protein 70 neutralization exerts potent antitumor effects in animal models of colon cancer and melanoma. Cancer Res 2006;66(8):4191–7.
88. Harst A, Lin H, Obermann WM. Aha1 competes with Hop, p50 and p23 for binding to the molecular chaperone Hsp90 and contributes to kinase and hormone receptor activation. Biochem J 2005;387(Pt 3):789.
89. Lu Z, Cyr DM. Protein folding activity of Hsp70 is modified differentially by the hsp40 co-chaperones Sis1 and Ydj1. J Biol Chem 1998;273(43):27824–30.
90. Yi F, Regan L. A novel class of small molecule inhibitors of Hsp90. ACS Chem Biol 2008;3(10):645–54.
91. Gurova KV, Hill JE, Guo C, et al. Small molecules that reactivate p53 in renal cell carcinoma reveal a NF-κB-dependent mechanism of p53 suppression in tumors. Proc Natl Acad Sci U S A 2005;102(48):17448–53.
92. Neznanov N, Gorbachev AV, Neznanova L, et al. Anti-malaria drug blocks proteotoxic stress response: anti-cancer implications. Cell Cycle 2009;8(23):3960–70.

93. Glazer ES, Curley SA. The ongoing history of thermal therapy for cancer. Surg Oncol Clin N Am 2011;20(2):229.

94. Dickson J, Calderwood S. Temperature range and selective sensitivity of tumors to hyperthermia: a critical review. Ann N Y Acad Sci 2006;335(1):180–205.

95. Wust P, Hildebrandt B, Sreenivasa G, et al. Hyperthermia in combined treatment of cancer. Lancet Oncol 2002;3(8):487–97.

96. Skitzki JJ, Repasky EA, Evans SS. Hyperthermia as an immunotherapy strategy for cancer. Curr Opin Investig Drugs 2009;10(6):550.

97. Hong K, Georgiades C. Radiofrequency ablation: mechanism of action and devices. J Vasc Interv Radiol 2010;21(8):S179–86.

Targeting Receptor Tyrosine Kinases in Solid Tumors

Jianliang Zhang, PhD, Steven N. Hochwald, MD*

KEYWORDS

- Tyrosine kinase inhibitors • Cancer • Solid tumors

KEY POINTS

- Hyperactivation of receptor tyrosine kinases (TK) is common in solid tumors.
- Inhibitors targeting TK signaling have been approved by the Food and Drug Administration to treat patients with primary and metastatic malignancies including cancers of the colon, lung, breast, pancreatic, and head and neck.
- Current advances in cancer-associated TK signaling, antibodies that block and neutralize receptor TK, and small-molecule drug targeting of TK signaling are evaluated and summarized.

INTRODUCTION
What are Tyrosine Kinase Inhibitors?

Animal tissues rely on cell-surface receptor tyrosine kinases (TK) to detect and respond to nutrients and growth factor hormones. Deregulated TK signaling, including overreaction to extracellular stimuli or autocrine activation, plays an important role in tumorigenesis. Hyperactivation of receptor TK caused by gene mutation, amplification, rearrangement, and transcriptional and translational deregulation is common in the tissues of solid tumors.[1] Better understanding of receptor TK signaling in the modulation of cell transformation, proliferation, apoptosis, angiogenesis, invasion, and migration can help the design of inhibitors to treat malignancies.

The TK family consists of 58 receptor and 32 nonreceptor or cytoplasmic TK.[2] Receptor TK span through the cell membrane with an extracellular and an intracellular domain. Stimuli such as growth factors bind to the extracellular domain, often leading to change and activation of TK conformation. The cytosolic kinase domain of TK catalyzes the transfer of a phosphor group from adenosine triphosphate (ATP) to the

Disclosures: The authors have nothing to disclose.
Department of Surgical Oncology, Roswell Park Cancer Institute, Elm and Carlton Streets, Buffalo, NY 14263, USA
* Corresponding author.
E-mail address: steven.hochwald@roswellpark.org

Surg Oncol Clin N Am 22 (2013) 685–703
http://dx.doi.org/10.1016/j.soc.2013.06.010
1055-3207/13/$ – see front matter © 2013 Elsevier Inc. All rights reserved.

tyrosine residues of substrate proteins. The chain activation of cascade kinases transmits microenvironmental cues to cellular growth, survival, or death. Deregulation of the outside-in signaling contributes to the abnormal survival and/or uncontrolled growth in tumorigenesis.

Inhibitors are designed to target specific receptor TK that are overactive because of insult-induced protein damage and/or genetic mutation-caused loss/gain of function in tumors. In comparison with classic cytotoxic chemotherapy, targeted treatment is expected to have fewer side effects or normal tissue injury, but higher selectivity or potency in inducing cancer cell death. Disadvantages of targeted therapies are: (1) the molecular, biochemical, and cellular information of dysfunctional TK must be available before TK inhibitors (TKI) can be designed[3]; (2) the outcomes of the targeted therapy can vary among patients because the signal alternations are varied even in the same tumor[4]; and (3) the effects of off-target inhibition can cause side effects.[5,6]

Current advances in novel technologies, disease models, and genetic manipulations allow identification of tumor-related signal pathways. TKI targeting such pathways have been developed. Searching the National Institutes of Health clinical trial database (clinicalTrial.gov) using the terms "tyrosine kinase inhibitors and cancer," 448 hits were revealed. Major targets include the epidermal growth factor receptor (EGFR), the human epidermal growth factor receptor 2 (HER2), the platelet-derived growth factor receptor (PDGFR), the vascular endothelial growth factor receptor (VEGFR), the fibroblast growth factor receptor (FGFR), c-Met (MET or MNNG HOS transforming gene) or the hepatocyte growth factor receptor (HGFR), and the insulin-like growth factor receptor (IGF-1R). Growth factor ligands bind and activate the receptor TK, inducing downstream signal transduction pathways including PI3K/Akt/mTOR, RAS/RAF/MEK/ERK, JAK/FAK/Src/STAT, and PLC/DAG/PKC signaling (**Fig. 1**). These pathways modulate cell-cycle progression, survival, differentiation, migration, and apoptosis. Deregulation caused by mutation, amplification, and overexpression or suppressed expression contributes to tumorigenesis.

TK SIGNALING AND SOLID TUMORS
EGFR Signaling in Proliferation and Migration of Cancer Cells

Function
EGFR belongs to a closely related ErbB subfamily that consists of EGFR (ErbB-1), HER2/c-neu (ErbB-2), HER3 (ErbB-3), and HER4 (ErbB-4). The gene symbol ErbB is derived from erythroblastic leukemia viral oncogene, to which these receptors are homologous. EGFR is located across the cell membrane, and its surface portion binds to extracellular protein ligands including epidermal growth factors (EGF) and transforming growth factor α. Ligand binding triggers the conformation change and dimerization of EGFR, leading to TK activity of its cytosolic domain. EGFR autophosphorylation at multiple sites such as Y992, Y1045, Y1068, Y1148, and Y1173 elicits downstream signaling through tyrosine phosphorylation of effectors including mitogen-activated protein kinase (MAPK), Akt, and JNK.[7] EGFR activation induces DNA synthesis and suppresses apoptosis, contributing to cell migration, adhesion, and proliferation (see **Fig. 1**).[8]

Tumorigenicity
Genetic mutations and/or insults that promote EGFR ligand binding, sustained activation, and receptor TK phosphorylation can enhance cell survival and abnormal growth. Overexpression, deregulation, and hyperactivation of EGFR or its family members are associated with cancers that are derived from epithelium.[9–12] Identification of

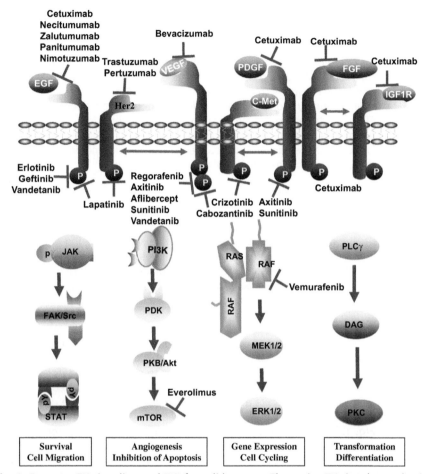

Fig. 1. Receptor TK signaling and TKI for solid tumors. The major TK signal transduction pathways that have led to the development of FDA-approved TKI are summarized. Growth factor ligand binding to their receptors induces dimerization, transphosphorylation, and activation of EGF receptor, HER2, PDGF receptor, VEGF receptor, c-Met, FGF receptor, and IGF receptor. Phosphorylation/stimulation of downstream effectors including JAK/FAK/Src/STAT, PI3K/PDK/Akt/mTOR, RAS/RAF/MEK/ERK, and PLC/DAG/PKC modulates cell survival, migration, angiogenesis, apoptosis, gene expression, cell-cycle progression, transformation, and differentiation. Monoclonal antibodies and small-molecule drugs inhibit the abnormal activity of receptor or effector TK, preventing tumor proliferation and growth. C-Met, MET or MNNG HOS transforming gene; EGF, epidermal growth factor; FGF, fibroblast growth factor; Her2, human epidermal growth factor receptor 2; IGF1R, insulin-like growth factor receptor; mTOR, mammalian target of rapamycin; PDGF, platelet-derived growth factor; PI3K, phosphatidylinositol-3-kinase; VEGF, vascular endothelial growth factor.

oncogenic EGFR has attracted great attention in the attempt to develop therapeutic interventions to treat EGFR hyperactive tumors. Receptor-neutralizing antibodies and small molecules are used to prevent ligand interactions, conformation changes or activation, and ATP binding.

HER2 and Cell Growth

HER2 is encoded by the *ERBB2* gene and belongs to the EGFR family. There is no known ligand that binds to HER2. It is a preferred binding partner of other EGFR members in forming heterodimers. Dimerization induces the autophosphorylation of the cytosolic kinase region, triggering several cascade events such as MAPK, PI3K/Akt, PPCγ, PKC, and STAT signal-transduction pathways (see **Fig. 1**).

EGFR signaling potently promotes cell proliferation and inhibits apoptosis. Hyperactivity of HER2 contributes to uncontrolled growth in tumorigenesis.[13,14] Overexpression and/or alterations of HER2 have been observed in breast, ovarian, stomach, and aggressive forms of uterine cancer, such as uterine serous endometrial carcinoma.[15] HER2 inhibition can prolong the survival of patients with cancer.[16]

VEGFR and Tumor Angiogenesis

Uncontrolled cell proliferation increases tumor size, leading to oxygen and nutrient deficiency due to perfusion limitations. Under hypoxic or nutrient-depleted conditions normal cells will die, but malignant cells live and survive. One of the adaptive responses of tumor cells is to release the vascular endothelial growth factor (VEGF). Endothelial cells line the blood vessels. The very end of the vasculature (capillary) consists of a single layer of endothelial cells that express VEGFR. In responding to VEGF, the endothelium expands or sprouts to form new vessels/branches to supply oxygen and nutrients.[17,18]

VEGF binding to its receptor induces VEGFR dimerization and activation through transphosphorylation. VEGF-A interacts and activates VEGFR1 (Flt-1) and VEGFR2 (KDR/Flk-1). VEGF-C and VEGF-D bind to VEGFR3. VEGFR2 is responsible for most VEGF-stimulated cellular responses. VEGFR1 seems to modulate VEGFR2 action as a decoy. A soluble form of VEGFR1 can be secreted, and serves as a decoy through binding to VEGF-A. VEGFR3 plays a role in lymphangiogenesis. TKI are designed to interrupt the VEGF binding, VEGFR transphosphorylation, and substrate-effector activation (see **Fig. 1**).[19,20] Preventing VEGF stimulation of angiogenesis or forming new blood vessels can cut off oxygen and nutrient supplies, often stopping tumor growth. However, some cancer cells can develop resistance to VEGFR inhibition through activation of alternative pathways.

PDGFR and Cell Differentiation and Proliferation

Phenotype changes are among the major hallmarks of malignancies. PDGFs play key roles in cell differentiation, proliferation, and growth. The PDGF family consists of PDGF-A, PDGF-B, PDGF-C, and PDGF-D, which can form homodimers or heterodimers: AA, BB, AB, CC, or DD. PDGFR-α and PDGFR-β are PDGF receptors encoded by different genes. On PDGF stimulation, the PDGFR can form αα, ββ, or αβ dimers. The combinations among PDGF and their receptors are varied in different cell types. Dimerization/transphosphorylation induces the PDGFR conformation change, resulting in kinase activation. Phosphorylation of downstream factors induces signaling cascades including RAS/MAPK and PI3K/PLCγ pathways (see **Fig. 1**). PDGFR overexpression and/or hyperactivity are common in solid tumors. For instance, the gene copy numbers of PDGFR are increased in non–small cell lung carcinoma (NSCLC).[21]

FGFR and Tumorigenesis

Four genes encode FGFR1, FGFR2, FGFR3, and FGFR4. Natural alterations of transcriptional splicing can generate 48 isoforms of FGFR.[22] There are 22 fibroblast growth factors (FGF), belonging to the largest family of growth factor ligands. Each ligand can bind to several FGFR that vary in properties. FGFR-mediated signaling contributes to cell proliferation, differentiation, survival, and invasion (see **Fig. 1**). Protein alterations, upregulation, and fusion caused by genetic mutation and rearrangements of FGFR genes are associated with many types of malignancies including prostate, lung, sarcoma, breast, bladder, melanoma, and moderately/poorly differentiated endometrial cancer.[23–25] Fewer studies have been performed on the development of TKI targeting FGFR in comparison with TKI targeting EGFR, VEGFR, PDGFR, and IGF-1R. Challenges are related to complexity of FGFR signaling pathways, the presence of fibroblasts in normal and tumor tissues, and a weak correlation between FGFR hyperactivity and tumor prognosis.

c-Met and Invasive Growth

The HGFR protein is encoded by c-Met. Posttranslational modifications of the precursor protein include cleavage and disulfide linking, resulting in the mature receptor. Hepatocyte growth factor is the only known ligand for HGFR, which is produced and released by cells of mesenchymal origin. HGFR is expressed in the cells of epithelial origin. On stimulation of hepatocyte growth factor, HGFR phosphorylates/activates downstream factors including PLCγ/PKC, PI3K/Akt, Ras/Raf/ERK, and FAK/Src (see **Fig. 1**). The activated cascades modulate invasive growth to generate new organs and tissues in embryonic development and tissue-wound healing.[26–28]

Cancer cells can hijack the HGFR-related growth process for their invasion and metastasis. C-Met overexpression contributes to apoptotic resistance of pancreatic and ovarian cancer.[29–31] Searching the ClinicalTrial.gov Web site (February 2013) revealed 10 studies on TKI targeting c-Met in advanced solid tumors, including lung and gastric cancer. Completion of these studies will help identify novel drugs to treat invasive and metastatic tumor.

IGF-1R and Tissue Overgrowth

The IGF-1R precursor is cleaved into 2 peptides (α and β subunits) and then linked via disulfide bonds to form a mature receptor. Its ligands, IGF-1 and IGF-2, are growth hormones with structural similarity to insulin, and bind to insulin receptors with low affinity. IGF-1R signaling promotes cell growth and tissue hypertrophy (see **Fig. 1**). Epithelial cells proliferate and expand to form duct and gland structures. After weaning, the epithelium disappears through apoptosis. In this process, IGF-1R is believed to promote differentiation and inhibits apoptosis.

Activation of IGF-1R signaling is correlated with primary and metastatic malignancies such as prostate, breast, pancreatic, and lung cancer.[32–35] The antiapoptosis property of IGF-1R–triggered kinase cascades contributes to cancer-cell resistance to cytotoxicity and vascularization. When EGFR pathways are blocked by inhibitors such as erlotinib, IGF-1R can resume EGFR-related signaling and promote survival in breast cancer. IGF-1R–enhanced angiogenesis is involved in tumor invasion and metastasis.[36–38]

Increased glucose uptake and metabolism are hallmarks of malignancies. Abnormal IGF-1R signaling can contribute to the tumor metabolism in several ways. First, IGF-1 binds to the insulin receptor, stimulating glucose uptake. Second, IGF-1R is associated with the insulin receptor. Hyperactivity of IGF-1R may enhance insulin receptor–induced glucose metabolism. Finally, IGF-1R signaling may promote the shift of cellular metabolism toward the generation of building materials to support proliferation. TKI targeting IGF-1R signaling can prevent abnormal glucose uptake and aerobic glycolysis.[39–43]

c-Kit and Cell Proliferation

Tyrosine protein kinase kit (c-Kit) or CD117 is the cellular homology of the feline sarcoma viral oncogene v-kit.[44] Hematopoietic stem cells, mast cells, skin melanocytes, and interstitial cells express c-Kit on the cellular surface. On binding to the stem-cell factor, c-Kit forms dimers and phosphorylates/activates effector proteins, modulating cell survival, proliferation, and differentiation.[45,46]

The activity and levels of c-Kit are increased in several types of solid tumors such as gastrointestinal stromal tumor,[47] seminoma,[48] breast cancer,[49] and lung adenocarcinoma.[50] For example, gain-of-function mutation of the KIT gene causes constitutive activation of the receptor even in the absence of its ligand, stem-cell factor, in human gastrointestinal stromal tumors.[51,52] Specific inhibitors have been developed to target hyperactivated c-Kit in these tumors, which marks the new era of targeted molecular therapy.[53] The TK inhibitor Gleevec (imatinib mesylate), has been approved by the Food and Drug Administration (FDA) to treat patients with tumors such as Philadelphia chromosome–positive chronic myeloid leukemia and KIT-positive unresectable and/ or metastatic malignant gastrointestinal stromal tumors.

Other Inhibitor-Targeted TK

The TK family consists of numerous members that are associated with tumorigenesis. Many TK have been studied for the development of inhibitors to treat malignancies according to the National Institutes of Health clinical trials database: estrogen receptor (ER), anaplastic lymphoma kinase (ALK), colony-stimulating factor 1 receptor (CSF1R), Raf/MAPK, PI3K/Akt, mTOR, JAK, and HSP90; they can be classified into receptor (ER, ALK, CSF-1R) and cytosolic (Raf/MAPK, PI3K/Akt, mTOR, JAK, and HSP90) TK families. Most cytosolic TK are downstream effectors of receptor TK. Overexpression, amplification, and fusion of the effector TK can result in their constitutive activation even in the absence of growth-factor stimulation. TKI targeting the effector kinases can block malignancy-associated overgrowth. However, the effector cascades are often shared by multiple receptor TK in responding to a variety of extracellular stimulation; they are essential for normal cell function, survival, and growth. TKI targeting downstream factors can be toxic to normal cells and can cause strong side effects.[54,55]

NEW TKI DRUGS APPROVED BY THE FDA

A molecular targeted therapeutic approach has the great advantage of specific inhibition of survival pathways in cancer. Intensive pharmaceutical research and development of TKI have led to the release of novel anticancer drugs. New TKI drugs, particularly FDA-approved anticancer TKI for solid tumors, are reviewed in this section. Basic information such as inhibitor types, targets, and FDA indications are summarized in **Table 1**. The most significant examples of new drugs targeting a particular pathway are briefly described.

Antibody-Based TKI

Targeting EGFR
Cetuximab (trade name: Erbitux) is a chimeric (mouse/human) monoclonal antibody (see **Table 1**). Cetuximab inhibits the activity of EGFR, which is highly expressed in metastatic colorectal cancer and squamous-cell carcinoma of the neck and head. Clinical trial results indicate that compared with capecitabine plus oxaliplatin treatment,[56] addition of cetuximab increases the median overall survival from 16.5 months to 20.5 months and the chance of response (61% vs 37%), and decreases the risk of

disease progression compared with FOLFOX-4 alone in patients with KRAS wild-type tumors.[57,58] The FDA has approved the use of cetuximab to treat patients with colorectal cancer in combination with chemotherapy or as a single agent after patients have failed oxaliplatin-based or irinotecan-based therapy. The assessment of metastasis, EGFR expression, and KRAS mutation are required for the use of cetuximab because Erbitux failed to benefit patients with nonmetastasized colorectal cancer and a KRAS mutation. EGFR activates downstream factors including KRAS. Patients with tumors possessing a KRAS mutation have sustained activation of downstream signaling, which is independent of EGFR stimulation. Thus, Erbitux inhibition of EGFR will not prevent KRAS-mediated cell proliferation and survival.

Cetuximab combined with standard cytotoxic chemotherapy increases overall survival rates when given as first-line treatment in patients with recurrent or metastatic squamous-cell carcinoma of the head and neck.[59] The FDA approved cetuximab in combination with platinum-based therapy plus 5-florouracil (5-FU) for the first-line treatment of patients with recurrent locoregional disease and/or metastatic squamous-cell carcinoma of the head and neck. Clinical studies have been conducted to assess the effects of cetuximab on breast cancer, carcinoma of the esophagus, and recurrent glioblastoma.[60–62] EGFR-pathway analysis is suggested because subtypes of patients respond to cetuximab.

New EGFR-targeting antibodies, including necitumumab, zalutumumab, panitumumab, and nimotuzumab, are being developed to provide more effective treatment. For example, necitumumab (IMC-11F8) is a fully humanized immunoglobulin G1 monoclonal antibody directed against EGFR. Necitumumab is associated with a statistically significant survival advantage in advanced NSCLC. Its potential benefits include low risk of hypersensitive reactivity and similar targeting cytotoxicity in comparison with cetuximab.[63,64] Ten clinical studies are currently being conducted to determine the toxicity and efficacy of Necitumumab in solid tumors, including lung and colon cancer (ClinicalTrials.gov, February 2013).

Panitumumab is a fully humanized monoclonal antibody specific to the EGFR (see **Table 1**). In 2006, the FDA approved panitumumab for the treatment of aggressive metastatic colorectal cancer. KRAS mutation is used as a predicative biomarker for panitumumab therapy. In 2009, the FDA relabeled the use of panitumumab and cetuximab for colon cancer to include KRAS mutation information. Investigations on the extended uses of panitumumab for the treatment of solid tumors, including lung, pancreatic, breast, and head and neck malignancies are actively being conducted, as there are 161 entries in the clinical trial database (ClinicalTrials.gov, February 2013).[65,66]

Targeting HER2 pathways

Gene amplification and overexpression result in increased HER2 levels in patients with aggressive breast cancer. HER2 inhibition improves survival of patients with HER2-positive metastatic breast cancer.[16,67–69] KRAS and EGFR/HER2 activation are common in pancreatic cancer, and dual inhibition of the receptor and downstream effectors prevents tumor growth.[70] Although HER2 was overexpressed in 11.7% of patients with operable gastric cancer, HER2 elevation was not correlated with survival.[71]

Trastuzumab emtansine (trade name: Kadcyla) is an antibody-drug conjugate targeting HER2 (see **Table 1**). The monoclonal antibody trastuzumab binds/neutralizes HER2/neu receptor. After release from the antibody, the cytotoxic agent mertansine enters cells and binds to tubulin, leading to cell death. The antibody-drug conjugation improves specificity because HER2 is overexpressed in tumor but only minimally in normal cells. About 22% of patients with advanced gastric cancer were found to

Table 1

New tyrosine kinase inhibitor drugs for solid tumors approved by the Food and Drug Administration (FDA) (2010–2013)

Name	Trade Name	Manufacturer	Type	Target	FDA Indication	Date
Cetuximab	Erbitux	Bristol-Myers Squibb & Eli Lilly	Mouse/human monoclonal antibody	EGFR	Squamous-cell carcinoma of the head and neck KRAS wild-type metastatic colorectal cancer Therascreen KRAS test	2006, 2008 2009 2012
Panitumumab	Vectibix	Amgen	Human monoclonal antibody	EGFR	EGFR-expressing metastatic colorectal cancer Relabeled for including KRAS detection	2006 2009
Trastuzumab emtansine	Kadcyla	Genentech/Roche	Antibody and toxin conjugate	HER2	HER2-positive metastatic breast cancer	2013
Pertuzumab	Perjeta	Genentech/Roche	Human monoclonal antibody	HER2	HER2-positive metastatic breast cancer	2012
Bevacizumab	Avastin	Genentech/Roche	Human monoclonal antibody	VEGFR	Colon cancer Lung cancer Breast cancer Renal and brain cancer	2004 2006 Approved 2008, revoked 2011 2009
Lapatinib	Tykerb/Tyverb	GSK	N-[3-Chloro-4-[(3-fluorophenyl)methoxy]phenyl]-6-[5-[(2-methylsulfonylethylamino)methyl]-2-furyl]quinazolin-4-amine	HER2, EGFR	Breast cancer HER2-positive metastatic breast cancer	2007 2010
Cabozantinib	Cometriq	Exelixis	N-(4-((6,7-Dimethoxyquinolin-4-yl)oxy)phenyl)-N-(4-fluorophenyl)cyclopropane-1,1-dicarboxamide	c-Met, VEGFR2	Medullary thyroid cancer	2012
Regorafenib	Stivarga	Bayer	4-[4-({[4-Chloro-3-(trifluoromethyl)phenyl]carbamoyl}amino)-3-fluorophenoxy]-N-methylpyridine-2-carboxamide hydrate	VEGFR2, Tie2	Metastatic colorectal cancer Advanced gastrointestinal stromal tumors	2012 2013

			Chemical name	Target	Indication	Year
Axitinib	Inlyta	Pfizer	N-Methyl-2-[[3-[(E)-2-pyridin-2-ylethenyl]-1H-indazol-6-yl]sulfanyl]benzamide	VEGFRs, PDGFR	Renal cell carcinoma	2012
Aflibercept	Zaltrap	Sanofi-Aventis and Regeneron Pharmaceuticals		VEGF-A/-B, PlGF	Metastatic colorectal cancer	2012
Crizotinib	Xalkori	Pfizer	3-[(1R)-1-(2,6-Dichloro-3-fluorophenyl)ethoxy]-5-(1-piperidin-4-ylpyrazol-4-yl)pyridin-2-amine		Non-small cell lung carcinoma	2011
Vemurafenib	Zelboraf	Plexxikon/Roche		B-Raf V600E	Late-stage melanoma	2011
Sunitinib	Sutent	Pfizer	N-(2-Diethylaminoethyl)-5-[(Z)-(5-fluoro-2-oxo-1H-indol-3-ylidene)methyl]-2,4-dimethyl-1H-pyrrole-3-carboxamide	PDGFR, VEGFR, c-Kit, Ret, CSFR, flt3	Renal and gastrointestinal stromal tumors Pancreatic neuroendocrine tumors	2006 2011
Vandetanib	Caprelsa	AstraZeneca	N-(4-Bromo-2-fluorophenyl)-6-methoxy-7-[(1-methylpiperidin-4-yl)methoxy]quinazolin-4-amine	EGFR, VEGFR, RET-TK	Metastatic medullary thyroid cancer	2011
Everolimus	Zortress	Novartis	Dihydroxy-12-[(2R)-1-[(1S,3R,4R)-4-(2-hydroxyethoxy)-3-methoxycyclohexyl]propan-2-yl]-19,30-dimethoxy-15,17,21,23,29,35-hexamethyl-11,36-dioxa-4-azatricyclo[30.3.1.04,9]hexatriaconta-16,24,26,28-tetraene-2,3,10,14,20-pentone	mTOR	Advanced kidney cancer Subependymal giant-cell astrocytoma Metastatic pancreatic neuroendocrine tumors Breast cancer	2009 2010 2011 2012
Erlotinib	Tarceva	Genentech/Roche	N-(3-Ethynylphenyl)-6,7-bis(2-methoxyethoxy) quinazolin-4-amine	EGFR	Lung cancer Pancreatic cancer	2004, 2009 2009

have tumors that overexpress human HER2. In a practice changing study, 594 patients with HER2-positive disease, who were identified after nearly 4000 patients with advanced gastric cancer were screened, received chemotherapy (most commonly cisplatin and capecitabine, but sometimes cisplatin and 5-FU) and half were randomized to also receive trastuzumab (6 mg/kg every 3 weeks until progression). The trial was stopped early (after a median follow-up of 17 months) because patients had significantly improved overall survival when trastuzumab (Herceptin) was added to chemotherapy, compared with chemotherapy alone.[72]

Trastuzumab improved survival by 5.8 months when used in combination with lapatinib and capecitabine on comparison with lapatinib and capecitabine alone in women with HER2-positive breast cancer who were resistant to trastuzumab alone.[67,73] In 2013, the FDA approved trastuzumab emtansine for the treatment of patients with HER2-positive, metastatic breast cancer who previously received trastuzumab and a taxane, separately or in combination.

Pertuzumab (trade name: Perjeta) is a humanized monoclonal antibody, which binds and prevents HER2 dimerization (see **Table 1**). HER2 activation requires dimerization with other HER2 receptors. Pertuzumab inhibition of HER2 dimerization blocks HER2-induced downstream signaling, leading to impaired growth and migration of HER2-positive tumor cells. Clinical studies show that the combination of the HER2 dimerization inhibitor, pertuzumab, with the receptor inhibitor, trastuzumab, is more active than monotherapy in HER2-positive progressive breast cancer.[74] The FDA warranted pertuzumab for the treatment of HER2-positive metastatic breast cancer in 2012.

Targeting VEGFR pathways

Release of VEGF to induce angiogenesis allows tumors to grow to large sizes and metastasize. Inhibition of VEGF receptors can attenuate cancer-induced formation of new blood vessels by blocking the supply of oxygen and nutrients to tumor.

Bevacizumab (trade name: Avastin) is the first anti–VEGF-A antibody to inhibit angiogenesis (see **Table 1**). In 2004, bevacizumab was approved by the FDA for combination use with other standard chemotherapy to treat metastatic colon cancer. Bevacizumab is also used to treat other cancers, including lung, breast, glioblastoma, kidney, and ovarian. Recent phase II/III clinical trials show both positive and negative effects of bevacizumab on different types of solid tumors. For example, maintenance Avastin after combination treatments of Avastin, pemetrexed, and carboplatin show antitumor activity with low toxicity.[75] Avastin in combination with either paclitaxel or capecitabine improved progression-free survival and response rate in phase II/III trials in metastatic breast cancer.[76,77] A phase II trial has shown antitumor activity in patients with recurrent glioblastoma.[78] The combination of Avastin with interferon-α improves progression-free survival when compared with interferon-α alone as a first-line treatment in patients with metastatic renal cell carcinoma.[79] Bevacizumab improves progression-free and overall survival in women with ovarian cancer, particularly those at high risk of disease progression.[80] However, bevacizumab has minimal effects on prostate cancer.[81,82]

Small-Molecule TKI

Small molecules are chemically manufactured active substances, still accounting for 90% of drugs on the market. Their small structure and composition often help them penetrate the cell membrane and reach almost any desired designation in the body. Small molecules targeting aberrant pathways in cancer cells have been actively developed, leading to the approval of many new drugs by the FDA. Those drugs approved for the treatment of solid tumors include gefitinib, erlotinib, lapatinib, cabozantinib, regorafenib, axitinib, aflibercept, crizotinib, vemurafenib, sunitinib, vandetanib, and everolimus (see **Table 1**).

Gefitinib (trade name: Iressa) is the first inhibitor of EGFR to interrupt ATP binding to the kinase domain. Blocking EGFR-induced activation of antiapoptotic Ras signaling cascades can lead to arrest of malignant growth. In 2003, the FDA approved gefitinib for the treatment of NSCLC after the failure of prior chemotherapy. However, the approval was withdrawn in 2005 after studies indicated that it did not extend survival. Additional studies demonstrate that gefitinib can benefit patients with lung cancer harboring EGFR mutation/activation.[83]

Erlotinib (trade name: Tarceva) reversibly inhibits EGFR through the competitive interaction with the ATP-binding site (see **Table 1**). Erlotinib extends the life of patients with lung cancer by 3.3 months.[84] KRAS wild type is associated with improved overall survival in erlotinib-treated patients with pancreatic cancer.[85] In 2004, the FDA approved erlotinib for the treatment of patients with metastatic NSCLC after failure of at least 1 prior chemotherapy. The second indication for erlotinib in the maintenance treatment of lung and pancreatic cancer was warranted by the FDA in 2009.

Regorafenib (commercial name: Stivarga) is an oral multikinase inhibitor that targets angiogenic, stromal, and oncogenic receptor TK (see **Table 1**). The antiangiogenic activity of regorafenib is associated with its dual inhibition of VEGFR2 and TIE2. Clinical studies demonstrate that regorafenib increases survival rates among patients with metastatic colorectal cancer.[86] In 2012, the FDA approved regorafenib for colon cancer,[87] and in 2013 the approval was extended to treat patients with advanced gastrointestinal stromal tumor that is refractory and nonresponsive to other treatments (FDA news release). Regorafenib significantly improves progression-free survival in these malignancies.[88]

Crizotinib (trade name: Xalkori) inhibits protein kinase activity by competitive binding within the ATP-interaction pocket of target kinases (see **Table 1**). Experimental data indicate that crizotinib inhibits ALK and c-Met/HGFR signaling.[89,90] Constitutive activation of ALK arising from a chromosome rearrangement occurs in about 4% of NSCLC.[91,92] ALK activation contributes to the malignant phenotype of 8% of neuroblastomas.[93] Clinical trial results indicate a 50% to 61% response rate among patients with ALK-rearranged NSCLC, which led to an accelerated approval of crizotinib by the FDA in 2011 for patients with metastatic ALK-positive NSCLC.[94]

Vemurafenib (trade name: Zelboraf) inhibits specific B-Raf mutation with valine (V) to glutamic acid (E) at amino acid 600, but not wild-type B-Raf. The B-Raf V600E mutation is common in melanoma cells (about 60%) (see **Table 1**). Vemurafenib inhibition of mutant B-Raf interrupts B-Raf/MEK/ERK signaling, leading to apoptosis of melanoma cells. Vemurafenib does not block but rather enhances wild-type B-Raf, likely promoting tumor growth. In a phase III clinical trial, 48% patients with melanoma responded to vemurafenib treatment compared with 5% who responded to dacarbazine.[95] Vemurafenib extended progression-free survival from 1.6 months to 5.3 months.[95,96] In 2012, the FDA approved vemurafenib for the treatment of patients with melanoma harboring the B-Raf V600E mutation.

Sunitinib (trade name: Sutent) is an oral, small-molecule, multitargeted receptor TKI (see **Table 1**). It has been shown that sunitinib inhibits several TK signal-transduction pathways including PDGFR, VEGFR, c-Kit, Ret, CSFR, and flt3. These pathways contribute to tumorigenesis, thus sunitinib has been shown to decrease tumor proliferation and shrink tumor size.[97,98] Sunitinib was the first anticancer drug that was simultaneously approved by the FDA in 2006 for the treatment of renal cell carcinoma and imatinib-resistant gastrointestinal stromal tumor. Phase I/III clinical trials demonstrate that sunitinib prolongs progression-free survival of patients with advanced pancreatic neuroendocrine tumors, leading to its FDA approval for the treatment of these tumors.[99–101] Clinical studies on the extended use of sunitinib to other types of solid tumors are actively being conducted.[98,102] Sunitinib targets many receptor TK that are essential for normal cell function and survival. It is understandable that sunitinib can cause many side effects, including the classic hand-foot syndrome, stomatitis, and other dermatologic toxicities.

Everolimus (trade name: Zortress) is a sirolimus derivative that inhibits mammalian target of rapamycin (mTOR) (see **Table 1**). It has been used as an immunosuppressant to prevent organ rejection and as an antitumor drug.[103] The FDA approved everolimus for the treatment of refractory metastatic renal cell cancer in 2009 because it increased median progression-free survival from 1.9 to 4.9 months in a phase III clinical trial.[104–107] Everolimus improved progression-free survival from 4.6 months to 11 months in RADIANT-3 and RADIANT-2 phase III trials in patients with pancreatic tumors.[108,109] The positive outcome led to the FDA approval of everolimus for the treatment of progressive or metastatic pancreatic neuroendocrine tumor not surgically removable.

POTENTIAL TARGETS FOR FUTURE DRUG DEVELOPMENT

Enthusiastic efforts in targeting therapeutics are leading to accelerated release of new TKI-based drugs to combat malignancies. The biggest advantage of TKI over classic chemotherapy is its ability to target signaling that contributes to tumorigenesis, resulting in high efficacy, low toxicity, and fewer side effects. However, evolutionary pressure often ensures that compensatory mechanisms are initiated when survival pathways are affected. Most, if not all, cancer-specific pathways are associated with cell proliferation and survival. It is often observed that tumors can develop resistance to TKI, contributing to the fact that most TKI-based drugs can only extend average disease progression-free survival by several months. This situation begs for the development of therapeutic interventions that target not only primary but also secondary/compensatory pathways. For example, cancer cells can develop resistance to cetuximab by activation of HER2 signaling. Cetuximab combined with lapatinib may inhibit primary and compensatory survival signaling, resulting in less resistance and longer survival. This multiple-targeting approach should be balanced by the possibility that completely diminishing a signal pathway may cause serious side effects because of normal cell death.

Malignancies are complex diseases for which an increased understanding has been recently countenanced.[110] First, the abnormalities can be at the levels of genomics (DNA modification, amplification, and rearrangements), transcription (overexpression, suppression, and siRNA/miRNA modulation), and translation (protein synthesis, modification, and degradation). Second, the same tumor can harbor more than 1 mutation or abnormality. Third, varied genes/pathways operate at different stages of the disease. Last but not the least, a similar type of tumor can behave or progress very differently in different patients. To overcome this obstacle, we may have to (1) find and inhibit the fundamental mechanisms that are essential for most types of tumors, (2) target multiple signaling pathways exposing the possibility of severe side effects, and (3) design drugs based on an individual's personal genomics and tumor signature for personalized medicine. Advances in these fields should allow for the development of more selective TKI-based drugs with minimal toxicities.

REFERENCES

1. Hamid O. Emerging treatments in oncology: focus on tyrosine kinase (erbB) receptor inhibitors. J Am Pharm Assoc (2003) 2004;44(1):52–8.

2. Robinson DR, Wu YM, Lin SF. The protein tyrosine kinase family of the human genome. Oncogene 2000;19(49):5548–57.
3. Sharma PS, Sharma R, Tyagi T. Receptor tyrosine kinase inhibitors as potent weapons in war against cancers. Curr Pharm Des 2009;15(7):758–76.
4. Cassier PA, Fumagalli E, Rutkowski P, et al. Outcome of patients with platelet-derived growth factor receptor alpha-mutated gastrointestinal stromal tumors in the tyrosine kinase inhibitor era. Clin Cancer Res 2012;18(16):4458–64.
5. Sivendran S, Liu Z, Portas LJ Jr, et al. Treatment-related mortality with vascular endothelial growth factor receptor tyrosine kinase inhibitor therapy in patients with advanced solid tumors: a meta-analysis. Cancer Treat Rev 2012;38(7):919–25.
6. Yang B, Papoian T. Tyrosine kinase inhibitor (TKI)-induced cardiotoxicity: approaches to narrow the gaps between preclinical safety evaluation and clinical outcome. J Appl Toxicol 2012;32(12):945–51.
7. Hartman Z, Zhao H, Agazie YM. HER2 stabilizes EGFR and itself by altering autophosphorylation patterns in a manner that overcomes regulatory mechanisms and promotes proliferative and transformation signaling. Oncogene 2012. [Epub ahead of print].
8. Dhomen NS, Mariadason J, Tebbutt N, et al. Therapeutic targeting of the epidermal growth factor receptor in human cancer. Crit Rev Oncog 2012; 17(1):31–50.
9. Ji H, Sharpless NE, Wong KK. EGFR targeted therapy: view from biological standpoint. Cell Cycle 2006;5(18):2072–6.
10. Lorenzo GD, Bianco R, Tortora G, et al. Involvement of growth factor receptors of the epidermal growth factor receptor family in prostate cancer development and progression to androgen independence. Clin Prostate Cancer 2003;2(1):50–7.
11. Franklin WA, Veve R, Hirsch FR, et al. Epidermal growth factor receptor family in lung cancer and premalignancy. Semin Oncol 2002;29(1 Suppl 4):3–14.
12. Maihle NJ, Baron AT, Barrette BA, et al. EGF/ErbB receptor family in ovarian cancer. Cancer Treat Res 2002;107:247–58.
13. Fassan M, Ludwig K, Pizzi M, et al. Human epithelial growth factor receptor 2 (HER2) status in primary and metastatic esophagogastric junction adenocarcinomas. Hum Pathol 2012;43(8):1206–12.
14. Kurebayashi J. Biological and clinical significance of HER2 overexpression in breast cancer. Breast Cancer 2001;8(1):45–51.
15. Tan M, Yu D. Molecular mechanisms of erbB2-mediated breast cancer chemoresistance. Adv Exp Med Biol 2007;608:119–29.
16. Nielsen DL, Kumler I, Palshof JA, et al. Efficacy of HER2-targeted therapy in metastatic breast cancer. Monoclonal antibodies and tyrosine kinase inhibitors. Breast 2013;22(1):1–12.
17. Jakobsson L, Franco CA, Bentley K, et al. Endothelial cells dynamically compete for the tip cell position during angiogenic sprouting. Nat Cell Biol 2010;12(10):943–53.
18. Gerhardt H, Golding M, Fruttiger M, et al. VEGF guides angiogenic sprouting utilizing endothelial tip cell filopodia. J Cell Biol 2003;161(6):1163–77.
19. Davis SL, Eckhardt SG, Messersmith WA, et al. The development of regorafenib and its current and potential future role in cancer therapy. Drugs Today (Barc) 2013;49(2):105–15.
20. Cabebe E, Wakelee H. Sunitinib: a newly approved small-molecule inhibitor of angiogenesis. Drugs Today (Barc) 2006;42(6):387–98.
21. Tsao AS, Wei W, Kuhn E, et al. Immunohistochemical overexpression of platelet-derived growth factor receptor-beta (PDGFR-beta) is associated with PDGFRB

gene copy number gain in sarcomatoid non-small-cell lung cancer. Clin Lung Cancer 2011;12(6):369–74.

22. Coutts JC, Gallagher JT. Receptors for fibroblast growth factors. Immunol Cell Biol 1995;73(6):584–9.

23. Turner N, Grose R. Fibroblast growth factor signalling: from development to cancer. Nat Rev Cancer 2010;10(2):116–29.

24. Wesche J, Haglund K, Haugsten EM. Fibroblast growth factors and their receptors in cancer. Biochem J 2011;437(2):199–213.

25. Cotton LM, O'Bryan MK, Hinton BT. Cellular signaling by fibroblast growth factors (FGFs) and their receptors (FGFRs) in male reproduction. Endocr Rev 2008; 29(2):193–216.

26. Sonnenberg E, Meyer D, Weidner KM, et al. Scatter factor/hepatocyte growth factor and its receptor, the c-met tyrosine kinase, can mediate a signal exchange between mesenchyme and epithelia during mouse development. J Cell Biol 1993;123(1):223–35.

27. Nusrat A, Parkos CA, Bacarra AE, et al. Hepatocyte growth factor/scatter factor effects on epithelia. Regulation of intercellular junctions in transformed and non-transformed cell lines, basolateral polarization of c-met receptor in transformed and natural intestinal epithelia, and induction of rapid wound repair in a transformed model epithelium. J Clin Invest 1994;93(5):2056–65.

28. Chmielowiec J, Borowiak M, Morkel M, et al. c-Met is essential for wound healing in the skin. J Cell Biol 2007;177(1):151–62.

29. Tang MK, Zhou HY, Yam JW, et al. c-Met overexpression contributes to the acquired apoptotic resistance of nonadherent ovarian cancer cells through a cross talk mediated by phosphatidylinositol 3-kinase and extracellular signal-regulated kinase 1/2. Neoplasia 2010;12(2):128–38.

30. Sawada K, Radjabi AR, Shinomiya N, et al. c-Met overexpression is a prognostic factor in ovarian cancer and an effective target for inhibition of peritoneal dissemination and invasion. Cancer Res 2007;67(4):1670–9.

31. Yu J, Ohuchida K, Mizumoto K, et al. Overexpression of c-met in the early stage of pancreatic carcinogenesis; altered expression is not sufficient for progression from chronic pancreatitis to pancreatic cancer. World J Gastroenterol 2006; 12(24):3878–82.

32. Moser C, Schachtschneider P, Lang SA, et al. Inhibition of insulin-like growth factor-I receptor (IGF-IR) using NVP-AEW541, a small molecule kinase inhibitor, reduces orthotopic pancreatic cancer growth and angiogenesis. Eur J Cancer 2008;44(11):1577–86.

33. Resnik JL, Reichart DB, Huey K, et al. Elevated insulin-like growth factor I receptor autophosphorylation and kinase activity in human breast cancer. Cancer Res 1998;58(6):1159–64.

34. Warshamana-Greene GS, Litz J, Buchdunger E, et al. The insulin-like growth factor-I receptor kinase inhibitor, NVP-ADW742, sensitizes small cell lung cancer cell lines to the effects of chemotherapy. Clin Cancer Res 2005;11(4):1563–71.

35. Putz T, Culig Z, Eder IE, et al. Epidermal growth factor (EGF) receptor blockade inhibits the action of EGF, insulin-like growth factor I, and a protein kinase A activator on the mitogen-activated protein kinase pathway in prostate cancer cell lines. Cancer Res 1999;59(1):227–33.

36. Ackermann M, Morse BA, Delventhal V, et al. Anti-VEGFR2 and anti-IGF-1R-Adnectins inhibit Ewing's sarcoma A673-xenograft growth and normalize tumor vascular architecture. Angiogenesis 2012;15(4):685–95.

37. Menu E, Jernberg-Wiklund H, De Raeve H, et al. Targeting the IGF-1R using picropodophyllin in the therapeutical 5T2MM mouse model of multiple myeloma: beneficial effects on tumor growth, angiogenesis, bone disease and survival. Int J Cancer 2007;121(8):1857–61.
38. Kucab JE, Dunn SE. Role of IGF-1R in mediating breast cancer invasion and metastasis. Breast Dis 2003;17:41–7.
39. Garg N, Thakur S, McMahan CA, et al. High fat diet induced insulin resistance and glucose intolerance are gender-specific in IGF-1R heterozygous mice. Biochem Biophys Res Commun 2011;413(3):476–80.
40. Olianas MC, Dedoni S, Onali P. delta-Opioid receptors stimulate GLUT1-mediated glucose uptake through Src- and IGF-1 receptor-dependent activation of PI3-kinase signalling in CHO cells. Br J Pharmacol 2011;163(3):624–37.
41. Shang Y, Mao Y, Batson J, et al. Antixenograft tumor activity of a humanized anti-insulin-like growth factor-I receptor monoclonal antibody is associated with decreased AKT activation and glucose uptake. Mol Cancer Ther 2008;7(9): 2599–608.
42. Zhong D, Xiong L, Liu T, et al. The glycolytic inhibitor 2-deoxyglucose activates multiple prosurvival pathways through IGF1R. J Biol Chem 2009;284(35): 23225–33.
43. Guha M, Srinivasan S, Biswas G, et al. Activation of a novel calcineurin-mediated insulin-like growth factor-1 receptor pathway, altered metabolism, and tumor cell invasion in cells subjected to mitochondrial respiratory stress. J Biol Chem 2007;282(19):14536–46.
44. Yarden Y, Kuang WJ, Yang-Feng T, et al. Human proto-oncogene c-kit: a new cell surface receptor tyrosine kinase for an unidentified ligand. EMBO J 1987; 6(11):3341–51.
45. Kapur R, Cooper R, Zhang L, et al. Cross-talk between alpha(4)beta(1)/alpha(5) beta(1) and c-Kit results in opposing effect on growth and survival of hematopoietic cells via the activation of focal adhesion kinase, mitogen-activated protein kinase, and Akt signaling pathways. Blood 2001;97(7):1975–81.
46. Broudy VC, Morgan DA, Lin N, et al. Stem cell factor influences the proliferation and erythroid differentiation of the MB-02 human erythroleukemia cell line by binding to a high-affinity c-kit receptor. Blood 1993;82(2):436–44.
47. Tuveson DA, Willis NA, Jacks T, et al. STI571 inactivation of the gastrointestinal stromal tumor c-KIT oncoprotein: biological and clinical implications. Oncogene 2001;20(36):5054–8.
48. Tsuura Y, Hiraki H, Watanabe K, et al. Preferential localization of c-kit product in tissue mast cells, basal cells of skin, epithelial cells of breast, small cell lung carcinoma and seminoma/dysgerminoma in human: immunohistochemical study on formalin-fixed, paraffin-embedded tissues. Virchows Arch 1994;424(2): 135–41.
49. Regan JL, Kendrick H, Magnay FA, et al. c-Kit is required for growth and survival of the cells of origin of Brca1-mutation-associated breast cancer. Oncogene 2012;31(7):869–83.
50. Micke P, Hengstler JG, Albrecht H, et al. c-kit expression in adenocarcinomas of the lung. Tumour Biol 2004;25(5–6):235–42.
51. Hirota S, Isozaki K, Moriyama Y, et al. Gain-of-function mutations of c-kit in human gastrointestinal stromal tumors. Science 1998;279(5350):577–80.
52. Taniguchi M, Nishida T, Hirota S, et al. Effect of c-kit mutation on prognosis of gastrointestinal stromal tumors. Cancer Res 1999;59(17):4297–300.

53. Demetri GD. Targeting c-kit mutations in solid tumors: scientific rationale and novel therapeutic options. Semin Oncol 2001;28(5 Suppl 17):19–26.

54. Lee DU, Jessen B. Off-target immune cell toxicity caused by AG-012986, a pan-CDK inhibitor, is associated with inhibition of p38 MAPK phosphorylation. J Biochem Mol Toxicol 2012;26(3):101–8.

55. Renninger JP, Murphy DJ, Morel DW. A selective Akt inhibitor produces hypotension and bradycardia in conscious rats due to inhibition of the autonomic nervous system. Toxicol Sci 2012;125(2):578–85.

56. Borner M, Koeberle D, Von Moos R, et al. Adding cetuximab to capecitabine plus oxaliplatin (XELOX) in first-line treatment of metastatic colorectal cancer: a randomized phase II trial of the Swiss Group for Clinical Cancer Research SAKK. Ann Oncol 2008;19(7):1288–92.

57. Bokemeyer C, Bondarenko I, Makhson A, et al. Fluorouracil, leucovorin, and oxaliplatin with and without cetuximab in the first-line treatment of metastatic colorectal cancer. J Clin Oncol 2009;27(5):663–71.

58. Dewdney A, Cunningham D, Tabernero J, et al. Multicenter randomized phase II clinical trial comparing neoadjuvant oxaliplatin, capecitabine, and preoperative radiotherapy with or without cetuximab followed by total mesorectal excision in patients with high-risk rectal cancer (EXPERT-C). J Clin Oncol 2012;30(14):1620–7.

59. Vermorken JB, Mesia R, Rivera F, et al. Platinum-based chemotherapy plus cetuximab in head and neck cancer. N Engl J Med 2008;359(11):1116–27.

60. Lv S, Teugels E, Sadones J, et al. Correlation of EGFR, IDH1 and PTEN status with the outcome of patients with recurrent glioblastoma treated in a phase II clinical trial with the EGFR-blocking monoclonal antibody cetuximab. Int J Oncol 2012;41(3):1029–35.

61. Carey LA, Rugo HS, Marcom PK, et al. TBCRC 001: randomized phase II study of cetuximab in combination with carboplatin in stage IV triple-negative breast cancer. J Clin Oncol 2012;30(21):2615–23.

62. Hurt CN, Nixon LS, Griffiths GO, et al. SCOPE1: a randomised phase II/III multicentre clinical trial of definitive chemoradiation, with or without cetuximab, in carcinoma of the oesophagus. BMC Cancer 2011;11:466.

63. Dienstmann R, Felip E. Necitumumab in the treatment of advanced non-small cell lung cancer: translation from preclinical to clinical development. Expert Opin Biol Ther 2011;11(9):1223–31.

64. Kuenen B, Witteveen PO, Ruijter R, et al. A phase I pharmacologic study of necitumumab (IMC-11F8), a fully human IgG1 monoclonal antibody directed against EGFR in patients with advanced solid malignancies. Clin Cancer Res 2010;16(6):1915–23.

65. Socinski MA. Antibodies to the epidermal growth factor receptor in non small cell lung cancer: current status of matuzumab and panitumumab. Clin Cancer Res 2007;13(15 Pt 2):s4597–601.

66. Weiner LM, Belldegrun AS, Crawford J, et al. Dose and schedule study of panitumumab monotherapy in patients with advanced solid malignancies. Clin Cancer Res 2008;14(2):502–8.

67. Boyraz B, Sendur MA, Aksoy S, et al. Trastuzumab emtansine (T-DM1) for HER2-positive breast cancer. Curr Med Res Opin 2013;29(4):405–14.

68. Dent S, Oyan B, Honig A, et al. HER2-targeted therapy in breast cancer: a systematic review of neoadjuvant trials. Cancer Treat Rev 2013;39(6):622–31.

69. Goss PE, Smith IE, O'Shaughnessy J, et al. Adjuvant lapatinib for women with early-stage HER2-positive breast cancer: a randomised, controlled, phase 3 trial. Lancet Oncol 2013;14(1):88–96.

70. Walters DM, Lindberg JM, Adair SJ, et al. Inhibition of the growth of patient-derived pancreatic cancer xenografts with the MEK inhibitor trametinib is augmented by combined treatment with the epidermal growth factor receptor/HER2 inhibitor lapatinib. Neoplasia 2013;15(2):143–55.

71. Aizawa M, Nagatsuma AK, Kitada K, et al. Evaluation of HER2-based biology in 1,006 cases of gastric cancer in a Japanese population. Gastric Cancer 2013. [Epub ahead of print].

72. Bang YJ, Van Cutsem E, Feyereislova A, et al. Trastuzumab in combination with chemotherapy versus chemotherapy alone for treatment of HER2-positive advanced gastric or gastro-oesophageal junction cancer (ToGA): a phase 3, open-label, randomised controlled trial. Lancet 2010;376(9742):687–97.

73. Verma S, Miles D, Gianni L, et al. Trastuzumab emtansine for HER2-positive advanced breast cancer. N Engl J Med 2012;367(19):1783–91.

74. Cortes J, Fumoleau P, Bianchi GV, et al. Pertuzumab monotherapy after trastuzumab-based treatment and subsequent reintroduction of trastuzumab: activity and tolerability in patients with advanced human epidermal growth factor receptor 2-positive breast cancer. J Clin Oncol 2012;30(14):1594–600.

75. Stevenson JP, Langer CJ, Somer RA, et al. Phase 2 trial of maintenance bevacizumab alone after bevacizumab plus pemetrexed and carboplatin in advanced, nonsquamous nonsmall cell lung cancer. Cancer 2012;118(22):5580–7.

76. Lang I, Brodowicz T, Ryvo L, et al. Bevacizumab plus paclitaxel versus bevacizumab plus capecitabine as first-line treatment for HER2-negative metastatic breast cancer: interim efficacy results of the randomised, open-label, non-inferiority, phase 3 TURANDOT trial. Lancet Oncol 2013;14(2):125–33.

77. Bisagni G, Musolino A, Panebianco M, et al. The Breast Avastin Trial: phase II study of bevacizumab maintenance therapy after induction chemotherapy with docetaxel and capecitabine for the first-line treatment of patients with locally recurrent or metastatic breast cancer. Cancer Chemother Pharmacol 2013;71(4):1051–7.

78. Kreisl TN, Kim L, Moore K, et al. Phase II trial of single-agent bevacizumab followed by bevacizumab plus irinotecan at tumor progression in recurrent glioblastoma. J Clin Oncol 2009;27(5):740–5.

79. Escudier B, Pluzanska A, Koralewski P, et al. Bevacizumab plus interferon alfa-2a for treatment of metastatic renal cell carcinoma: a randomised, double-blind phase III trial. Lancet 2007;370(9605):2103–11.

80. Perren TJ, Swart AM, Pfisterer J, et al. A phase 3 trial of bevacizumab in ovarian cancer. N Engl J Med 2011;365(26):2484–96.

81. Ogita S, Tejwani S, Heilbrun L, et al. Pilot phase II trial of bevacizumab monotherapy in nonmetastatic castrate-resistant prostate cancer. ISRN Oncol 2012; 2012:242850.

82. Kelly WK, Halabi S, Carducci M, et al. Randomized, double-blind, placebo-controlled phase III trial comparing docetaxel and prednisone with or without bevacizumab in men with metastatic castration-resistant prostate cancer: CALGB 90401. J Clin Oncol 2012;30(13):1534–40.

83. Mok TS, Wu YL, Thongprasert S, et al. Gefitinib or carboplatin-paclitaxel in pulmonary adenocarcinoma. N Engl J Med 2009;361(10):947–57.

84. Cohen MH, Johnson JR, Chattopadhyay S, et al. Approval summary: erlotinib maintenance therapy of advanced/metastatic non-small cell lung cancer (NSCLC). Oncologist 2010;15(12):1344–51.

85. Heinemann V, Vehling-Kaiser U, Waldschmidt D, et al. Gemcitabine plus erlotinib followed by capecitabine versus capecitabine plus erlotinib followed by

gemcitabine in advanced pancreatic cancer: final results of a randomised phase 3 trial of the 'Arbeitsgemeinschaft Internistische Onkologie' (AIO-PK0104). Gut 2013;62(5):751–9.

86. Grothey A. Regorafenib in metastatic colorectal cancer. Clin Adv Hematol Oncol 2012;10(5):324–5.

87. FDA approves regorafenib (Stivarga) for metastatic colorectal cancer. Oncology (Williston Park) 2012;26(10):896.

88. George S, Wang Q, Heinrich MC, et al. Efficacy and safety of regorafenib in patients with metastatic and/or unresectable GI stromal tumor after failure of imatinib and sunitinib: a multicenter phase II trial. J Clin Oncol 2012;30(19):2401–7.

89. Cui JJ, Tran-Dube M, Shen H, et al. Structure based drug design of crizotinib (PF-02341066), a potent and selective dual inhibitor of mesenchymal-epithelial transition factor (c-MET) kinase and anaplastic lymphoma kinase (ALK). J Med Chem 2011;54(18):6342–63.

90. Rodig SJ, Shapiro GI. Crizotinib, a small-molecule dual inhibitor of the c-Met and ALK receptor tyrosine kinases. Curr Opin Investig Drugs 2010;11(12):1477–90.

91. Wallander ML, Geiersbach KB, Tripp SR, et al. Comparison of reverse transcription-polymerase chain reaction, immunohistochemistry, and fluorescence in situ hybridization methodologies for detection of echinoderm microtubule-associated proteinlike 4-anaplastic lymphoma kinase fusion-positive non-small cell lung carcinoma: implications for optimal clinical testing. Arch Pathol Lab Med 2012;136(7):796–803.

92. O'Bryant CL, Wenger SD, Kim M, et al. Crizotinib: a new treatment option for ALK-positive non-small cell lung cancer. Ann Pharmacother 2013;47(2):189–97.

93. George RE, Sanda T, Hanna M, et al. Activating mutations in ALK provide a therapeutic target in neuroblastoma. Nature 2008;455(7215):975–8.

94. Trial watch: success for crizotinib in ALK-driven cancer. Nat Rev Drug Discov 2010;9(12):908.

95. Patrawala S, Puzanov I. Vemurafenib (RG67204, PLX4032): a potent, selective BRAF kinase inhibitor. Future Oncol 2012;8(5):509–23.

96. Chapman PB, Hauschild A, Robert C, et al. Improved survival with vemurafenib in melanoma with BRAF V600E mutation. N Engl J Med 2011;364(26):2507–16.

97. Hiles JJ, Kolesar JM. Role of sunitinib and sorafenib in the treatment of metastatic renal cell carcinoma. Am J Health Syst Pharm 2008;65(2):123–31.

98. Faivre S, Zappa M, Vilgrain V, et al. Changes in tumor density in patients with advanced hepatocellular carcinoma treated with sunitinib. Clin Cancer Res 2011;17(13):4504–12.

99. Raymond E, Dahan L, Raoul JL, et al. Sunitinib malate for the treatment of pancreatic neuroendocrine tumors. N Engl J Med 2011;364(6):501–13.

100. Delbaldo C, Faivre S, Dreyer C, et al. Sunitinib in advanced pancreatic neuroendocrine tumors: latest evidence and clinical potential. Ther Adv Med Oncol 2012;4(1):9–18.

101. Blumenthal GM, Cortazar P, Zhang JJ, et al. FDA approval summary: sunitinib for the treatment of progressive well-differentiated locally advanced or metastatic pancreatic neuroendocrine tumors. Oncologist 2012;17(8):1108–13.

102. Harvey RD, Owonikoko TK, Lewis CM, et al. A phase 1 Bayesian dose selection study of bortezomib and sunitinib in patients with refractory solid tumor malignancies. Br J Cancer 2013;108(4):762–5.

103. Gabardi S, Baroletti SA. Everolimus: a proliferation signal inhibitor with clinical applications in organ transplantation, oncology, and cardiology. Pharmacotherapy 2010;30(10):1044–56.

104. Anandappa G, Hollingdale A, Eisen T. Everolimus—a new approach in the treatment of renal cell carcinoma. Cancer Manag Res 2010;2:61–70.
105. Oudard S, Thiam R, Fournier LS, et al. Optimisation of the tumour response threshold in patients treated with everolimus for metastatic renal cell carcinoma: analysis of response and progression-free survival in the RECORD-1 study. Eur J Cancer 2012;48(10):1512–8.
106. Calvo E, Escudier B, Motzer RJ, et al. Everolimus in metastatic renal cell carcinoma: subgroup analysis of patients with 1 or 2 previous vascular endothelial growth factor receptor-tyrosine kinase inhibitor therapies enrolled in the phase III RECORD-1 study. Eur J Cancer 2012;48(3):333–9.
107. Grunwald V, Karakiewicz PI, Bavbek SE, et al. An international expanded-access programme of everolimus: addressing safety and efficacy in patients with metastatic renal cell carcinoma who progress after initial vascular endothelial growth factor receptor-tyrosine kinase inhibitor therapy. Eur J Cancer 2012; 48(3):324–32.
108. Yao JC, Shah MH, Ito T, et al. Everolimus for advanced pancreatic neuroendocrine tumors. N Engl J Med 2011;364(6):514–23.
109. Pavel ME, Hainsworth JD, Baudin E, et al. Everolimus plus octreotide long-acting repeatable for the treatment of advanced neuroendocrine tumours associated with carcinoid syndrome (RADIANT-2): a randomised, placebo-controlled, phase 3 study. Lancet 2011;378(9808):2005–12.
110. Zhang J, Francois R, Iyer R, et al. Current understanding of the molecular biology of pancreatic neuroendocrine tumors (PanNETs). J Natl Cancer Inst 2013;105(14):1005–17.

Targeting the NF-κB Pathway in Cancer Therapy

Derek J. Erstad, MD[a], James C. Cusack Jr, MD[b],*

KEYWORDS

- NF-κB inhibitor • IKK inhibitor • Targeting NF-κB • Chemoresistance
- Radioresistance • Apoptosis

KEY POINTS

- NF-κB comprises a family of transcription factors that stimulate tumor promotion and progression, chemoresistance, and radioresistance.
- Hundreds of NF-κB inhibitors have been documented that target 3 main pathway sites of signaling integration: the IKK complex, IκBs and NF-κB transcription factors.
- Most NF-κB inhibitors such as synthetic IKKβ inhibitors, interfering RNAs, and gene therapy are not yet in clinical trial.
- Targeting NF-κB is limited by intrinsic pathway complexity, cross-talk with other pathways, lack of biomarkers, poor drug specificity, drug resistance, and drug delivery limitations.
- Future NF-κB targeting will be improved by better understanding of the pathway, more specific inhibitors, and multimodality therapies, which will reduce resistance and increase efficacy.

INTRODUCTION

The NF-κB pathway, which is ubiquitous in nature and evolutionarily conserved in most cell types,[1] controls the expression of genes involved in multiple physiologic processes, including development, immune regulation, acute and chronic inflammation, cytoskeletal remodeling, cellular adhesion, survival, and apoptosis. Constitutive NF-κB activity drives chronic inflammation, which is essential to the development, maintenance, and progression of multiple diseases, including cancer, arthritis, atherosclerosis, inflammatory bowel disease (IBD), degenerative disorders, and autoimmune processes. In cancer, NF-κB has been linked to tumor promotion and progression, as well as chemotherapy and radiotherapy resistance, and is therefore a promising

Disclosures: No financial disclosures.
[a] Department of Surgery, Massachusetts General Hospital, 55 Fruit Street, Boston, MA 02114, USA; [b] Division of Surgical Oncology, Harvard Medical School, Massachusetts General Hospital, 55 Fruit Street, Boston, MA 02114, USA
* Corresponding author.
E-mail address: jcusack@partners.org

therapeutic target. Hundreds of NF-κB pathway inhibitors have been documented, affecting multiple signaling components of the pathway. First, the NF-κB pathway and its function in tumor development, chemoresistance, and radioresistance are discussed. Secondly, relevant NF-κB inhibitors are reviewed, the challenges and shortcomings of targeting NF-κB are evaluated, and the future directions for NF-κB inhibition in cancer therapy are presented.

THE NF-κB SIGNALING PATHWAY

The NF-κB transcription factors include RelA (p65), RelB, C-Rel, NFKB1 (p50 and its precursor p105), and NFKB2 (p52 and its precursor p100), all of which form homodimers and heterodimers.[2] They are related through a shared Rel homology domain, and are further categorized into 2 classes based on C-terminal structures. Class I includes p105 and p100, which undergo proteasomal processing before localizing to the nucleus, and class II includes RelA, RelB, and c-Rel. Class II factors contain a transcription activation domain, which endows them with transcriptional capability, whereas class I factors can only competitively bind DNA in a manner that represses class II transcription. NF-κB is sequestered to the cytoplasm by the IκB proteins, which include IκBα, IκBβ, IκBγ, IκBε, Bcl-3, p100, and p105. Sequestration is a key regulatory step that basally inhibits NF-κB.[3,4] Context-dependent differences in expression, activation, and interaction of NF-κB factors contribute to the highly variable nature of NF-κB target gene expression.[5,6]

NF-κB signaling occurs through 2 main pathways known as the classic or canonical and the alternative or noncanonical (**Fig. 1**). The classic pathway is activated by many receptor types, including tumor necrosis factor receptors(TNFRs), toll-like receptors, and interleukin 1 β (IL-1β), which relay cytoplasmic signals that activate the p50/p65 heterodimer, resulting in expression of genes encoding regulators of innate and adaptive immune responses, prosurvival signals, and development genes.[7–9] The alternative pathway is activated by a subset of TNFR family receptors including CD40, lymphotoxin β (LTβR), B-cell activating factor (BAFF), as well as human T-cell leukemia virus (HTLV), and Epstein-Barr virus (EBV), which activate the p52/RelB heterodimer, resulting in expression of genes that are vital to lymphoid organogenesis and B-cell maturation and survival.[10–12]

The classic pathway relies on IKKβ, IKKγ, and IκB proteins for activation, whereas the alternative pathway relies on IKKα and NIK. In classic signaling, IKKα and IKKβ dimerize and bind IKKγ, also called NEMO, to form the IKK complex.[13] The IKK complex phosphorylates IκBα, the main inhibitor of p65/p50, targeting the protein for K-48 polyubiquitination and degradation by the 26S proteasome.[14] This process liberates NF-κB, which translocates to the nucleus and transcribes target genes.[15] In alternative signaling, NIK activates IKKα, which then phosphorylates p100, targeting it for ubiquitination and proteasomal processing to p52, which is required for p52/RelB nuclear translocation and activation.[12,16,17]

Once NF-κB localizes to the nucleus, it must undergo a series of posttranslational modifications, including phosphorylation, acetylation, and methylation for transcriptional activation, adding another layer of pathway regulation. In classic signaling, protein kinase A (PKA) and mitogen and stress-activated protein kinases 1/2 (MSK1/2) phosphorylate p65, which is necessary for subsequent acetylation by the cyclic adenosine monophosphate response element binding protein (CREB) binding protein (CBP).[18,19] Once acetylated, p65 is capable of initiating transcriptional activation. NF-κB activation in the nucleus is an area of active research, and other known players include p53, IKKα, SMRT, and GSK3β.[20,21]

In addition to canonical and noncanonical signaling, NF-κB is atypically activated by intermediates that cross-talk with the NF-κB pathway at 3 main sites of signaling integration: the IKK complex, the IκBs, and the NF-κB transcription factors. NF-κB is activated by endoplasmic reticulum stress, reactive oxygen species, and genotoxic stress, which have all been associated with malignancies. NF-κB may also be overactivated by oncogenic mutations in parallel pathways including epidermal growth factor receptor (EGFR), RAS, and phosphatidylinositol 3′-kinase-AKT (PI3K-AKT), which cross-talk with NF-κB at various levels in the pathway (**Fig. 2**). Atypical activation complicates targeting of NF-κB, because portions of the pathway may be bypassed, conferring intrinsic resistance to certain classes of inhibitors, but it also broadens the mechanisms by which NF-κB may be constitutively activated in cancers.

A key function of NF-κB is the orchestration of inflammation, which involves the expression of cytokines and chemokines at sites of cellular injury that then recruit macrophages, leukocytes, and fibroblasts to the site of damaged tissue to promote healing. Within injured cells, NF-κB transcribes target genes involved in evasion of apoptosis, growth regulation, cell cycle promotion, and angiogenesis to support the recovery process.[22] There is a conversion to an antiinflammatory phase, in which cellular proliferation slows, apoptosis increases, immune cells emigrate, and the involved tissue returns to baseline function.[23]

The resolution of inflammation is poorly understood, although several mechanisms have thus far been elucidated. Most relate to inactivation of p65 activity, which seems to be the main driver of proinflammatory signaling. p65 transcribes IκBα in a negative autofeedback mechanism.[24] Similarly, p65 also upregulates A20, a deubiquitinase that attenuates tumor necrosis factor α (TNFα)-mediated and IL-1-mediated canonical signaling.[25] There is evidence that p65 is phosphorylated by the copper metabolism MURR1 domain containing 1 (COMMD-1) protein, which targets it for ubiquitination by SOCS-1 and subsequent proteasomal degradation.[26,27] In addition, p65 expression decreases, whereas p50 expression increases, and p50 homodimers competitively inhibit p65 transcription of proinflammatory target genes through binding the same κB DNA promoter sites.[28] Other contributing factors include upregulation of protein-tyrosine phosphatases[29] and alteration in transforming growth factor β (TGF-β) signaling.[30]

THE ROLE OF NF-κB IN CANCER

Appreciation for the role of NF-κB in cancer was initially delayed because the pathway rarely contains mutations. However, interest in NF-κB increased with the discovery that the avian viral oncogene, v-Rel, which is associated with aggressive leukemias and lymphomas in chickens, has structural homology to the NF-κB Rel transcription factors.[31] Over the last 2 decades, NF-κB has come to be appreciated as a key integrator of immunity, inflammation, and oncogenesis. Constitutive activation of the pathway has been shown in most cancers that are preceded by chronic inflammation, such as gastric cancer driven by *Helicobacter pylori* infection, and this activity supports many of the tumorigenic processes highlighted in Weinberg's characteristics of cancer, including survival, evasion of apoptosis, proliferation, angiogenesis, invasion, and metastases.[32]

Several studies have directly linked NF-κB activity to tumor promotion and progression in inflammatory cancers, providing evidence that NF-κB may be a promising drug target. The first of these studies used a mouse colitis-associated cancer model, and selectively inactivated IKKβ in enterocytes, thereby preventing NF-κB activation. This change resulted in 80% reduction in tumor incidence but had no effect on mutation rate or tumor size, suggesting that IKKβ was important for early tumor promotion

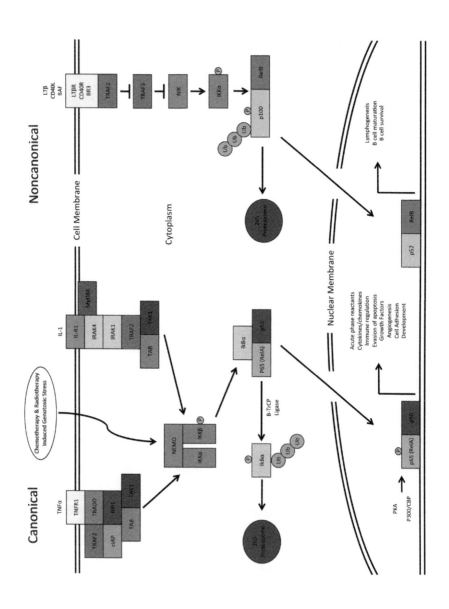

but not initiation or progression. Researchers also inactivated IKKβ in the myeloid cells of these mice, with the belief that the inflammation was initially driven by macrophages in the lamina propria, highlighting the role of immunity in oncogenesis. This practice resulted in only 50% reduction of tumor incidence but a significant reduction in tumor size, providing evidence that classic NF-κB signaling in the surrounding intestinal stroma is important for tumor promotion and progression. This study, in addition to validating the role of NF-κB in tumor development, suggests that tumor survival and growth rely on inflammatory signaling not only in the neoplastic cells but also the surrounding stromal leukocytes and macrophages.[33]

A second important study linking NF-κB to tumor development used the multidrug-resistant 2 transporter knockout mouse model, in which transporter deletion induces accumulation of bile acids and phospholipids in hepatocytes, resulting in inflammation and hepatocellular cancer formation around 9 to 10 months of life. In this model, IκB-super repressor, a nondegradable IκB, inserted into a constitutively active promoter site abrogated tumor formation via inhibition of IKKβ-dependent classic signaling. Treatment in the first 7 months of life had no effect on tumor initiation or promotion, but treatment later had an effect on tumor incidence and size, indicating that in this model, NF-κB is important for tumor promotion and progression but not initiation.[34] Taken together, both studies provide evidence that NF-κB activity is a strong driver of tumor promotion and progression in certain inflammatory cancers.

Subsequent studies have explored the mechanism by which NF-κB induces tumor promotion through expression of target genes involved in evasion of apoptosis and cell cycle progression. NF-κB uses multiple antiapoptotic mechanisms, including inhibition and downregulation of death receptors, inhibition and degradation of caspases, induction of IAPs and Bcl2 family members, inhibition of p53 activity, and production of antioxidant molecules to mitigate cellular damage by reactive oxygen species (ROS). NF-κB promotes cell cycle progression through upregulation of cyclins D1, D2, D3, E, and c-Myc. Documented target genes and their mechanisms are shown in **Table 1**.

NF-κB activity supports tumor progression by several mechanisms, including decreasing tumor surveillance, stimulating angiogenesis and promoting expression of proteases and adhesion molecules needed for tumor invasion. NF-κB induces the expression of inflammatory cytokines by tumor-associated macrophages (TAMs) in the stroma surrounding a neoplasm, which act to suppress nearby dendritic cell maturation and adaptive immune responses that are needed for tumor rejection.[35] NF-κB activity within tumor cells stimulates angiogenesis by promoting expression of CXCR4 and CXCL8,[36] which then promote expression of VEGF.[37] NF-κB also targets genes that promote destruction of surrounding extracellular structures necessary for

---

Fig. 1. Canonical and noncanonical NF-κB signaling pathways. NF-κB signals through 2 main pathways: the canonical (*left*) and the noncanonical (*right*). Extracellular ligands including TNF-α, IL-1, and LTβ bind their respective receptors at the cellular membrane, inducing intracellular recruitment of proximal adaptor proteins. Signal propagation to IKK proteins occurs through TRAF, RIP, and NEMO for the canonical pathway, and TRAF and NIK for the noncanonical pathway. IKK activation leads to phosphorylation, ubiquitination, and proteasomal degradation of IκBs in canonical signaling, whereas in noncanonical it leads to proteasomal processing of p100 to p52. These steps free NF-κB dimers to cross the nuclear membrane and induce transcription of target genes. cIAP, cellular inhibitor of apoptosis protein; IRAK1/4, IL-1 receptor associated kinase 1/4; MyD88, myeloid differentiation primary response gene 88; RIP1, receptor-interacting protein 1; TAB, TAK-binding protein; TAK1, TGF-β–activated protein kinase 1; TNF-α, tumor necrosis factor α; TNFR1, tumor necrosis factor receptor 1; TRAF2/3, TNFR-associated factor 2/3; TRADD, tumor necrosis factor receptor type 1-associated DEATH domain.

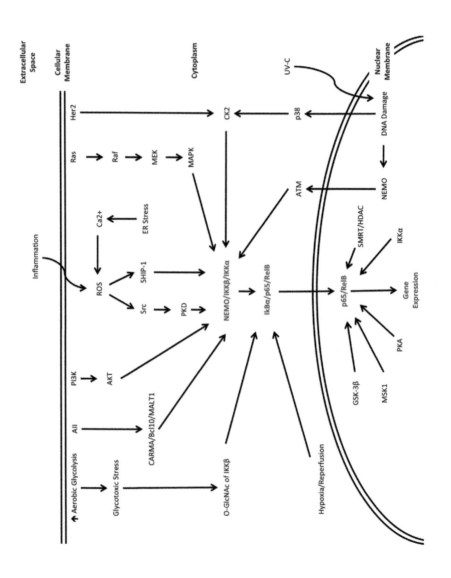

Table 1
Documented mechanisms of evasion of apoptosis targeted by the NF-κB pathway

Category	Mechanism
Inhibition and degradation of death receptors and caspases	Upregulation of FLIP, which competes with caspases 8 and 10 for binding with DISC, and inhibits protease-dependent activation of apoptosis[244]
	Downregulation of TRAIL receptors DR4 and DR5[245]
	Upregulation of DcR1, which competes for TRAIL binding with death receptors[246]
	Downregulation of caspase-8[245]
Induction of IAPs (XIAP, c-IAP1, c-IAP2, survivin)[247]	XIAP, c-IAP1, c-IAP2 inhibit activation and activity of caspases 3, 7, and 9[248–250]
	XIAP K48 ubiquitinates COMMD1, targeting for proteasomal degradation and abrogating repression of p65-mediated gene expression[251]
	XIAP ubiquitinates TAK1, leading to inhibition of JNK and TGF-β–dependent apoptotic signaling[252]
	Survivin binds and inhibits caspases 3 and 7; inhibits Fas-mediated and bax-mediated apoptosis[253]
Induction of Bcl-2 family members (Bcl-xL, Bfl-1/A1, Bcl-2)[254–257]	Members inhibit apoptosis by competition with proapoptotic Bcl family members[258]
Inhibition of p53 activity	NF-κB transcription factors directly compete with p53 for CBP and subsequent transcriptional activity[259]
	Upregulation of Mdm2, the E3 ligase for p53, which leads to p53 destabilization and enhanced degradation[70]
Induction of antioxidant enzymes	Upregulation of MnSOD[260] and FHC,[261] leading to decreased ROS levels and subsequent prevention of JNK-mediated apoptosis[80]

Abbreviations: bax, Bcl-2-associated X; Bcl-2/xL, B-cell lymphoma/leukemia-2/xL; c-IAP1/2, cellular inhibitor of apoptosis 1/2; DcR1, decoy of TNF-related apoptosis-inducing ligand (TRAIL) receptor 1; DISC, death-inducing signaling complex; FHC, ferritin heavy chain; FLIP, FLICE-like inhibitor protein; JNK, c-Jun N-terminal kinase; Mdm2, mouse double minute 2; MnSOD, manganese superoxide dismutase; TAK1, TGF-β–activated protein kinase 1; TRAIL, TNF-α–related apoptosis-inducing ligand; XIAP, x-linked inhibitor of apoptosis.

tumor invasion, including heparanase, matrix metalloproteinases (MMPs), and ROS via iNOS expression.[38–40] NF-κB induces expression of adhesion molecules including ICAM-1 within malignant cells to facilitate their migration to distant sites of metastases.[41] The impact of these processes can be seen in certain cancers, including gastric

---

Fig. 2. Activation of the NF-κB pathway may result through interaction with a wide range of signaling pathways. Multiple pathways stimulate NF-κB activity through cross-talk at 1 of 3 main sites of signaling integration (IKKs, IκBs, or NF-κB transcription factors). Pathways include Her2,[187,231] UV-C/p38/CK2,[232] ATM/NEMO,[233] Ras,[234–236] ER stress/Ca2+,[237] SHIP-1,[238] Src/PKD,[239] PI3K-AKT,[240] AII,[241] glycotoxic stress,[242] and hypoxia/reperfusion.[243] AII, angiotensin II; ATM, ataxia telangiectasia mutated; Bcl10, B-cell lymphoma/leukemia 10; CARMA, CARD-containing MAGUK protein; CK2, casein kinase 2; ER, endoplasmic reticulum; GSK-3β, glycogen synthase kinase-3 β; HDAC, histone deacetylase; Her2, human epidermal growth factor receptor 2; MALT1, mucosa-associated lymphoid tissue lymphoma translocation protein 1; MAPK, mitogen-activated protein kinase; MEK, MAPK/ERK kinase; O-GlcNac, O-linked N-acetylglucosamine; PKD, protein kinase D; Raf, rapidly accelerated fibrosarcoma; SHIP-1, Src homology-2 domain containing inositol 5-phosphatase-1; SMRT, silencing mediator for retinoid or thyroid-hormone receptors; UV-C, ultraviolet subtype C.

and ovarian, in which greater NF-κB activity has been shown to correlate with more severe local invasion and greater likelihood of developing distant disease, conferring a worse prognosis.[42,43]

Targeting NF-κB is contingent on understanding how the pathway is constitutively activated, which can be through a variety of mechanisms, including viruses, mutations in the pathway, and processes that upregulate the expression or activity of NF-κB signaling components. Certain viral oncoproteins have a unique ability to bypass the classic and alternative pathways and directly stimulate p65 activation, as seen with the HTLV-1 virus transforming oncoprotein, tax1.[44,45] Activating mutations in the NF-κB pathway are rare and account for only a few inflammatory cancers, mainly some liquid malignancies (**Table 2**). Instead, most cancers with constitutive NF-κB activity rely on upstream pathway stimulation through a variety of mechanisms, including autocrine and paracrine secretion of inflammatory cytokines by tumor cells and TAMs; upregulation of signaling intermediates; inactivating mutations of inhibitory tumor suppressors; and activating mutations in oncogenes that cross-talk with NF-κB (see **Fig. 2**). **Table 3** shows several examples of constitutive NF-κB activation in different cancers.

Table 2
Mutations in the NF-κB pathway documented in different cancers

Cancer Type	Mutated Gene	Mechanism
Diffuse large B-cell lymphoma, primary B-cell lymphoma	c-Rel	Amplification, role in cancer undetermined[262]
MALTOMA	cIAP2	T(11;18)(q21;q21) translocation creates a chimera of MALT1 and c-IAP2, which has the ability to activate RelB/p50 heterodimers[263]
B-cell lymphocytic leukemia	Bcl-3	T(14;19)(q32;q13) translocation results in increased expression of Bcl-3 and upregulation of targets, including cyclin D1[264]
Hodgkin lymphoma	IκBα	Mutation in IκBα, resulting in high constitutive canonical pathway function found in Reed-Sternberg cells[265]
Multiple myeloma	NF-κB1, NF-κB2, NIK, CD40, LTβR, TACI TRAF2, TRAF3, c-IAP1, c-IAP2, CYLD	Gain for function mutations found in 20% of cases that upregulate NF-κB signaling[266,267] Loss of function mutations that derepress NF-κB signaling[266,267]
B-cell and T-cell lymphoma, multiple myeloma	NF-κB2	T(10;14)(q24;q32) results in loss of regulatory C-terminal ankyrin repeat, leading to constitutive p52 activity[268]
Breast cancer	IKKε	Identified as breast cancer oncogene,[269] phosphorylates CYLD which is essential to transformation[270]

Abbreviations: Bcl-3, B-cell lymphoma/leukemia-3; cIAP2, cellular inhibitor of apoptosis 2; MALT1, mucosa-associated lymphoid tissue lymphoma translocation protein 1; TACI, transmembrane activator and CAML interactor; TRAF2/3, TNFR-associated factor 2/3.

Table 3
Mechanisms of constitutive NF-κB activation in different cancers

Cancer	Gene Involved	Mechanism of NF-κB Activation
Chronic myeloid leukemia	BCR-ABL	Chimera upregulates NF-κB activity, which may contribute to oncogenesis[271]
Acute myeloid leukemia	RTK, Flt3, K-RAS, N-RAS	Activating mutations that cross-talk with NF-κB[272]
Multiple myeloma	Raf	Activating mutation that increases Ras-mediated NF-κB activation[267]
Brain cancer	ING4	Normally repressed p65; inactivating mutation leads to NF-κB activation and subsequent tumor survival, growth, and angiogenesis[273]
Head and neck squamous cell carcinoma	H-RAS, K-RAS, PI3K, Akt, mTOR	Activating mutations that cross-talk with NF-κB[274–277]
	PTEN	Inactivating mutation liberates p65 transcriptional activity[276]
Breast carcinoma	c-Rel	Overexpression in transgenic mouse associated with 31% tumor incidence and upregulation of NF-κB target genes cyclin D1, c-myc, and Bcl-xL[278]
	BRCA1	Normally interacts with p65, magnifying the transcription of Fas ligand, enhancing apoptosis[279]
	Her2	Increases upstream stimulation of NF-κB pathway[280]
Lung cancers	EGFR, ERBB2, BRAF, K-RAS, Myc, PI3K	Activating mutations that cross-talk with NF-κB[281–284]
	P53, RB, PTEN, STK11	Inactivating mutations that increase NF-κB transcriptional activity[285]
Gastric carcinoma	IL-1	Polymorphism that increases NF-κB transcription. RelA levels correlate with lymphatic invasion, depth of invasion, peritoneal metastases, and tumor size[42]
Pancreatic adenocarcinoma	TGF-β	Increases NF-κB activity, which leads to decreased PTEN expression[286]
	GSK3β	Inactivation mutation leads to decreased inhibitory phosphorylation of p65[287]
Colorectal adenocarcinoma	K-RAS	Associated with increased NF-κB activity[288]
Prostate adenocarcinoma	EGFR, Her2, mTOR	Induces PI3K-Akt-mediated activation of NF-κB[289,290]
Melanoma	IKKβ	Knockout in mice abrogates tumor formation[291]
	NIK	Direct NF-κB pathway upregulation[292]

Abbreviations: Bcl-xL, B-cell lymphoma/leukemia-xL; BRCA1, breast cancer type 1 susceptibility protein; Flt3, FMS-like tyrosine kinase 3; GSK3β, glycogen synthase kinase 3 β; Her2, human epidermal growth factor receptor 2; ING4, inhibitor of growth protein 4; mTOR, mammalian target of rapamycin; PTEN, phosphatase and tensin homolog; RTK, receptor tyrosine kinase; STK11, serine/threonine kinase 11.

The IKK proteins, in addition to being activated by cross-talk with parallel pathways, have also been shown to target oncogenic pathways other than NF-κB. In certain breast cancers, IKKβ phosphorylates TSC1, the inhibitor of mammalian target of rapamycin (mTOR), targeting it for degradation. This liberates mTOR to initiate downstream signaling, which has been implicated in tumor development and angiogenesis.[46] IKKβ also phosphorylates the tumor suppressor FOXO3A, targeting it for degradation and thereby promoting tumor initiaton,[47] and Dok1, a scaffolding protein that downregulates tyrosine kinase signaling, altering the activity of the protein to support cell migration.[48] IKKβ directly phosphorylates the p105/TPL-2 complex, targeting p105 for degradation and liberating the MAP kinase pathway to promote proliferation.[49] IKKβ also targets CYLD, a deubiquitinating enzyme that inhibits NF-κB signaling, for degradation.[50] IKKβ has been shown to directly phosphorylate p65, increasing nuclear translocation of the transcription factor.[51]

IKKα also stimulates several non–NF-κB targets. For example, IKKα has been shown to phosphorylate β-catenin, preventing this transcription factor from ubiquitination and degradation. β-catenin activity, which is a downstream target of the Wnt pathway, supports cellular survival by producing cell cycle promoters, including cyclin D1.[52] IKKα also interacts with CBP in 2 important ways. First it directly binds CBP, and the complex phosphorylates histone 3 (H3), augmenting H3 activity in a manner that increases the expression of inflammatory NF-κB target genes on cytokine stimulation. Second, IKKα directly phosphorylates CBP, and this has been shown to increase CBP affinity for NF-κB, increase NF-κB–dependent gene expression, and inhibit p53-dependent gene expression.[53] NEMO has been shown to activate the interferon regulatory factor 3 and 7 pathways as well as 2 IKK-related kinases, TANK-binding kinase-1 and IKKε, via its interaction with TANK.[54] Other more recently discovered IKK-related proteins, including IKKε and TANK-binding protein 1 (TBK1), also have off-target oncogenic roles, which have been well described in previous reviews.[55] We are just starting to appreciate the complexity of NF-κB signaling in different cancers, which can both stimulate and be stimulated by other oncogenic pathways.

NF-κB IN CHEMOTHERAPY AND RADIOTHERAPY RESISTANCE

Recent evidence suggests that the NF-κB pathway may also contribute to the development of chemotherapy and radiotherapy resistance, which is the cause of treatment failure and mortality in most cancers. The mechanisms of chemoresistance and radioresistance have been well documented in previous reviews,[56,57] and are briefly summarized in **Table 4**. Resistance may precede treatment, as commonly seen with chemoresistance in pancreatic cancers or non–small cell lung cancers (NSCLC) that have high multidrug resistance expression,[58] or resistance may be acquired after therapy, as seen with cisplatin use in colorectal cancer. Resistant cancers often show more aggressive growth potential and have worse prognosis, although it is not entirely

Table 4
Mechanisms of resistance to chemotherapy and radiotherapy

Chemotherapy	Radiotherapy
Reduced intracellular drug concentration via transporter proteins	Redistribution of cells to a quiescent phase of the cell cycle where they are less vulnerable to DNA damage from ionizing radiation
Reduced drug activation or increased detoxification	Improved DNA damage repair mechanisms
Increased repair or reproduction of damaged drug target	Upregulation of cell cycle checkpoint proteins
Change in binding affinity of drug target Evasion of apoptosis or cell cycle arrest	Increased expression of ROS scavengers

understood how resistance and growth relate. One possibility is that both phenotypes require the shared activity of specific signaling mechanisms that are selected for when tumor cells are exposed to chemical and radiation stressors. Therefore, although chemotherapy and radiotherapy may provide temporary suppression of cancer progression, the remaining cells that survive these stressors are particularly resilient and aggressive, making future treatment more difficult.

There are several lines of evidence to support the role of NF-κB in chemotherapy and radiotherapy resistance. First, treatment with chemotherapy and radiotherapy induces constitutive NF-κB activation in certain cancers.[59–61] Second, constitutive activation of NF-κB is associated with the development of both chemoresistance and radioresistance.[62–65] Third, and most significantly, inhibition of NF-κB activity in resistant cancers is associated with resensitization, shown by increased apoptosis after treatment with both radiation and chemotherapy.[66–69] Proposed mechanisms of NF-κB activation, depending on the cancer type and treatment used, include the classic pathway,[70] the alternative pathway,[71] DNA-damage–mediated activation,[72] and activation by other pathways at sites of signaling integration.[73] NF-κB overcomes apoptotic stimuli from chemotherapy and radiotherapy by stimulating genes involved in evasion of apoptosis,[74] cell cycle promotion,[75] cellular adhesion, and production of antioxidants,[76] similar to those that also contribute to tumor promotion and progression. Given this evidence, simultaneously inhibiting NF-κB with chemotherapy and radiotherapy may be of great value in counteracting intrinsic, acquired, or induced resistance mechanisms.

INHIBITORS OF NF-κB
Antioxidant Therapy

Dysregulated activation of redox-sensitive transcription factors including NF-κB, activator protein 1, and hypoxia inducible factor have been found to contribute to oncogenesis by promoting uncontrolled cell growth, evasion from apoptosis and angiogenesis. Antioxidants may serve as therapeutic NF-κB inhibitors based on evidence that ROS and reactive nitrogen species (RNS), which are created and destroyed by NF-κB target genes, also activate NF-κB through multiple mechanisms (see **Fig. 2**). Oxidative stress affects cells in a dose-dependent manner, in which minimal ROS generation is easily managed with upregulation of antioxidant enzymes, but intermediate levels, albeit survivable, induce NF-κB activity and the cellular stress response, and may result in lipid peroxidation, protein cross-links, DNA base-pair alterations and double-strand breaks. High levels of oxidative stress overwhelm compensatory mechanisms, override NF-κB survival programs, damage mitochondria, disrupt electron transport, and induce cell death, often through JNK-mediated apoptosis.[77,78] ROS generation may be deliberate, as seen with macrophages during acute inflammation, or it may be incidental with natural errors in electron transport or exposure to cigarette smoke and ionizing radiation. NF-κB is capable of regulating oxidation states by promoting both ROS-generating and RNS-generating enzymes such as cyclooxygenase[79] and iNOS,[40] respectively, and antioxidant enzymes like MnSOD.[80] Although not yet established, it may be that in certain cancers, NF-κB regulates ROS in a manner that supports continued NF-κB activity and prevents apoptosis. Radiotherapy and some chemotherapies rely on ROS generation to induce cell killing, therefore, NF-κB-mediated regulation of oxidative stress may contribute to resistance for both modalities. In premalignant cells, controlled but increased ROS formation during chronic inflammation may also contribute to genetic mutations that support tumor initiation.

More than 30 antioxidant compounds have been shown to inhibit the NF-κB pathway at various sites,[81] although most are not in clinical use. Some of the more notable agents include curcumin, diferoxamine, disulfuram, flavonoids, L-cystein, melatonin, quercitin, rotenanone, and vitamins C and E. For most compounds, the mechanism of NF-κB inhibition is unclear, but presumably involves ROS scavenging or prevention, or stimulation of antioxidant enzymes. For example, studies on N-acetylcysteine, which functions by reducing the principal native antioxidant, glutathione (GSH), have shown that this compound inhibits TNF-α–mediated NF-κB activation, but has no effect on IKK activity or IκBα phosphorylation, indicating that its affect is likely upstream, perhaps involving the affinity of TNF-α for its receptor or the receptor complex itself.[82] Conversely, GSH has been shown to directly inhibit IκBα phosphorylation and degradation.[83] Although a third mechanism is seen with caffeic acid phenethyl ester, which may directly inhibit NF-κB DNA binding by augmenting the nuclear redox state.[84]

Continued research on several aspects of antioxidants is needed before they have broader clinical applicability. First, better understanding is needed of antioxidant mechanisms of NF-κB inhibition, because it is unclear whether some agents are truly antioxidant in nature and at what level of the NF-κB pathway they involve. Better understanding is also needed of how ROS promotes pro-oncogenic phenotypes and in which cancers oxidative stress is a relevant target. Because most antioxidants are studied in vitro or in animal models, clinical trials are needed to determine the safety and efficacy of attaining the drug concentrations necessary for achieving true antioxidant effects in humans.

Proteasome Inhibitors

The final cytoplasmic step in NF-κB activation involves the phosphorylation, ubiquitination, and degradation of IκBα by the 26S proteasome, making proteasome inhibitors attractive therapeutic agents. The 26S proteasome is a multisubunit, adenosine triphosphate (ATP)-dependent complex that contains several different catalytic sites, including chymotrypsinlike (B5), trypsinlike (B2), and caspaselike (B1) proteases, which are the main targets for most inhibitors.[85,86] There are 8 major classes of proteasome inhibitors (aldehydes, boronic acid compounds, expoxyketones, α-ketoaldehyde, vinyl sulfones, β-lactones, syrbactins and bacteria-specific compounds), which may be categorized by several criteria, including whether they form a covalent or noncovalent bond with the active site, whether they are an artificial or natural compound, drug target site, and compound structure.[87]

Proteasome inhibitors, which were initially designed as antiinflammatories, were incidentally discovered to preferentially kill transformed cells with minimal effect on normal cells. Since this discovery, proteasomal inhibition has become a promising field of cancer therapy that has rapidly progressed over the last decade. Bortezomib (PS-341) is front-line therapy for treatment of multiple myeloma, although it has been shown to be cytotoxic against a range of human tumor cell lines, including brain,[88] pancreatic,[89] colorectal,[90] lung,[91] breast,[92] and prostate.[93] There are multiple other proteasome inhibitors in clinical trials, including other boronic acid compounds, epoxyketones and β-lactones.[87]

Bortezomib has been shown to enhance chemotherapy and radiotherapy sensitivity in an NF-κB–dependent manner for a variety of cancers. In 1 study, LoVo colorectal cancer cells in culture and xenograft were treated with increasing quantities of ionizing radiation. Pretreatment with either bortezomib or IκBα-SR similarly resulted in significantly increased apoptosis and reduced tumor size, suggesting that bortezomib may be a useful radiosensitizing agent in colorectal cancers.[94] In melanoma, in vitro cells treated simultaneously with camptothecin and either bortezomib or the kinase inhibitor of NF-κB-1 had significantly greater apoptosis, decreased cell growth, and invasion through an artificial basement than with camptothecin alone. In the same study, in mice injected with B16F10 melanoma cells and similarly treated, those receiving either type of NF-κB inhibitor had fewer pulmonary metastases, suggesting that bortezomib may be an effective chemosensitizing agent in melanomas.[95] Another example of bortezomib chemosenzitization is from studies on pancreatic cancer. Mice xenografted with intraperitoneal injections of the p53 −/− AsPC-1 pancreatic cancer cell line experienced significantly reduced local tumor growth when treated with bortezomib and gemcitabine compared with gemcitibine alone. Bortezomib therapy was associated with increased levels of p21 and p27, indicating that it may prevent antiapoptotic mechanisms with gemcitabine therapy.[96] In another study using H157 and A459 NSCLC lines, bortezomib was shown to prevent gemcitabine-induced NF-κB activity, thereby showing a potential role for this drug in preventing chemoresistance.[97]

Recent evidence suggests that the anticancer effects of bortezomib and other proteasome inhibitors are more complex than solely NF-κB inhibition. This finding was first observed in multiple myeloma, in which it was shown that direct inhibition of NF-κB using the IKKβ inhibitor PS-1145 had a milder effect on cell death than bortezomib.[98] It was subsequently found that myeloma cells, which produce large amounts of IgG or IgA proteins, are particularly sensitive to the unfolded protein response, making bortezomib a uniquely fitting anticancer agent.[99] The proteasome has also been shown to regulate degradation of key cell cycle regulators and apoptotic factors, which may independently contribute to bortezomib efficacy in certain cancers. Degraded proteins include: cyclins A,[100] B,[101] D,[102] E[103]; cyclin-dependent kinases inhibitors p21 and p27[104]; phosphatases Cdc25A and Cdc25C[105]; p53[106] and Bcl-2 family members, and IAPs including XIAP and CIAP.[107] On proteasomal dysregulation in certain cancers, stabilization of tumor suppressors such as p53, p21, and p27 may initiate apoptosis.

Proteasome inhibitors will continue to advance in several ways. First, more inhibitors will likely continue to be discovered or developed, adding to the diversity of target sites. Recently published compounds include hydroxyureas,[108] allosteric inhibitors,[109] and nonspecific inhibitors like tea polyphenols[110] and triterpenoids.[111] Several agents are in clinical trial and will likely be in use in the near future. We are also starting to appreciate mechanisms of bortezomib resistance, which may eventually be counteracted by using other agents, combination therapy or possibly even prevented. Bortezomib has also shown promise as a component in multidrug therapy, which will continue to be optimized for multiple cancer types. As more cancers are shown to both have constitutive NF-κB activity and tightly rely on proteasome function for survival and growth, the application of bortezomib and other proteasome inhibitors should continue to expand into different cancers.

Nonsteroidal Antiinflammatory Drugs

Nonsteroidal antiinflammatory drugs (NSAIDs) such as ibuprofen, naproxen, aspirin, indomethacin, and sulindac may serve as useful therapeutics for a range of inflammatory cancers. The mechanism by which NSAIDs prevent tumor formation and development is not firmly established, although it likely in part involves cyclooxygenase 2 (COX-2) inhibition, and as an indirect consequence of dampening inflammatory signaling, decreased NF-κB activity. Both NF-κB and COX-2 promote activation of each other in a feedforward fashion. NF-κB regulates the COX-2 promoter, and inhibition of NF-κB with curcumin decreased COX-2 activity and synthesis in human colon epithelia cells.[112] Similarly, prostaglandin E_2, a key inflammatory product of COX-2, primarily activates the E2 and E4 receptors, which have been shown to upregulate inflammatory cytokines, which recruit immune cells and promote NF-κB activation.[113] However, most studies have viewed COX-2 and prostaglandins as independent variables without controlling for NF-κB activity. Therefore, with NSAIDs, it is undetermined how much of the anticancer function is contingent on NF-κB downregulation.

Prostaglandins, through their stimulation of G-coupled EP receptors, have been implicated in multiple oncogenic processes, including angiogenesis, mitogenic signaling, tumor invasion, and metastases. A recent study showed that celecoxib inhibition of COX-2 in HT-29 colorectal carcinoma xenografts resulted in significantly reduced local tumor growth and decreased metastases to lymph nodes and lungs in a dose-dependent manner. This finding was associated with decreased prostaglandin E_2 synthesis, decreased VEGF expression and angiogenesis, and increased tumor cell apoptosis.[114] In Lewis lung carcinoma lung cancer cells, prostaglandin E_2 activation of the EP3 receptor induced expression of MMP-9 and VEGF, proteins that are commonly implicated in tumor invasion and angiogenesis, respectively, which was abrogated by COX-2 inhibition with aspirin or NS-398.[115] The role of prostaglandin E_2 in tumor angiogenesis was also validated in breast cancer progression, in which treatment of COX-2 overexpressing transgenic mice with indomethacin or celecoxib strongly inhibited microvessel density and tumor progression.[116] The role of COX-2 in mitogenic signaling was validated in normal gastric epithelial cells (RGM1) and multiple colon cancer lines, including Caco-2, LoVo, and HT-29, in which prostaglandin E_2 rapidly phosphorylates the EGFR and triggers extracellular signal-regulated kinase 2, stimulating mitogenic signals that support cellular proliferation.[117] Similarly, in certain prostate cancer cell lines, it was shown that prostaglandin E_2 stimulation of EP2 and EP4 receptors was sufficient to activate EGFR and β_3 integrin, leading to activation of AP-1 and expression of VEGF.[118] COX-2 inhibition has also been shown to increase the cytoplasmic concentration of arachidonic acid, the inflammatory precursor of prostanoids, to levels that can stimulate apoptosis.[119]

Salicylates and aspirin have been shown to directly compete with ATP for IKKβ, inhibiting IKKβ function and preventing NF-κB activation. Researchers quantified the inhibitory effect of aspirin, showing that IKKβ activity was decreased by 50% after 30 minutes exposure to aspirin at a concentration of 50 μM.[120] This same group performed another study for sulindac, showing that it prevented IκBα degradation, which was associated with significantly increased apoptosis in HCT-15 colon cancer cells at concentrations of 100 μM. HCT-15 cells lack prostaglandins, indicating that the cell death in this study was mediated in a COX-2–independent fashion. Researchers found no apoptosis with ibuprofen or indomethacin; however, in a different study, ibuprofen was shown to inhibit IKKα and constitutive NF-κB activity in androgen-independent prostate cancer cells.[121] These data suggest that the effect of NSAIDs on NF-κB activation is drug and cell type–specific.

Recently, aspirin therapy in colorectal cancer has received publicity after a study showed that patients with PI3K mutations (15%–20% of colon cancers) treated with daily aspirin had a 64% reduction in overall mortality and an 82% reduction in cancer-specific mortality. PI3K has been shown to upregulate COX-2 and prostaglandin E_2 synthesis, and the antitumor effect of aspirin was not so pronounced in cancers lacking this mutation.[122] Although the NF-κB pathway integrates with both PI3K and COX-2, its role was not established in this study. The evidence suggests that NSAID use for cancer prevention and therapy holds great promise. Their mechanisms of function need more clarity, but the advantage of this drug class is availability: they are well studied and safe in humans, therefore their application in novel scenarios of cancer treatment can be expedited.

Sulfasalazine

Sulfasalazine, which contains salicylate covalently linked to sulfapyridine through an azo bond, is another type of antiinflammatory agent that is commonly used in ulcerative colitis and rheumatoid arthritis. Sulfasalazine was shown to inhibit NF-κB activation by TNF-α, lipopolysaccharide (LPS), and phorbol ester in SW620 colon cancer cells at micromolar concentrations.[123] It was later shown that sulfasalazine directly inhibits both IKKα and IKKβ in Jurkat T cells and SW620 colon cancer cells.[124] Sulfasalazine has been shown to attenuate growth in multiple cancer types, including breast,[125] brain,[126] colon,[127] lymphoma,[128] and leukemia.[129] This effect is in part caused by NF-κB inhibition, although its contribution is not well established relative to that of other pharmacologic properties such as ROS sensitization.[130,131]

Sulfasalazine may also be an effective chemosensitizing agent in certain cancers. In pancreatic cancer, sulfasalazine was shown to enhance the cytotoxic effects of etoposide chemotherapy through inhibition of NF-κB activity.[132] In a similar study, sulfasalazine and MG132, a type of proteasome inhibitor, were shown to sensitize BxPc-3, Capan-1, and PancTu-1 pancreatic cancer cell lines to gemcitibine-mediated apoptosis, and they also prevented gemcitibine-induced NF-κB activation.[133] Sulfasalazine-mediated chemosenzitization has also been observed in lung and brain cancers.

Glucocorticoids

Glucocorticoids (GCs) are another widely prescribed class of drugs commonly used for treatment of leukemias, lymphomas, and myelomas. GCs exert a strong antiinflammatory effect by downregulating proinflammatory cytokines, stimulating transcriptional activity of GC receptors (GRs) and by directly inhibiting the NF-κB pathway. Dexamethasone (DEX), a synthetic GC, was shown to activate the endogenous GR, which inhibits NF-κB DNA binding and transcriptional activation. It was shown that the zinc-finger component of activated GR is capable of directly binding and inhibiting p65 in the nucleus. In the same study, DEX was also shown to induce transcription of IκBα in a manner sufficient to attenuate nuclear translocation of NF-κB, although this was limited to certain cell types.[134] More recently, it was shown that the CBP binds both GR and p65 in the nucleus, integrating their physical interaction and thereby enhancing their mutual antagonism.[135]

GCs have been used as effective chemosensitizing agents, particularly in liquid malignancies, although they have shown function in tumors as well. In SiHa cervical carcinoma cells, DEX therapy enhanced cisplatin-induced cytoxicity, which correlated with GR-mediated prevention of cisplatin-dependent NF-κB activation.[136] Pretreatment with DEX in a mouse model for breast cancer resulted in significantly enhanced cytotoxicity with adriamycin treatment. This finding was associated with decreased IL-1β and VEGF expression, adriamycin cytoplasmic accumulation, and NF-κB inhibition.[137] In another study by the same group,[138] DEX pretreatment was an effective chemosensitizer for carboplatin and gemcitabine in multiple mouse xenograft models, including colon, lung, breast, and brain cancers. However, not all GCs are equally effective, and 1 study reported that triamcinolone, clobetasol, DEX, and betamethasone were the most effective compounds at inducing GR target genes, promoting lymphocyte apoptosis, and inhibiting NF-κB activity.[139]

GC resistance is a common but poorly understood problem in cancer therapy. Although GCs inhibit NF-κB activity, refractory NF-κB function may be a key regulator of GC resistance.[140–142] This topic has been well studied in steroid-resistant IBD, in which epithelial NF-κB activity is strongly associated with resistance.[143] In a recent study, U37 and THP1 monocytic cells resistant to GCs were chronically exposed to sulfasalazine, which attenuated the constitutive NF-κB activity and resensitized both lines to steroid-induced cell killing. mTOR dysfunction, and its promotion of NF-κB, may also play a role in GC resistance. In a study on myeloid immune cells, mTOR inactivation by rapamycin abrogated the ability of steroids to inhibit NF-κB activity, to downregulate the expression of inflammatory cytokines, and to prevent the promotion of the Th1 response. In the same study, it was also shown that long-term inflammation in monocytes induced by LPS exposure upregulates TSC2, the main endogenous inhibitor of mTOR.[144] Based on these data, mTOR-dependent suppression of NF-κB may be required for GC sensitivity in certain cell types. Alternative splicing may be another mechanism of GC resistance based on a study showing that certain resistant osteosarcoma cells express a GR isoform that lacks N-terminal residues, rendering the protein incapable of inhibiting NF-κB and antiapoptotic genes.[145] GC resistance in certain cancers may also be independent of NF-κB, as was shown in PreB 697 acute lymphoblastic leukemia cells.[140] In such cases, decreased expression or mutations in GR may contribute.[146] More research is needed to understand how NF-κB can override GC suppression, and to establish alternative mechanisms of resistance for cancers in which NF-κB may be irrelevant.

To more widely apply GCs as cancer therapy, more research is needed to determine in which cancers GC therapy may be of use. Although GCs may initially be advantageous with respect to tumor suppression, this may change with continued use or refractory disease. More research on the mechanisms of GC resistance may help to salvage this therapy both as a cytotoxic agent and chemosensitizer.

IKKβ Inhibitors

On the early recognition that IKKβ was a key driver of classic NF-κB signaling, pharmaceutical companies invested heavily in developing inhibitors. Multiple small molecule inhibitors have been designed, although none is in clinical use and only several have published results. They all preferentially inhibit IKKβ, although some also have decreased affinity for IKKα. Most compounds are either competitors of ATP-binding, which is required for IKKβ activation, or they possess allosteric qualities that decrease IKK activity.[147] Several synthetic inhibitors that have been tried in human cancer lines include SU6668, PS-1145, ML120B, and BMS-345541. SU6668, an indoline-based tyrosine kinase inhibitor capable of inhibiting VEGF, has completed phase I clinical trials as an antiangiogenic agent.[148] SU6668 has also shown inhibition of TBK1, which is capable of liberating NF-κB from IκBα similar to the IKKs, and therefore may also be a useful NF-κB inhibitor.[149] PS-1145 (Millennium Pharmaceuticals) is a β-carbolin compound originally shown to have an antiproliferative effect in myeloma.[98] In DU145 prostate cancer cells, PS-1145 inhibited basal and induced NF-κB activity, sensitized cells to caspase 3/7-dependent apoptosis and attenuated proliferation. These responses were associated with decreased cyclins, inflammatory interleukins, and antiapoptotic factors.[150] In another study,[151] PS-1145 resensitized leukemic cells resistant to imatinib-induced cytotoxicity from patients with CML.

BMS-345541 and ML120B are less well studied in human cancers. BMS-345541, a quinoxaline compound capable of allosterically inhibiting IKKβ, has shown proapoptotic effects in melanoma cells.[152] ML120B (Millennium Pharmaceuticals), a B-carboline based ATP-mimetic, has been shown to enhance vincristine-induced cytotoxicity and prevent induction of NF-κB activity in follicular and diffuse large cell lymphoma lines.[153]

Two other synthetic agents, BAY 11-7082 and BAY 11-7085, are standard NF-κB inhibitors used in the laboratory setting, which have been used in multiple human cancer lines with promising results. BAY 11-7082 strongly inhibits IKKβ and prevents the activation and translocation of the p65/p50 dimer.[154,155] It has also been shown to decrease the ATP-ase activity of the inflammasome,[156] to downregulate TNF-α–mediated ICAM-1 expression,[157] to decrease nuclear translocation of the inflammatory transcription factor AP-1, and to inhibit JAK/STAT signaling.[158] BAY 11-7082 is cytotoxic to myeloma, lymphoma, and myeloid leukemia cells.[98,159] It has shown radiosensitizing capability in thyroid and nasopharyngeal cancer cells,[160,161] and chemosensitizing function in PC-3 prostate cancer cells resistant to docetaxel.[162] BAY 11-7085, which is similar in structure to BAY11-7082, is cytotoxic to multiple cancers, including lymphoma,[163] leukemia,[164] renal,[165] breast,[166] and colon.[167] It has been shown to chemosensitize NSCLC cells and ovarian cancer cells to histone deacetylase inhibitors and paclitaxel, respectively.[168] As more studies are performed, both agents inevitably show cytotoxic, chemosensitizing, and radiosensitizing capability in other cancer types that have constitutive NF-κB activity. However, before a BAY-like agent can be evaluated in humans, more research is needed to determine their off-target effects and toxicities.

A novel approach to IKK inhibition involves targeting protein-protein interactions within the IKK complex by designing highly selective peptides.[147] One successful example is a hexapeptide targeting the NEMO-binding domain (NBD), which has been used in in vitro and in vivo models for oral squamous cell carcinoma. This agent has shown the ability to increase apoptosis, decrease proliferation, and attenuate local bone invasion in SCCVII cells.[169] In a breast cancer model, NBD peptide was shown to prevent NF-κB activation, induce apoptosis, and attenuate proliferation in nonresting ER-negative, ErbB2-positive SKBr3 cells.[170] This peptide is relatively unstable, thereby limiting its commercial attractiveness.

Several other drugs have been shown to inhibit IKKβ activity, including arsenic trioxide, manumycin, and celastol. Arsenic trioxide, a thiol-reactive compound, induced apoptosis in several cancers, including brain,[171] colon,[172] liver,[173] leukemia,[174] neuroblastoma,[175] Ewing sarcoma,[176] and fibrosarcoma.[177] Arsenic trioxide has also been shown to be an effective chemosensitizing agent for multiple chemicals in a variety of cancers. In glioma, arsenic trioxide was able to overcome cisplatin resistance and potentiate doxorubicin-induced cell killing.[171] In CaSki cervical carcinoma cells, arsenic trioxide was sufficient to prevent radiotherapy-induced MMPs, decreasing the metastatic potential of cells.[178] Manumycin, a farnesyltransferase inhibitor originally designed to inhibit Ras, is another agent with IKKβ inhibitory capability. This molecule was shown to induce apoptosis in hepatocellular carcinoma HepG2 cells, which was associated with NF-κB inhibition.[179] Celastol, a quinone methide triterpine, inhibits both IKKα and IKKβ[180] and has been shown to decrease NF-κB activation, induce apoptosis, and chemosensitize cells to a variety of agents in multiple cancers, including myeloma,[181] melanoma,[182] prostate,[183] and breast.[184]

For clinical application, IKKβ inhibitors must advance in several ways. More research is needed to determine the spectrum of different IKK isoform functions in normal physiology and immune regulation, which will help to anticipate unwanted toxicity. NF-κB variably regulates the expression of target genes in a manner that is dependent on multiple factors, including upstream adaptors and the particular NF-κB transcription factor dimer, but the IKK complex may also contribute. Therefore, better understanding is needed of the structural configurations at the IKK level that support tumor activity, particularly when designing protein-protein inhibitory peptides. Although all IKK isoforms have been implicated in cancer, their relevance is cell specific, and needs more clarification. There are few specific inhibitors for IKKα,[185] which has been shown to regulate cell cycle progression and contribute to tumorigenesis in skin,[186] breast,[187] liver,[188] prostate,[189] and colon[190] cancers. For most IKKβ inhibitors that are of the ATP-mimetic form, these agents have good oral bioavailability but they have shown multiple off-target effects, which are perhaps expected given the broad use of ATP by cells. The consequences of this lower selectivity need to be more fully evaluated.[191]

Natural Compounds

Spice-derived neutraceuticals and other phytochemicals from medical plants have shown promising anticancer functions through a variety of mechanisms. These compounds are unique in their regular human consumption, giving them the advantage of potentially expedited use in cancer prevention and therapy. Many agents have been shown to potentially inhibit NF-κB activity, including capsaicin, cardamonin, diosgenin, gamboic acid, [6]-gingerol, resveratrol, thymoquinone, ursolic acid, and xanthohumol. The anticancer characteristics of capsaicin, curcumin, and resveratrol, 3 regularly consumed compounds that have been extensively studied in multiple cancer lines, animal models and clinical trials, are described in more detail in **Table 5**.

Statins

Statins, which are fungal antimicrobials originally used to inhibit 3-hydroxy-3-methylglutaryl coenzyme A reductase and reduce cholesterol synthesis, were subsequently found to also reduce cardiovascular events in patients with increased C-reactive protein levels in the JUPITER trial, showing an antiinflammatory effect.[192] More recently, a clinical trial from Denmark showed that statin users, when compared with nonstatin users, have a multivariate-adjusted hazard ratio for death from cancer of 0.85.[193] The mechanism of the anticancer effects of statin is not fully understood but likely in part involves inhibition of the NF-κB pathway. In MDA-MB-231 breast cancer cells, cerivastatin was shown to reduce NF-κB activation and subsequently downregulate expression of MMP-9 and urokinase, both of which are involved in tumor cell migration.[194] In a different study, cerivastatin was shown to inhibit NF-κB activity by decreasing transcription factor DNA binding, and this was associated with direct cytotoxicity to colorectal cancer cells. In this study, cerivastatin also resensitized resistant cells to 5-fluorouracil–mediated killing.[195] Lovastatin was shown to decrease ionizing radiation-induced E-selectin in colon cancer cells, thereby decreasing the unwanted enhancement of metastatic potential induced by radiotherapy.[196] Simvastatin showed a novel anticancer effect in EBV-transformed lymphoblastoid cell lines by binding to the inserted domain of leukocyte function antigen 1, disrupting lipid raft formation and downstream NF-κB activation, resulting in the induction of apoptosis.[197] Simvastatin was also shown to inhibit TNF-α–induced activation of IKKβ in KBM-5 myeloid cells, decreasing IκBα degradation and NF-κB activation. This finding was associated with downregulation of genes involved in evasion of apoptosis, tumor invasion, and metastasis, including VEGF, MMP-9, and ICAM-1, respectively.[198] More recently, in MDA-MB-231 breast cancer cells, simvastatin decreased NF-κB activation, resulting in derepression of the tumor suppressor PTEN, which was sufficient to attenuate breast cancer cell growth.[199]

Clinical trials for statins in cancer therapy are still mostly in early phases and have shown mixed results. A recent phase II study of gefitinib plus simvastatin versus gefitinib alone in previously treated patients with advanced NSCLC[200] showed that simvastin significantly increased the response rate and progression-free survival ($P = .027$). However, in another phase II study of irinotecan, cisplatin, and simvastatin for untreated extensive-disease small cell lung cancer,[201] simvastatin showed no benefit. In a phase II clinical trial for patients with advanced gastric cancer, the

Table 5
Natural compounds with anti-NF-κB activity

Agent	Common Use	Proposed Functions	Anti-NF-κB Mechanism	Advantage	Limitation
Capsaicin (quinone phytochemical)	Principal pungent agent in chili peppers	Chemotherapeutic,[293] chemopreventative	Downregulation of proinflammatory cytokines,[294] blocks degradation of IκBα,[295] inhibits nuclear translocation of NF-κB dimers,[296] antioxidant[297]	Safe human consumption safety record	Minimal clinical trial data
Curcumin (polyphenol)	Foods, dyes, herbal remedy	Antiinflammatory,[298] antioxidant,[299] antiamyloid,[300] antiangiogenic,[301] antimetastatic,[302] chemopreventative,[303] antichemoresistance, anti-radioresistance, and chemotherapeutic[304]	Antioxidant via inhibition of TNF-α,[305] phorbol ester[306] and hydrogen peroxide; downregulation of IL-1, IL-6, IL-8, IFN-γ, and TNF-α[307]	Multimodal targeting of NF-κB; safe human consumption safety record	Poor bioavailability; unpredictable serum concentrations; limited late-phase clinical trial data
Resveratrol (polyphenol)	Red wine	Antioxidant,[308] antiinflammatory,[309] antiangiogenic,[310] chemopreventative,[311] chemotherapeutic,[312] and chemosenzitizing[313]	Inhibition of IκBα degradation, p65 nuclear translocation, and DNA binding through inhibition of the proteasome,[314] p65 deacetylation,[315] antioxidant[316]	Safe human consumption safety record	Poor bioavailability; limited clinical trial data

Abbreviations: IκBα, inhibitor of kappa b alpha; IFN-γ, interferon γ.

addition of pravastatin to epirubicin, cisplatin, and capecitabine therapy had no benefit on outcome.[202] Simvastatin has also had mixed results in multiple myeloma. In a phase II trial for patients with myeloma with cancers resistant to bortezomib and bendamustine, cotreatment with simvastatin for cycles 3/4 resulted in reduced resistance compared with controls.[203] However, in a separate myeloma phase II trial, administration of high-dose simvastatin had no effect on resistance to vincristine, adriamycin, and dexamethasone.[204]

Statins are the most widely prescribed drug worldwide, and their side effect profiles, particularly liver and muscle toxicity, are well studied and can be easily managed. Over the last decade, hundreds of studies have documented the multiple anticancer effects of statins, some of which have been summarized, including chemopreventive, chemotherapeutic, antiangiogenic, antimetastatic, and chemosensitizing qualities. Unlike the poor bioavailability of curcumin and resveratrol, with statins the serum concentrations needed to obtain anticancer effects are achievable through oral administration. More research is needed to establish the anticancer mechanisms of statins, and to more clearly determine which portions of the NF-κB pathway these compounds inhibit, which may include multiple sites. Understanding statin anticancer mechanisms may also help explain their variable efficacy in different clinical trials for cancers. It is conceivable that depending on the basal activity of NF-κB and other oncogenic pathways, variable doses of statins are needed to overcome these signals, in which case, underdosing may explain their lack of effect in certain instances. Statins hold significant promise for cancer therapy, and continued clinical trials for the treatment of specific cancers, both independently and in combination with other chemotherapies and radiotherapy, are greatly needed, particularly as we try to better understand the relevance of these drugs for different malignancies.

Gene Therapy

Gene therapy using viral delivery of NF-κB inhibitors to tumor cells may one day be a viable clinical resource. Adenoviral delivery of IκBα-super repressor (IκBα-SR), a synthetic nondegradable IκBα, in LoVo colorectal cancer cells abrogated NF-κB activation and sensitized previously resistant cells to both TNF-α and CPT-11 induced killing.[66] Adenoviral delivery of IκBα-SR has also been effective in squamous cell lung cancer cells, abrogating p65 nuclear translocation and resensitizing the cells to TNF-α–mediated cell killing.[205] In HT29 and HCT-15 colorectal cancer cells, pretreatment with adenoviral delivery of IκBα-SR resulted in significantly increased sensitivity to radiotherapy both in vitro and in mouse xenografts.[206] IκBα-SR gene therapy has been effective at directly inducing cell death or sensitizing cells to cytotoxic agents for several other cancer types, including oral squamous cell,[207] glioma,[208] and hepatocellular carcinoma.[209] A dominant negative IKKβ, which directly inhibits IKK, has also been delivered via adenovirus and has been shown to sensitize breast[210] and prostate[211] cancer cells to TNF-α–related apoptosis-inducing ligand (TRAIL)-mediated apoptosis. Multiple phase I clinical trials for the adenoviral delivery of the E1A gene have been performed for breast, ovarian, and head and neck cancers.[212,213] However, delivery of IκBα-SR or IKKβ dominant negative NF-κB inhibitors has not been tried in humans. Viral specificity for targeting only tumor cells is a developing technology, and therefore we need to establish a more thorough understanding of the implications of off-target abrogation of NF-κB in healthy cells when using this modality.

RNA Interference

Antisense oligonucleotides targeting mRNA for NF-κB signaling intermediates including IKKα, IKKβ, and IKKγ present another modality for NF-κB inhibition. IKKβ

RNAi attenuated NF-κB activity and suppressed growth of pancreatic cancer cells in vitro.[214] Liposomal transfection or nanoparticle vehicles could be used for the local delivery of these small molecules to the tumor.

Biologics

Monoclonal antibody (mAb) inhibitors of key inflammatory cytokines, including Il-1, Il-6, and TNF-α, have been tried with limited success in several clinical trials for different cancers. Infliximab, a TNF-α mAb, was given to patients with advanced prostate cancer complicated by bony metastases. A few patients experienced transient improvement in pain that was associated with decreased serum IL-6 concentration, but all patients developed disease progression.[215] In a phase II trial, patients with advanced renal cell carcinoma experienced no benefit from dual treatment with infliximab and sorafenib compared with sorafenib alone.[216] Etanercept, a recombinant fusion protein containing the TNFR, has been shown to have some benefit in breast cancer,[217] ovarian cancer,[218] myelodysplastic syndrome,[219] chronic lymphocytic leukemia, and small lymphocytic lymphoma.[220] Rituximab, a chimeric anti-CD20 antibody, has been used in multiple clinical trials for hematologic malignancies. In drug-resistant non-Hodgkin lymphoma cells lines, this biologic was shown to abrogate constitutive NF-κB activation, resensitizing these cells to paclitaxel-mediated apoptosis. The drug resistance was mediated by increased expression of Bcl family proteins, expressed by NF-κB transcription factors.[221] Siltuximab, an IL-6 mAb, has been tested in clinical trial for prostate, ovarian, and renal cancers. In phase II clinical trials for castration-resistant prostate cancer, siltuximab provided no benefit in outcome.[222] In a phase II trial for patients with metastatic renal cell carcinoma, siltuximab stabilized progressive disease in greater than 50% of patients, showing some initial promise as an immunotherapy for this disease.[223] In a phase II clinical trial for patients with platinum-resistant ovarian cancer, only 1 of 18 patients had a partial response, although 7 others experienced transient disease stabilization.[224] Generally, biologics have been studied in patients with advanced disease and found to have limited benefit, although it is not well established what they contribute in earlier stages of disease.

CURRENT LIMITATIONS AND FUTURE DIRECTIONS FOR TARGETING NF-κB IN CANCER
NF-κB Pathway Complexity

New insights into NF-κB signaling have helped reveal the difficulty of targeting this pathway. Novel signaling intermediates have been discovered, such as ELKs and HSP70, and posttranslational modifications, including phosphorylation, ubiquitination, and methylation, have been found to play significant roles in pathway regulation. Atypical activation of NF-κB through ER stress, DNA damage, and ROS formation, as well as cross-talk with parallel oncogenic pathways, including EGFR, RAS, and PI3K/Akt, have revealed new insights into constitutive NF-κB activation in cancers. In addition, it has been found that the different NF-κB transcription factor subunits are variably expressed and have different intrinsic and modifiable activity levels, but their regulation is poorly understood. Despite hundreds of NF-κB target genes, only certain sets of genes are expressed at any given time, which is likely determined by multiple factors, including the unique pairing of NF-κB dimer pairs, posttranslational modifications of NF-κBs, expression of transcriptional coactivators, chromatin remodeling, and other epigenetic factors. NF-κB gene expression may thereby induce different phenotypes, but it is unclear how to specifically inhibit oncogenic traits, which may be expressed by multiple Rel family members depending on these modifying factors.

These nuances may in part explain how target genes are selectively expressed, as well as the inherent or acquired ineffectiveness of certain inhibitors. Knockout or mutant models for specific NF-κB subunits and the study of posttranslational states may thereby provide valuable insight. Development of inhibitors specific to NF-κB subunits, which has not been undertaken, may be of value by protecting desired NF-κB functions, limiting side effects, and blocking only those functions contributing to malignancy.

Specificity

As with NF-κB subunits, lack of specificity is a limitation in targeting this pathway. The mechanism of NF-κB inhibition for most drugs is not well established, and multiple sites of intervention are often proposed. This finding is partly because of our limited ability to observe only key steps in the pathway including the presence or absence of IκBα, IκBα phosphorylation status, NF-κB nuclear translocation, and NF-κB DNA binding. As more is learned about posttranslational modifications for signaling intermediates, measurement of these changes will add more specificity to observations of NF-κB activity. In addition, for most cancers, the mechanism of constitutive NF-κB activation is also unknown. Genetic sequencing of tumors can be used to reveal oncogenic mutations linked to NF-κB activation, such as mutations in Ras, PI3K/Akt, or EGFR. These oncogenes may themselves be targetable, but there should be a library of NF-κB inhibitors that are highly specific for different pathway components, including upstream activators, IKK, IκB, and NF-κB subunits. This library will also be expanded through targeting of novel signaling intermediates, regulators of posttranslational modifications, parallel pathway mediators, and transcriptional coactivators. Protein assays will also be useful to detect increased expression or activity of these signaling components that contribute to NF-κB activity, especially if they are not mutated.

Multimodal Therapy

Most NF-κB inhibitors have limited intrinsic chemotherapeutic effect, and are instead best used as sensitizers for other cytotoxic agents; this combination approach represents the current paradigm. Given that there are likely multiple simultaneous mechanisms contributing to NF-κB constitutive activation, multi-targeted NF-κB inhibition may be most effective. Therapy would be adjusted based on genetic and proteomic findings to maximize inhibition of pathways that most contribute to NF-κB activation in a given tumor, and may evolve over time. Similar to HAART (highly active antiretroviral therapy) for human immunodeficiency virus, it may be desirable to have an NF-κB cocktail. For example, in a relevant cancer, the simultaneous application of a proteasome inhibitor, aspirin, or statin therapy, and an Akt inhibitor may be sufficient to prevent NF-κB induction. This approach ideally maximizes NF-κB inhibition, particularly after stimulation by chemotherapy and radiotherapy, thereby improving sensitivity to cell-killing agents and limiting the contribution NF-κB to tumor promotion and progression.

Biomarkers

Another limitation to targeting NF-κB is the lack of biomarkers to diagnose, augment therapy, and prognosticate. Tumors are constantly evolving, and there is no method to detect the success or failure of NF-κB inhibition. This finding is particularly important with respect to chemotherapy and radiotherapy, which induce NF-κB activity and can enhance tumor aggressiveness. Genetic and protein studies can lead to biomarker discovery, but these tests need to be designed and then ways found to incorporate them into clinical trials.

NF-κB Inhibitor Resistance

Resistance to NF-κB inhibitors may occur through several mechanisms. In the case of the proteasome inhibitor bortezomib, mutations in proteasomal subunits may decrease drug binding, but new inhibitors are being designed to overcome this resistance by targeting different catalytic sites.[87] Atypical pathways, depending on the level of signaling integration, may bypass segments of the NF-κB pathway, causing intrinsic or acquired ineffectiveness of NF-κB inhibitors acting upstream. This situation may also contribute to chemotherapy and radiotherapy resistance. Biomarker development would allow for detection of NF-κB inhibitor resistance, whereas improved knowledge of the different mechanisms of action for inhibitors would allow for more tailored therapy.

Delivery

Delivery is an issue for certain classes of NF-κB inhibitors, including IKKβ synthetics, NEMO-binding peptides, and interfering RNA oligonucleotides. Nanoparticle technology may eventually provide vehicles targeting tumor cells that can effectively transport these agents. Delivery is also an issue for curcumin, resveratrol, and other phytoalexins, which have poor oral bioavailability. A recent phase I clinical trial showed that a novel nanoparticle curcumin (Theracurmin), which has increased water solubility, safely increased curcumin serum concentration with minimal toxicity.[225] Multiple structural analogues for curcumin and other natural compounds are in development, which may improve their usefulness as anticancer agents.[226,227]

Unexplored Targets

Most IKK inhibitors are highly selective for the β isoform, and there are few IKKα-specific inhibitors. Historically, IKKβ activation of RelA/p65 has been seen as the main driver of oncogenic phenotypes, but IKKα-mediated activity has also been implicated in certain cancers. In addition, IKKα enhances RelA/p65 activity, adding incentive to target this protein. Another potential target involves ubiquitin, which has been found to play an important role in NF-κB signaling. Targeting of both E3 ligases (ie, TRAFs and LUBAC) and deubiquitinating enzymes (ie, CYLD and A20) may contribute to NF-κB inhibition. As new inhibitors are developed, the ideal features include specificity, reversibility, and minimal toxicity. A limitation of inhibiting signaling intermediates like ubiquitin-regulating enzymes is that their functions are often broad within a cell, which may lead to detrimental adverse effects. In addition, simultaneously targeting oncogenic pathways that activate NF-κB, including EGFR, PI3K/Akt, and Ras, will be of additional usefulness for cancers that contain these mutations, and several of these oncogenes already have multiple inhibitors.

Prevention Versus Treatment

NF-κB regulates multiple functions, including immune regulation, development, and cell cycle control, and it can be presumed that indefinite and complete NF-κB inhibition may predispose patients to immunosuppression and unforeseen adverse effects. For most agents, their potency or effectiveness at inhibiting NF-κB is not known. Instead, the focus of treatment should be on the primary causes of inflammation, including infections (ie, *Helicobacter* pylori) and chronic inflammatory disorders (ie, ulcerative colitis). In addition, the timing and duration of NF-κB inhibition should depend on the therapy, because they have different therapeutic profiles and adverse effects. For immunosuppressive agents, including TNF-α mAbs, treatment should be transient because patients are at risk for developing hematologic malignancies, demyelinating disorders, and severe infections. Similarly, chronic GC use can result in immunosuppression, hypertension, and diabetes. Conversely, aspirin and statins are used daily with documented chemoprevention and minimal toxicity.[122,193] Dietary choices such as regular consumption of curcumin may be associated with decreased risk of colorectal cancers.[228] Exercise and normal body mass index have antiinflammatory benefit and are believed to be associated with reduced risk of cardiovascular disease and certain cancers.[229,230] Each of these preventive strategies likely involves multiple molecular mechanisms, but NF-κB inhibition in part contributes to their effect.

SUMMARY

Since its discovery nearly 3 decades ago, NF-κB has become a central focus in the study of cancer and other inflammatory diseases. This pathway is a key driver of tumor promotion, progression, chemoresistance, and radioresistance in many malignancies. Hundreds of NF-κB inhibitors have been described in the literature, most of which target 1 of 3 main pathway sites of signaling integration: the IKK complex, IκB proteins, and NF-κB transcription factors. Several main classes of inhibitors are described and future directions proposed for their application to human disease, including antioxidants, antiinflammatory compounds (NSAIDs, GCs, sulfasalazine), natural compounds (capsaicin, curcumin, resveratrol), statins, proteasome inhibitors, IKKβ inhibitors, biologics, gene therapies, and RNA interference. Pathway complexity, lack of biomarkers, poor drug specificity, drug resistance, and limitations with drug delivery complicate targeting of NF-κB. Improvement on these limitations, as well as development of new drug targets and clinical application of multimodality NF-κB inhibition, are key steps to optimizing clinical targeting of this pathway.

REFERENCES

1. Wang XW, Tan NS, Ho B, et al. Evidence for the ancient origin of the NF-kappaB/IkappaB cascade: its archaic role in pathogen infection and immunity. Proc Natl Acad Sci U S A 2006;103:4204–9.
2. Urban MB, Schreck R, Baeuerle PA. NF-kappa B contacts DNA by a heterodimer of the p50 and p65 subunit. EMBO J 1991;10:1817–25.
3. Baeuerle PA, Baltimore D. I kappa B: a specific inhibitor of the NF-kappa B transcription factor. Science 1988;242:540–6.
4. Yamazaki S, Muta T, Takeshige K. A novel IkappaB protein, IkappaB-zeta, induced by proinflammatory stimuli, negatively regulates nuclear factor-kappaB in the nuclei. J Biol Chem 2001;276:27657–62.
5. Perkins ND, Schmid RM, Duckett CS, et al. Distinct combinations of NF-kappa B subunits determine the specificity of transcriptional activation. Proc Natl Acad Sci U S A 1992;89:1529–33.
6. Lernbecher T, Muller U, Wirth T. Distinct NF-kappa B/Rel transcription factors are responsible for tissue-specific and inducible gene activation. Nature 1993;365: 767–70.
7. Lai JH, Horvath G, Subleski J, et al. RelA is a potent transcriptional activator of the CD28 response element within the interleukin 2 promoter. Mol Cell Biol 1995; 15:4260–71.

8. Beg AA, Sha WC, Bronson RT, et al. Embryonic lethality and liver degeneration in mice lacking the RelA component of NF-kappa B. Nature 1995;376:167–70.

9. Ivanov VN, Lee RK, Podack ER, et al. Regulation of Fas-dependent activation-induced T cell apoptosis by cAMP signaling: a potential role for transcription factor NF-kappa B. Oncogene 1997;14:2455–64.

10. Schiemann B, Gommerman JL, Vora K, et al. An essential role for BAFF in the normal development of B cells through a BCMA-independent pathway. Science 2001;293:2111–4.

11. Pomerantz JL, Baltimore D. Two pathways to NF-kappaB. Mol Cell 2002;10: 693–5.

12. Senftleben U, Cao Y, Xiao G, et al. Activation by IKKalpha of a second, evolutionary conserved, NF-kappa B signaling pathway. Science 2001;293:1495–9.

13. May MJ, D'Acquisto F, Madge LA, et al. Selective inhibition of NF-kappaB activation by a peptide that blocks the interaction of NEMO with the IkappaB kinase complex. Science 2000;289:1550–4.

14. Palombella VJ, Rando OJ, Goldberg AL, et al. The ubiquitin-proteasome pathway is required for processing the NF-kappa B1 precursor protein and the activation of NF-kappa B. Cell 1994;78:773–85.

15. Ghosh S, Baltimore D. Activation in vitro of NF-kappa B by phosphorylation of its inhibitor I kappa B. Nature 1990;344:678–82.

16. Chiao PJ, Miyamoto S, Verma IM. Autoregulation of I kappa B alpha activity. Proc Natl Acad Sci U S A 1994;91:28–32.

17. Woronicz JD, Gao X, Cao Z, et al. IkappaB kinase-beta: NF-kappaB activation and complex formation with IkappaB kinase-alpha and NIK. Science 1997; 278:866–9.

18. Zhong H, Voll RE, Ghosh S. Phosphorylation of NF-kappa B p65 by PKA stimulates transcriptional activity by promoting a novel bivalent interaction with the coactivator CBP/p300. Mol Cell 1998;1:661–71.

19. Joo JH, Jetten AM. NF-kappaB-dependent transcriptional activation in lung carcinoma cells by farnesol involves p65/RelA(Ser276) phosphorylation via the MEK-MSK1 signaling pathway. J Biol Chem 2008;283:16391–9.

20. Hoberg JE, Popko AE, Ramsey CS, et al. IkappaB kinase alpha-mediated derepression of SMRT potentiates acetylation of RelA/p65 by p300. Mol Cell Biol 2006;26:457–71.

21. Grimes CA, Jope RS. CREB DNA binding activity is inhibited by glycogen synthase kinase-3 beta and facilitated by lithium. J Neurochem 2001;78: 1219–32.

22. Li F, Sethi G. Targeting transcription factor NF-kappaB to overcome chemoresistance and radioresistance in cancer therapy. Biochim Biophys Acta 2010; 1805:167–80.

23. Lawrence T, Willoughby DA, Gilroy DW. Anti-inflammatory lipid mediators and insights into the resolution of inflammation. Nat Rev Immunol 2002;2:787–95.

24. Ito CY, Kazantsev AG, Baldwin AS Jr. Three NF-kappa B sites in the I kappa B-alpha promoter are required for induction of gene expression by TNF alpha. Nucleic Acids Res 1994;22:3787–92.

25. Collett GP, Campbell FC. Overexpression of p65/RelA potentiates curcumin-induced apoptosis in HCT116 human colon cancer cells. Carcinogenesis 2006;27:1285–91.

26. Rodrigues L, Filipe J, Seldon MP, et al. Termination of NF-kappaB activity through a gammaherpesvirus protein that assembles an EC5S ubiquitin-ligase. EMBO J 2009;28:1283–95.

27. de Bie P, van de Sluis B, Burstein E, et al. Characterization of COMMD protein-protein interactions in NF-kappaB signalling. Biochem J 2006;398:63–71.

28. Udalova IA, Richardson A, Denys A, et al. Functional consequences of a polymorphism affecting NF-kappaB p50-p50 binding to the TNF promoter region. Mol Cell Biol 2000;20:9113–9.

29. Yang J, Fan GH, Wadzinski BE, et al. Protein phosphatase 2A interacts with and directly dephosphorylates RelA. J Biol Chem 2001;276:47828–33.

30. Arsura M, Wu M, Sonenshein GE. TGF beta 1 inhibits NF-kappa B/Rel activity inducing apoptosis of B cells: transcriptional activation of I kappa B alpha. Immunity 1996;5:31–40.

31. Ballard DW, Walker WH, Doerre S, et al. The v-rel oncogene encodes a kappa B enhancer binding protein that inhibits NF-kappa B function. Cell 1990;63:803–14.

32. Hanahan D, Weinberg RA. The hallmarks of cancer. Cell 2000;100:57–70.

33. Greten FR, Eckmann L, Greten TF, et al. IKKbeta links inflammation and tumorigenesis in a mouse model of colitis-associated cancer. Cell 2004;118:285–96.

34. Pikarsky E, Porat RM, Stein I, et al. NF-kappaB functions as a tumour promoter in inflammation-associated cancer. Nature 2004;431:461–6.

35. Pollard JW. Tumour-educated macrophages promote tumour progression and metastasis. Nat Rev Cancer 2004;4:71–8.

36. Bobrovnikova-Marjon EV, Marjon PL, Barbash O, et al. Expression of angiogenic factors vascular endothelial growth factor and interleukin-8/CXCL8 is highly responsive to ambient glutamine availability: role of nuclear factor-kappaB and activating protein-1. Cancer Res 2004;64:4858–69.

37. Martin D, Galisteo R, Gutkind JS. CXCL8/IL8 stimulates vascular endothelial growth factor (VEGF) expression and the autocrine activation of VEGFR2 in endothelial cells by activating NFkappaB through the CBM (Carma3/Bcl10/Malt1) complex. J Biol Chem 2009;284:6038–42.

38. Wu W, Pan C, Meng K, et al. Hypoxia activates heparanase expression in an NF-kappaB dependent manner. Oncol Rep 2010;23:255–61.

39. Bond M, Fabunmi RP, Baker AH, et al. Synergistic upregulation of metalloproteinase-9 by growth factors and inflammatory cytokines: an absolute requirement for transcription factor NF-kappa B. FEBS Lett 1998;435:29–34.

40. Xie QW, Kashiwabara Y, Nathan C. Role of transcription factor NF-kappa B/Rel in induction of nitric oxide synthase. J Biol Chem 1994;269:4705–8.

41. Tomonaga M, Hashimoto N, Tokunaga F, et al. Activation of nuclear factor-kappa B by linear ubiquitin chain assembly complex contributes to lung metastasis of osteosarcoma cells. Int J Oncol 2012;40:409–17.

42. Sasaki N, Morisaki T, Hashizume K, et al. Nuclear factor-kappaB p65 (RelA) transcription factor is constitutively activated in human gastric carcinoma tissue. Clin Cancer Res 2001;7:4136–42.

43. Kleinberg L, Dong HP, Holth A, et al. Cleaved caspase-3 and nuclear factor-kappaB p65 are prognostic factors in metastatic serous ovarian carcinoma. Hum Pathol 2009;40:795–806.

44. Harhaj EW, Good L, Xiao G, et al. Gene expression profiles in HTLV-I-immortalized T cells: deregulated expression of genes involved in apoptosis regulation. Oncogene 1999;18:1341–9.

45. Lamsoul I, Lodewick J, Lebrun S, et al. Exclusive ubiquitination and sumoylation on overlapping lysine residues mediate NF-kappaB activation by the human T-cell leukemia virus tax oncoprotein. Mol Cell Biol 2005;25:10391–406.

46. Lee DF, Kuo HP, Chen CT, et al. IKK beta suppression of TSC1 links inflammation and tumor angiogenesis via the mTOR pathway. Cell 2007;130:440–55.

47. Hu MC, Lee DF, Xia W, et al. IkappaB kinase promotes tumorigenesis through inhibition of forkhead FOXO3a. Cell 2004;117:225–37.

48. Lee S, Andrieu C, Saltel F, et al. IkappaB kinase beta phosphorylates Dok1 serines in response to TNF, IL-1, or gamma radiation. Proc Natl Acad Sci U S A 2004;101:17416–21.

49. Gantke T, Sriskantharajah S, Sadowski M, et al. IkappaB kinase regulation of the TPL-2/ERK MAPK pathway. Immunol Rev 2012;246:168–82.

50. Reiley W, Zhang M, Wu X, et al. Regulation of the deubiquitinating enzyme CYLD by IkappaB kinase gamma-dependent phosphorylation. Mol Cell Biol 2005;25: 3886–95.

51. Mattioli I, Sebald A, Bucher C, et al. Transient and selective NF-kappa B p65 serine 536 phosphorylation induced by T cell costimulation is mediated by I kappa B kinase beta and controls the kinetics of p65 nuclear import. J Immunol 2004;172:6336–44.

52. Lamberti C, Lin KM, Yamamoto Y, et al. Regulation of beta-catenin function by the IkappaB kinases. J Biol Chem 2001;276:42276–86.

53. Yamamoto Y, Verma UN, Prajapati S, et al. Histone H3 phosphorylation by IKK-alpha is critical for cytokine-induced gene expression. Nature 2003;423: 655–9.

54. Zhao T, Yang L, Sun Q, et al. The NEMO adaptor bridges the nuclear factor-kappaB and interferon regulatory factor signaling pathways. Nat Immunol 2007;8:592–600.

55. Lee DF, Hung MC. Advances in targeting IKK and IKK-related kinases for cancer therapy. Clin Cancer Res 2008;14:5656–62.

56. Stavrovskaya AA. Cellular mechanisms of multidrug resistance of tumor cells. Biochemistry (Mosc) 2000;65:95–106.

57. Moncharmont C, Levy A, Gilormini M, et al. Targeting a cornerstone of radiation resistance: cancer stem cell. Cancer Lett 2012;322:139–47.

58. Shen DW, Fojo A, Chin JE, et al. Human multidrug-resistant cell lines: increased mdr1 expression can precede gene amplification. Science 1986;232:643–5.

59. Cusack JC, Liu R, Baldwin AS. NF- kappa B and chemoresistance: potentiation of cancer drugs via inhibition of NF- kappa B. Drug Resist Updat 1999;2:271–3.

60. Nakanishi C, Toi M. Nuclear factor-kappaB inhibitors as sensitizers to anticancer drugs. Nat Rev Cancer 2005;5:297–309.

61. Brach MA, Hass R, Sherman ML, et al. Ionizing radiation induces expression and binding activity of the nuclear factor kappa B. J Clin Invest 1991;88:691–5.

62. Weldon CB, Burow ME, Rolfe KW, et al. NF-kappa B-mediated chemoresistance in breast cancer cells. Surgery 2001;130:143–50.

63. Arlt A, Vorndamm J, Muerkoster S, et al. Autocrine production of interleukin 1beta confers constitutive nuclear factor kappaB activity and chemoresistance in pancreatic carcinoma cell lines. Cancer Res 2002;62:910–6.

64. Chen X, Shen B, Xia L, et al. Activation of nuclear factor kappaB in radioresistance of TP53-inactive human keratinocytes. Cancer Res 2002;62:1213–21.

65. Fan M, Ahmed KM, Coleman MC, et al. Nuclear factor-kappaB and manganese superoxide dismutase mediate adaptive radioresistance in low-dose irradiated mouse skin epithelial cells. Cancer Res 2007;67:3220–8.

66. Wang CY, Cusack JC Jr, Liu R, et al. Control of inducible chemoresistance: enhanced anti-tumor therapy through increased apoptosis by inhibition of NF-kappaB. Nat Med 1999;5:412–7.

67. Cusack JC Jr, Liu R, Baldwin AS Jr. Inducible chemoresistance to 7-ethyl-10-[4-(1-piperidino)-1-piperidino]-carbonyloxycamptothecin (CPT-11) in colorectal

cancer cells and a xenograft model is overcome by inhibition of nuclear factor-kappaB activation. Cancer Res 2000;60:2323–30.

68. Patel NM, Nozaki S, Shortle NH, et al. Paclitaxel sensitivity of breast cancer cells with constitutively active NF-kappaB is enhanced by IkappaBalpha super-repressor and parthenolide. Oncogene 2000;19:4159–69.

69. Munshi A, Kurland JF, Nishikawa T, et al. Inhibition of constitutively activated nuclear factor-kappaB radiosensitizes human melanoma cells. Mol Cancer Ther 2004;3:985–92.

70. Tergaonkar V, Pando M, Vafa O, et al. p53 stabilization is decreased upon NFkappaB activation: a role for NFkappaB in acquisition of resistance to chemotherapy. Cancer Cell 2002;1:493–503.

71. Bednarski BK, Ding X, Coombe K, et al. Active roles for inhibitory kappaB kinases alpha and beta in nuclear factor-kappaB-mediated chemoresistance to doxorubicin. Mol Cancer Ther 2008;7:1827–35.

72. Janssens S, Tinel A, Lippens S, et al. PIDD mediates NF-kappaB activation in response to DNA damage. Cell 2005;123:1079–92.

73. Grandage VL, Gale RE, Linch DC, et al. PI3-kinase/Akt is constitutively active in primary acute myeloid leukaemia cells and regulates survival and chemoresistance via NF-kappaB, Mapkinase and p53 pathways. Leukemia 2005;19:586–94.

74. Notarbartolo M, Poma P, Perri D, et al. Antitumor effects of curcumin, alone or in combination with cisplatin or doxorubicin, on human hepatic cancer cells. Analysis of their possible relationship to changes in NF-kB activation levels and in IAP gene expression. Cancer Lett 2005;224:53–65.

75. Meinel FG, Mandl-Weber S, Baumann P, et al. The novel, proteasome-independent NF-kappaB inhibitor V1810 induces apoptosis and cell cycle arrest in multiple myeloma and overcomes NF-kappaB-mediated drug resistance. Mol Cancer Ther 2010;9:300–10.

76. Josson S, Xu Y, Fang F, et al. RelB regulates manganese superoxide dismutase gene and resistance to ionizing radiation of prostate cancer cells. Oncogene 2006;25:1554–9.

77. Tonks NK. Redox redux: revisiting PTPs and the control of cell signaling. Cell 2005;121:667–70.

78. Shen HM, Liu ZG. JNK signaling pathway is a key modulator in cell death mediated by reactive oxygen and nitrogen species. Free Radic Biol Med 2006;40:928–39.

79. Fang IM, Yang CH, Yang CM, et al. Linoleic acid-induced expression of inducible nitric oxide synthase and cyclooxygenase II via p42/44 mitogen-activated protein kinase and nuclear factor-kappaB pathway in retinal pigment epithelial cells. Exp Eye Res 2007;85:667–77.

80. Delhalle S, Deregowski V, Benoit V, et al. NF-kappaB-dependent MnSOD expression protects adenocarcinoma cells from TNF-alpha-induced apoptosis. Oncogene 2002;21:3917–24.

81. Epinat JC, Gilmore TD. Diverse agents act at multiple levels to inhibit the Rel/NF-kappaB signal transduction pathway. Oncogene 1999;18:6896–909.

82. Hayakawa M, Miyashita H, Sakamoto I, et al. Evidence that reactive oxygen species do not mediate NF-kappaB activation. EMBO J 2003;22:3356–66.

83. Cho S, Urata Y, Iida T, et al. Glutathione downregulates the phosphorylation of I kappa B: autoloop regulation of the NF-kappa B-mediated expression of NF-kappa B subunits by TNF-alpha in mouse vascular endothelial cells. Biochem Biophys Res Commun 1998;253:104–8.

84. Natarajan K, Singh S, Burke TR Jr, et al. Caffeic acid phenethyl ester is a potent and specific inhibitor of activation of nuclear transcription factor NF-kappa B. Proc Natl Acad Sci U S A 1996;93:9090–5.
85. Eytan E, Ganoth D, Armon T, et al. ATP-dependent incorporation of 20S protease into the 26S complex that degrades proteins conjugated to ubiquitin. Proc Natl Acad Sci U S A 1989;86:7751–5.
86. Tanaka K, Mizushima T, Saeki Y. The proteasome: molecular machinery and pathophysiological roles. Biol Chem 2012;393:217–34.
87. Kisselev AF, van der Linden WA, Overkleeft HS. Proteasome inhibitors: an expanding army attacking a unique target. Chem Biol 2012;19:99–115.
88. Yin D, Zhou H, Kumagai T, et al. Proteasome inhibitor PS-341 causes cell growth arrest and apoptosis in human glioblastoma multiforme (GBM). Oncogene 2005;24:344–54.
89. Shah SA, Potter MW, McDade TP, et al. 26S proteasome inhibition induces apoptosis and limits growth of human pancreatic cancer. J Cell Biochem 2001;82:110–22.
90. Coquelle A, Mouhamad S, Pequignot MO, et al. Cell cycle-dependent cytotoxic and cytostatic effects of bortezomib on colon carcinoma cells. Cell Death Differ 2006;13:873–5.
91. Ling YH, Liebes L, Jiang JD, et al. Mechanisms of proteasome inhibitor PS-341-induced G(2)-M-phase arrest and apoptosis in human non-small cell lung cancer cell lines. Clin Cancer Res 2003;9:1145–54.
92. Adams J. The proteasome as a novel target for the treatment of breast cancer. Breast Dis 2002;15:61–70.
93. Williams S, Pettaway C, Song R, et al. Differential effects of the proteasome inhibitor bortezomib on apoptosis and angiogenesis in human prostate tumor xenografts. Mol Cancer Ther 2003;2:835–43.
94. Russo SM, Tepper JE, Baldwin AS Jr, et al. Enhancement of radiosensitivity by proteasome inhibition: implications for a role of NF-kappaB. Int J Radiat Oncol Biol Phys 2001;50:183–93.
95. Amschler K, Schon MP, Pletz N, et al. NF-kappaB inhibition through proteasome inhibition or IKKbeta blockade increases the susceptibility of melanoma cells to cytostatic treatment through distinct pathways. J Invest Dermatol 2010;130: 1073–86.
96. Awasthi N, Schwarz MA, Schwarz RE. Combination effects of bortezomib with gemcitabine and EMAP II in experimental pancreatic cancer. Cancer Biol Ther 2010;10:99–107.
97. Denlinger CE, Rundall BK, Keller MD, et al. Proteasome inhibition sensitizes non-small-cell lung cancer to gemcitabine-induced apoptosis. Ann Thorac Surg 2004;78:1207–14 [discussion: 14].
98. Hideshima T, Chauhan D, Richardson P, et al. NF-kappa B as a therapeutic target in multiple myeloma. J Biol Chem 2002;277:16639–47.
99. Obeng EA, Carlson LM, Gutman DM, et al. Proteasome inhibitors induce a terminal unfolded protein response in multiple myeloma cells. Blood 2006;107: 4907–16.
100. Yam CH, Siu WY, Lau A, et al. Degradation of cyclin A does not require its phosphorylation by CDC2 and cyclin-dependent kinase 2. J Biol Chem 2000;275: 3158–67.
101. Sudakin V, Ganoth D, Dahan A, et al. The cyclosome, a large complex containing cyclin-selective ubiquitin ligase activity, targets cyclins for destruction at the end of mitosis. Mol Biol Cell 1995;6:185–97.

102. Diehl JA, Zindy F, Sherr CJ. Inhibition of cyclin D1 phosphorylation on threonine-286 prevents its rapid degradation via the ubiquitin-proteasome pathway. Genes Dev 1997;11:957–72.

103. Clurman BE, Sheaff RJ, Thress K, et al. Turnover of cyclin E by the ubiquitin-proteasome pathway is regulated by cdk2 binding and cyclin phosphorylation. Genes Dev 1996;10:1979–90.

104. Pagano M, Tam SW, Theodoras AM, et al. Role of the ubiquitin-proteasome pathway in regulating abundance of the cyclin-dependent kinase inhibitor p27. Science 1995;269:682–5.

105. Chen F, Zhang Z, Bower J, et al. Arsenite-induced Cdc25C degradation is through the KEN-box and ubiquitin-proteasome pathway. Proc Natl Acad Sci U S A 2002;99:1990–5.

106. Scheffner M, Werness BA, Huibregtse JM, et al. The E6 oncoprotein encoded by human papillomavirus types 16 and 18 promotes the degradation of p53. Cell 1990;63:1129–36.

107. Yang Y, Fang S, Jensen JP, et al. Ubiquitin protein ligase activity of IAPs and their degradation in proteasomes in response to apoptotic stimuli. Science 2000;288:874–7.

108. Gallastegui N, Beck P, Arciniega M, et al. Hydroxyureas as noncovalent proteasome inhibitors. Angew Chem Int Ed Engl 2012;51:247–9.

109. Tan X, Osmulski PA, Gaczynska M. Allosteric regulators of the proteasome: potential drugs and a novel approach for drug design. Curr Med Chem 2006;13:155–65.

110. Nam S, Smith DM, Dou QP. Ester bond-containing tea polyphenols potently inhibit proteasome activity in vitro and in vivo. J Biol Chem 2001;276:13322–30.

111. Chauhan D, Li G, Podar K, et al. The bortezomib/proteasome inhibitor PS-341 and triterpenoid CDDO-Im induce synergistic anti-multiple myeloma (MM) activity and overcome bortezomib resistance. Blood 2004;103:3158–66.

112. Plummer SM, Holloway KA, Manson MM, et al. Inhibition of cyclo-oxygenase 2 expression in colon cells by the chemopreventive agent curcumin involves inhibition of NF-kappaB activation via the NIK/IKK signalling complex. Oncogene 1999;18:6013–20.

113. Harris SG, Padilla J, Koumas L, et al. Prostaglandins as modulators of immunity. Trends Immunol 2002;23:144–50.

114. Ninomiya I, Nagai N, Oyama K, et al. Antitumor and anti-metastatic effects of cyclooxygenase-2 inhibition by celecoxib on human colorectal carcinoma xenografts in nude mouse rectum. Oncol Rep 2012;28:777–84.

115. Amano H, Ito Y, Suzuki T, et al. Roles of a prostaglandin E-type receptor, EP3, in upregulation of matrix metalloproteinase-9 and vascular endothelial growth factor during enhancement of tumor metastasis. Cancer Sci 2009;100:2318–24.

116. Chang SH, Liu CH, Conway R, et al. Role of prostaglandin E2-dependent angiogenic switch in cyclooxygenase 2-induced breast cancer progression. Proc Natl Acad Sci U S A 2004;101:591–6.

117. Pai R, Soreghan B, Szabo IL, et al. Prostaglandin E2 transactivates EGF receptor: a novel mechanism for promoting colon cancer growth and gastrointestinal hypertrophy. Nat Med 2002;8:289–93.

118. Jain S, Chakraborty G, Raja R, et al. Prostaglandin E2 regulates tumor angiogenesis in prostate cancer. Cancer Res 2008;68:7750–9.

119. Chen Q, Galleano M, Cederbaum AI. Cytotoxicity and apoptosis produced by arachidonic acid in Hep G2 cells overexpressing human cytochrome P4502E1. J Biol Chem 1997;272:14532–41.

120. Yin MJ, Yamamoto Y, Gaynor RB. The anti-inflammatory agents aspirin and salicylate inhibit the activity of I(kappa)B kinase-beta. Nature 1998;396:77–80.
121. Palayoor ST, Youmell MY, Calderwood SK, et al. Constitutive activation of Ikappa-paB kinase alpha and NF-kappaB in prostate cancer cells is inhibited by ibuprofen. Oncogene 1999;18:7389–94.
122. Liao X, Lochhead P, Nishihara R, et al. Aspirin use, tumor PIK3CA mutation, and colorectal-cancer survival. N Engl J Med 2012;367:1596–606.
123. Wahl C, Liptay S, Adler G, et al. Sulfasalazine: a potent and specific inhibitor of nuclear factor kappa B. J Clin Invest 1998;101:1163–74.
124. Weber CK, Liptay S, Wirth T, et al. Suppression of NF-kappaB activity by sulfasalazine is mediated by direct inhibition of IkappaB kinases alpha and beta. Gastroenterology 2000;119:1209–18.
125. Narang VS, Pauletti GM, Gout PW, et al. Suppression of cystine uptake by sulfasalazine inhibits proliferation of human mammary carcinoma cells. Anticancer Res 2003;23:4571–9.
126. Robe PA, Bentires-Alj M, Bonif M, et al. In vitro and in vivo activity of the nuclear factor-kappaB inhibitor sulfasalazine in human glioblastomas. Clin Cancer Res 2004;10:5595–603.
127. Ryan BM, Russel MG, Langholz E, et al. Aminosalicylates and colorectal cancer in IBD: a not-so bitter pill to swallow. Am J Gastroenterol 2003;98:1682–7.
128. Gout PW, Simms CR, Robertson MC. In vitro studies on the lymphoma growth-inhibitory activity of sulfasalazine. Anticancer Drugs 2003;14:21–9.
129. Habens F, Srinivasan N, Oakley F, et al. Novel sulfasalazine analogues with enhanced NF-kB inhibitory and apoptosis promoting activity. Apoptosis 2005; 10:481–91.
130. Linares V, Alonso V, Domingo JL. Oxidative stress as a mechanism underlying sulfasalazine-induced toxicity. Expert Opin Drug Saf 2011;10:253–63.
131. Chung WJ, Sontheimer H. Sulfasalazine inhibits the growth of primary brain tumors independent of nuclear factor-kappaB. J Neurochem 2009;110:182–93.
132. Muerkoster S, Arlt A, Witt M, et al. Usage of the NF-kappaB inhibitor sulfasalazine as sensitizing agent in combined chemotherapy of pancreatic cancer. Int J Cancer 2003;104:469–76.
133. Arlt A, Gehrz A, Muerkoster S, et al. Role of NF-kappaB and Akt/PI3K in the resistance of pancreatic carcinoma cell lines against gemcitabine-induced cell death. Oncogene 2003;22:3243–51.
134. Scheinman RI, Gualberto A, Jewell CM, et al. Characterization of mechanisms involved in transrepression of NF-kappa B by activated glucocorticoid receptors. Mol Cell Biol 1995;15:943–53.
135. McKay LI, Cidlowski JA. CBP (CREB binding protein) integrates NF-kappaB (nuclear factor-kappaB) and glucocorticoid receptor physical interactions and antagonism. Mol Endocrinol 2000;14:1222–34.
136. Lu YS, Yeh PY, Chuang SE, et al. Glucocorticoids enhance cytotoxicity of cisplatin via suppression of NF-{kappa}B activation in the glucocorticoid receptor-rich human cervical carcinoma cell line SiHa. J Endocrinol 2006;188: 311–9.
137. Wang H, Wang Y, Rayburn ER, et al. Dexamethasone as a chemosensitizer for breast cancer chemotherapy: potentiation of the antitumor activity of adriamycin, modulation of cytokine expression, and pharmacokinetics. Int J Oncol 2007;30:947–53.
138. Wang H, Li M, Rinehart JJ, et al. Pretreatment with dexamethasone increases antitumor activity of carboplatin and gemcitabine in mice bearing human cancer

xenografts: in vivo activity, pharmacokinetics, and clinical implications for cancer chemotherapy. Clin Cancer Res 2004;10:1633–44.

139. Hofmann TG, Hehner SP, Bacher S, et al. Various glucocorticoids differ in their ability to induce gene expression, apoptosis and to repress NF-kappaB-dependent transcription. FEBS Lett 1998;441:441–6.

140. Nicholson L, Hall AG, Redfern CP, et al. NFkappaB modulators in a model of glucocorticoid resistant, childhood acute lymphoblastic leukemia. Leuk Res 2010;34:1366–73.

141. Oerlemans R, Vink J, Dijkmans BA, et al. Sulfasalazine sensitises human monocytic/macrophage cells for glucocorticoids by upregulation of glucocorticoid receptor alpha and glucocorticoid induced apoptosis. Ann Rheum Dis 2007;66:1289–95.

142. Chauhan D, Auclair D, Robinson EK, et al. Identification of genes regulated by dexamethasone in multiple myeloma cells using oligonucleotide arrays. Oncogene 2002;21:1346–58.

143. Bantel H, Domschke W, Schulze-Osthoff K, et al. Abnormal activation of transcription factor NF-kappaB involved in steroid resistance in chronic inflammatory bowel disease. Am J Gastroenterol 2000;95:1845–6.

144. Weichhart T, Haidinger M, Katholnig K, et al. Inhibition of mTOR blocks the anti-inflammatory effects of glucocorticoids in myeloid immune cells. Blood 2011;117:4273–83.

145. Gross KL, Oakley RH, Scoltock AB, et al. Glucocorticoid receptor alpha isoform-selective regulation of antiapoptotic genes in osteosarcoma cells: a new mechanism for glucocorticoid resistance. Mol Endocrinol 2011;25:1087–99.

146. Schmidt S, Irving JA, Minto L, et al. Glucocorticoid resistance in two key models of acute lymphoblastic leukemia occurs at the level of the glucocorticoid receptor. FASEB J 2006;20:2600–2.

147. Gamble C, McIntosh K, Scott R, et al. Inhibitory kappa B kinases as targets for pharmacological regulation. Br J Pharmacol 2012;165:802–19.

148. Sessa C, Vigano L, Grasselli G, et al. Phase I clinical and pharmacological evaluation of the multi-tyrosine kinase inhibitor SU006668 by chronic oral dosing. Eur J Cancer 2006;42:171–8.

149. Godl K, Gruss OJ, Eickhoff J, et al. Proteomic characterization of the angiogenesis inhibitor SU6668 reveals multiple impacts on cellular kinase signaling. Cancer Res 2005;65:6919–26.

150. Yemelyanov A, Gasparian A, Lindholm P, et al. Effects of IKK inhibitor PS1145 on NF-kappaB function, proliferation, apoptosis and invasion activity in prostate carcinoma cells. Oncogene 2006;25:387–98.

151. Cilloni D, Messa F, Arruga F, et al. The NF-kappaB pathway blockade by the IKK inhibitor PS1145 can overcome imatinib resistance. Leukemia 2006;20:61–7.

152. Wen D, Nong Y, Morgan JG, et al. A selective small molecule IkappaB kinase beta inhibitor blocks nuclear factor kappaB-mediated inflammatory responses in human fibroblast-like synoviocytes, chondrocytes, and mast cells. J Pharmacol Exp Ther 2006;317:989–1001.

153. Al-Katib A, Arnold AA, Aboukameel A, et al. I-kappa-kinase-2 (IKK-2) inhibition potentiates vincristine cytotoxicity in non-Hodgkin's lymphoma. Mol Cancer 2010;9:228.

154. Meng X, Martinez MA, Raymond-Stintz MA, et al. IKK inhibitor bay 11-7082 induces necroptotic cell death in precursor-B acute lymphoblastic leukaemic blasts. Br J Haematol 2010;148:487–90.

155. Garcia MG, Alaniz L, Lopes EC, et al. Inhibition of NF-kappaB activity by BAY 11-7082 increases apoptosis in multidrug resistant leukemic T-cell lines. Leuk Res 2005;29:1425–34.
156. Juliana C, Fernandes-Alnemri T, Wu J, et al. Anti-inflammatory compounds parthenolide and Bay 11-7082 are direct inhibitors of the inflammasome. J Biol Chem 2010;285:9792–802.
157. Lee H, Lin CI, Liao JJ, et al. Lysophospholipids increase ICAM-1 expression in HUVEC through a Gi- and NF-kappaB-dependent mechanism. Am J Physiol Cell Physiol 2004;287:C1657–66.
158. Lee J, Rhee MH, Kim E, et al. BAY 11-7082 is a broad-spectrum inhibitor with anti-inflammatory activity against multiple targets. Mediators Inflamm 2012; 2012:416036.
159. Frelin C, Imbert V, Griessinger E, et al. Targeting NF-kappaB activation via pharmacologic inhibition of IKK2-induced apoptosis of human acute myeloid leukemia cells. Blood 2005;105:804–11.
160. Meng Z, Lou S, Tan J, et al. Nuclear factor-kappa B inhibition can enhance therapeutic efficacy of (131)I on the in vivo management of differentiated thyroid cancer. Life Sci 2012;91:1236–41.
161. Ma X, Yang L, Xiao L, et al. Down-regulation of EBV-LMP1 radio-sensitizes nasal pharyngeal carcinoma cells via NF-kappaB regulated ATM expression. PLoS One 2011;6:e24647.
162. O'Neill AJ, Prencipe M, Dowling C, et al. Characterisation and manipulation of docetaxel resistant prostate cancer cell lines. Mol Cancer 2011; 10:126.
163. Bavi P, Uddin S, Bu R, et al. The biological and clinical impact of inhibition of NF-kappaB-initiated apoptosis in diffuse large B cell lymphoma (DLBCL). J Pathol 2011;224:355–66.
164. Hu X, Janssen WE, Moscinski LC, et al. An IkappaBalpha inhibitor causes leukemia cell death through a p38 MAP kinase-dependent, NF-kappaB-independent mechanism. Cancer Res 2001;61:6290–6.
165. Sourbier C, Danilin S, Lindner V, et al. Targeting the nuclear factor-kappaB rescue pathway has promising future in human renal cell carcinoma therapy. Cancer Res 2007;67:11668–76.
166. Domingo-Domenech J, Pippa R, Tapia M, et al. Inactivation of NF-kappaB by proteasome inhibition contributes to increased apoptosis induced by histone deacetylase inhibitors in human breast cancer cells. Breast Cancer Res Treat 2008;112:53–62.
167. Scaife CL, Kuang J, Wills JC, et al. Nuclear factor kappaB inhibitors induce adhesion-dependent colon cancer apoptosis: implications for metastasis. Cancer Res 2002;62:6870–8.
168. Rundall BK, Denlinger CE, Jones DR. Combined histone deacetylase and NF-kappaB inhibition sensitizes non-small cell lung cancer to cell death. Surgery 2004;136:416–25.
169. Furuta H, Osawa K, Shin M, et al. Selective inhibition of NF-kappaB suppresses bone invasion by oral squamous cell carcinoma in vivo. Int J Cancer 2012;131: E625–35.
170. Biswas DK, Shi Q, Baily S, et al. NF-kappa B activation in human breast cancer specimens and its role in cell proliferation and apoptosis. Proc Natl Acad Sci U S A 2004;101:10137–42.
171. Zanotto-Filho A, Braganhol E, Schroder R, et al. NFkappaB inhibitors induce cell death in glioblastomas. Biochem Pharmacol 2011;81:412–24.

172. Lee HR, Cheong HJ, Kim SJ, et al. Sulindac enhances arsenic trioxide-mediated apoptosis by inhibition of NF-kappaB in HCT116 colon cancer cells. Oncol Rep 2008;20:41–7.

173. Ma Y, Wang J, Liu L, et al. Genistein potentiates the effect of arsenic trioxide against human hepatocellular carcinoma: role of Akt and nuclear factor-kappaB. Cancer Lett 2011;301:75–84.

174. Mahieux R, Pise-Masison C, Gessain A, et al. Arsenic trioxide induces apoptosis in human T-cell leukemia virus type 1- and type 2-infected cells by a caspase-3-dependent mechanism involving Bcl-2 cleavage. Blood 2001; 98:3762–9.

175. Woo SY, Lee MY, Jung YJ, et al. Arsenic trioxide inhibits cell growth in SH-SY5Y and SK-N-AS neuroblastoma cell lines by a different mechanism. Pediatr Hematol Oncol 2006;23:231–43.

176. Mathieu J, Besancon F. Clinically tolerable concentrations of arsenic trioxide induce p53-independent cell death and repress NF-kappa B activation in Ewing sarcoma cells. Int J Cancer 2006;119:1723–7.

177. Park MJ, Lee JY, Kwak HJ, et al. Arsenic trioxide (As2O3) inhibits invasion of HT1080 human fibrosarcoma cells: role of nuclear factor-kappaB and reactive oxygen species. J Cell Biochem 2005;95:955–69.

178. Wei LH, Lai KP, Chen CA, et al. Arsenic trioxide prevents radiation-enhanced tumor invasiveness and inhibits matrix metalloproteinase-9 through downregulation of nuclear factor kappaB. Oncogene 2005;24:390–8.

179. Zhou JM, Zhu XF, Pan QC, et al. Manumycin induces apoptosis in human hepatocellular carcinoma HepG2 cells. Int J Mol Med 2003;12:955–9.

180. Salminen A, Lehtonen M, Paimela T, et al. Celastrol: molecular targets of thunder god vine. Biochem Biophys Res Commun 2010;394:439–42.

181. Kannaiyan R, Hay HS, Rajendran P, et al. Celastrol inhibits proliferation and induces chemosensitization through down-regulation of NF-kappaB and STAT3 regulated gene products in multiple myeloma cells. Br J Pharmacol 2011;164: 1506–21.

182. Chen M, Rose AE, Doudican N, et al. Celastrol synergistically enhances temozolomide cytotoxicity in melanoma cells. Mol Cancer Res 2009;7:1946–53.

183. Dai Y, Desano J, Tang W, et al. Natural proteasome inhibitor celastrol suppresses androgen-independent prostate cancer progression by modulating apoptotic proteins and NF-kappaB. PLoS One 2010;5:e14153.

184. Kim Y, Kang H, Jang SW, et al. Celastrol inhibits breast cancer cell invasion via suppression of NF-kB-mediated matrix metalloproteinase-9 expression. Cell Physiol Biochem 2011;28:175–84.

185. Pletz N, Schon M, Ziegelbauer K, et al. Doxorubicin-induced activation of NF-kappaB in melanoma cells is abrogated by inhibition of IKKbeta, but not by a novel IKKalpha inhibitor. Exp Dermatol 2012;21:301–4.

186. Alameda JP, Moreno-Maldonado R, Fernandez-Acenero MJ, et al. Increased IKKalpha expression in the basal layer of the epidermis of transgenic mice enhances the malignant potential of skin tumors. PLoS One 2011;6:e21984.

187. Merkhofer EC, Cogswell P, Baldwin AS. Her2 activates NF-kappaB and induces invasion through the canonical pathway involving IKKalpha. Oncogene 2010;29: 1238–48.

188. Liu M, Lee DF, Chen CT, et al. IKKalpha activation of NOTCH links tumorigenesis via FOXA2 suppression. Mol Cell 2012;45:171–84.

189. Mahato R, Qin B, Cheng K. Blocking IKKalpha expression inhibits prostate cancer invasiveness. Pharm Res 2011;28:1357–69.

190. Charalambous MP, Lightfoot T, Speirs V, et al. Expression of COX-2, NF-kappaB-p65, NF-kappaB-p50 and IKKalpha in malignant and adjacent normal human colorectal tissue. Br J Cancer 2009;101:106–15.
191. Garber K. The second wave in kinase cancer drugs. Nat Biotechnol 2006;24: 127–30.
192. Ridker PM, Danielson E, Fonseca FA, et al. Rosuvastatin to prevent vascular events in men and women with elevated C-reactive protein. N Engl J Med 2008;359:2195–207.
193. Nielsen SF, Nordestgaard BG, Bojesen SE. Statin use and reduced cancer-related mortality. N Engl J Med 2012;367:1792–802.
194. Denoyelle C, Vasse M, Korner M, et al. Cerivastatin, an inhibitor of HMG-CoA reductase, inhibits the signaling pathways involved in the invasiveness and metastatic properties of highly invasive breast cancer cell lines: an in vitro study. Carcinogenesis 2001;22:1139–48.
195. Wang W, Collie-Duguid E, Cassidy J. Cerivastatin enhances the cytotoxicity of 5-fluorouracil on chemosensitive and resistant colorectal cancer cell lines. FEBS Lett 2002;531:415–20.
196. Nubel T, Dippold W, Kaina B, et al. Ionizing radiation-induced E-selectin gene expression and tumor cell adhesion is inhibited by lovastatin and all-trans retinoic acid. Carcinogenesis 2004;25:1335–44.
197. Katano H, Pesnicak L, Cohen JI. Simvastatin induces apoptosis of Epstein-Barr virus (EBV)-transformed lymphoblastoid cell lines and delays development of EBV lymphomas. Proc Natl Acad Sci U S A 2004;101:4960–5.
198. Ahn KS, Sethi G, Aggarwal BB. Simvastatin potentiates TNF-alpha-induced apoptosis through the down-regulation of NF-kappaB-dependent antiapoptotic gene products: role of IkappaBalpha kinase and TGF-beta-activated kinase-1. J Immunol 2007;178:2507–16.
199. Ghosh-Choudhury N, Mandal CC, Ghosh Choudhury G. Simvastatin induces derepression of PTEN expression via NFkappaB to inhibit breast cancer cell growth. Cell Signal 2010;22:749–58.
200. Han JY, Lee SH, Yoo NJ, et al. A randomized phase II study of gefitinib plus simvastatin versus gefitinib alone in previously treated patients with advanced non-small cell lung cancer. Clin Cancer Res 2011;17:1553–60.
201. Han JY, Lim KY, Yu SY, et al. A phase 2 study of irinotecan, cisplatin, and simvastatin for untreated extensive-disease small cell lung cancer. Cancer 2011; 117:2178–85.
202. Konings IR, van der Gaast A, van der Wijk LJ, et al. The addition of pravastatin to chemotherapy in advanced gastric carcinoma: a randomised phase II trial. Eur J Cancer 2010;46:3200–4.
203. Schmidmaier R, Baumann P, Bumeder I, et al. First clinical experience with simvastatin to overcome drug resistance in refractory multiple myeloma. Eur J Haematol 2007;79:240–3.
204. van der Spek E, Bloem AC, Sinnige HA, et al. High dose simvastatin does not reverse resistance to vincristine, adriamycin, and dexamethasone (VAD) in myeloma. Haematologica 2007;92:e130–1.
205. Batra RK, Guttridge DC, Brenner DA, et al. IkappaBalpha gene transfer is cytotoxic to squamous-cell lung cancer cells and sensitizes them to tumor necrosis factor-alpha-mediated cell death. Am J Respir Cell Mol Biol 1999;21:238–45.
206. Mukogawa T, Koyama F, Tachibana M, et al. Adenovirus-mediated gene transduction of truncated I kappa B alpha enhances radiosensitivity in human colon cancer cells. Cancer Sci 2003;94:745–50.

207. Chen S, Fribley A, Wang CY. Potentiation of tumor necrosis factor-mediated apoptosis of oral squamous cell carcinoma cells by adenovirus-mediated gene transfer of NF-kappaB inhibitor. J Dent Res 2002;81:98–102.
208. Weaver KD, Yeyeodu S, Cusack JC Jr, et al. Potentiation of chemotherapeutic agents following antagonism of nuclear factor kappa B in human gliomas. J Neurooncol 2003;61:187–96.
209. Lee WP, Tai DI, Tsai SL, et al. Adenovirus type 5 E1A sensitizes hepatocellular carcinoma cells to gemcitabine. Cancer Res 2003;63:6229–36.
210. Sanlioglu AD, Dirice E, Aydin C, et al. Surface TRAIL decoy receptor-4 expression is correlated with TRAIL resistance in MCF7 breast cancer cells. BMC Cancer 2005;5:54.
211. Sanlioglu AD, Koksal IT, Karacay B, et al. Adenovirus-mediated IKKbetaKA expression sensitizes prostate carcinoma cells to TRAIL-induced apoptosis. Cancer Gene Ther 2006;13:21–31.
212. Hortobagyi GN, Ueno NT, Xia W, et al. Cationic liposome-mediated E1A gene transfer to human breast and ovarian cancer cells and its biologic effects: a phase I clinical trial. J Clin Oncol 2001;19:3422–33.
213. Villaret D, Glisson B, Kenady D, et al. A multicenter phase II study of tgDCC-E1A for the intratumoral treatment of patients with recurrent head and neck squamous cell carcinoma. Head Neck 2002;24:661–9.
214. Ochiai T, Saito Y, Saitoh T, et al. Inhibition of IkappaB kinase beta restrains oncogenic proliferation of pancreatic cancer cells. J Med Dent Sci 2008;55:49–59.
215. Diaz LA Jr, Messersmith W, Sokoll L, et al. TNF-blockade in patients with advanced hormone refractory prostate cancer. Invest New Drugs 2011;29:192–4.
216. Larkin JM, Ferguson TR, Pickering LM, et al. A phase I/II trial of sorafenib and infliximab in advanced renal cell carcinoma. Br J Cancer 2010;103:1149–53.
217. Madhusudan S, Foster M, Muthuramalingam SR, et al. A phase II study of etanercept (Enbrel), a tumor necrosis factor alpha inhibitor in patients with metastatic breast cancer. Clin Cancer Res 2004;10:6528–34.
218. Madhusudan S, Muthuramalingam SR, Braybrooke JP, et al. Study of etanercept, a tumor necrosis factor-alpha inhibitor, in recurrent ovarian cancer. J Clin Oncol 2005;23:5950–9.
219. Scott BL, Ramakrishnan A, Storer B, et al. Prolonged responses in patients with MDS and CMML treated with azacitidine and etanercept. Br J Haematol 2010;148:944–7.
220. Woyach JA, Lin TS, Lucas MS, et al. A phase I/II study of rituximab and etanercept in patients with chronic lymphocytic leukemia and small lymphocytic lymphoma. Leukemia 2009;23:912–8.
221. Jazirehi AR, Huerta-Yepez S, Cheng G, et al. Rituximab (chimeric anti-CD20 monoclonal antibody) inhibits the constitutive nuclear factor-{kappa}B signaling pathway in non-Hodgkin's lymphoma B-cell lines: role in sensitization to chemotherapeutic drug-induced apoptosis. Cancer Res 2005;65:264–76.
222. Fizazi K, De Bono JS, Flechon A, et al. Randomised phase II study of siltuximab (CNTO 328), an anti-IL-6 monoclonal antibody, in combination with mitoxantrone/prednisone versus mitoxantrone/prednisone alone in metastatic castration-resistant prostate cancer. Eur J Cancer 2012;48:85–93.
223. Rossi JF, Negrier S, James ND, et al. A phase I/II study of siltuximab (CNTO 328), an anti-interleukin-6 monoclonal antibody, in metastatic renal cell cancer. Br J Cancer 2010;103:1154–62.

224. Coward J, Kulbe H, Chakravarty P, et al. Interleukin-6 as a therapeutic target in human ovarian cancer. Clin Cancer Res 2011;17:6083–96.
225. Kanai M, Imaizumi A, Otsuka Y, et al. Dose-escalation and pharmacokinetic study of nanoparticle curcumin, a potential anticancer agent with improved bioavailability, in healthy human volunteers. Cancer Chemother Pharmacol 2012;69:65–70.
226. Steward WP, Gescher AJ. Curcumin in cancer management: recent results of analogue design and clinical studies and desirable future research. Mol Nutr Food Res 2008;52:1005–9.
227. Szekeres T, Fritzer-Szekeres M, Saiko P, et al. Resveratrol and resveratrol analogues–structure-activity relationship. Pharm Res 2010;27:1042–8.
228. Johnson JJ, Mukhtar H. Curcumin for chemoprevention of colon cancer. Cancer Lett 2007;255:170–81.
229. Mahabir S, Leitzmann MF, Pietinen P, et al. Physical activity and renal cell cancer risk in a cohort of male smokers. Int J Cancer 2004;108:600–5.
230. Kirkegaard H, Johnsen NF, Christensen J, et al. Association of adherence to lifestyle recommendations and risk of colorectal cancer: a prospective Danish cohort study. BMJ 2010;341:c5504.
231. Romieu-Mourez R, Landesman-Bollag E, Seldin DC, et al. Protein kinase CK2 promotes aberrant activation of nuclear factor-kappaB, transformed phenotype, and survival of breast cancer cells. Cancer Res 2002;62:6770–8.
232. Kato T Jr, Delhase M, Hoffmann A, et al. CK2 is a C-terminal IkappaB kinase responsible for NF-kappaB activation during the UV response. Mol Cell 2003; 12:829–39.
233. Wu ZH, Wong ET, Shi Y, et al. ATM- and NEMO-dependent ELKS ubiquitination coordinates TAK1-mediated IKK activation in response to genotoxic stress. Mol Cell 2010;40:75–86.
234. Ling J, Kang Y, Zhao R, et al. KrasG12D-induced IKK2/beta/NF-kappaB activation by IL-1alpha and p62 feedforward loops is required for development of pancreatic ductal adenocarcinoma. Cancer Cell 2012;21:105–20.
235. Basseres DS, Ebbs A, Levantini E, et al. Requirement of the NF-kappaB subunit p65/RelA for K-Ras-induced lung tumorigenesis. Cancer Res 2010;70: 3537–46.
236. Birkenkamp KU, Geugien M, Schepers H, et al. Constitutive NF-kappaB DNA-binding activity in AML is frequently mediated by a Ras/PI3-K/PKB-dependent pathway. Leukemia 2004;18:103–12.
237. Amma H, Naruse K, Ishiguro N, et al. Involvement of reactive oxygen species in cyclic stretch-induced NF-kappaB activation in human fibroblast cells. Br J Pharmacol 2005;145:364–73.
238. Gloire G, Charlier E, Rahmouni S, et al. Restoration of SHIP-1 activity in human leukemic cells modifies NF-kappaB activation pathway and cellular survival upon oxidative stress. Oncogene 2006;25:5485–94.
239. Storz P, Doppler H, Toker A. Activation loop phosphorylation controls protein kinase D-dependent activation of nuclear factor kappaB. Mol Pharmacol 2004;66: 870–9.
240. Beraud C, Henzel WJ, Baeuerle PA. Involvement of regulatory and catalytic subunits of phosphoinositide 3-kinase in NF-kappaB activation. Proc Natl Acad Sci U S A 1999;96:429–34.
241. McAllister-Lucas LM, Ruland J, Siu K, et al. CARMA3/Bcl10/MALT1-dependent NF-kappaB activation mediates angiotensin II-responsive inflammatory signaling in nonimmune cells. Proc Natl Acad Sci U S A 2007;104:139–44.

242. Kawauchi K, Araki K, Tobiume K, et al. Loss of p53 enhances catalytic activity of IKKbeta through O-linked beta-N-acetyl glucosamine modification. Proc Natl Acad Sci U S A 2009;106:3431–6.

243. Rupec RA, Baeuerle PA. The genomic response of tumor cells to hypoxia and reoxygenation. Differential activation of transcription factors AP-1 and NF-kappa B. Eur J Biochem 1995;234:632–40.

244. Mezzanzanica D, Balladore E, Turatti F, et al. CD95-mediated apoptosis is impaired at receptor level by cellular FLICE-inhibitory protein (long form) in wild-type p53 human ovarian carcinoma. Clin Cancer Res 2004;10:5202–14.

245. Chen X, Kandasamy K, Srivastava RK. Differential roles of RelA (p65) and c-Rel subunits of nuclear factor kappa B in tumor necrosis factor-related apoptosis-inducing ligand signaling. Cancer Res 2003;63:1059–66.

246. Bernard D, Quatannens B, Vandenbunder B, et al. Rel/NF-kappaB transcription factors protect against tumor necrosis factor (TNF)-related apoptosis-inducing ligand (TRAIL)-induced apoptosis by up-regulating the TRAIL decoy receptor DcR1. J Biol Chem 2001;276:27322–8.

247. Wang CY, Mayo MW, Korneluk RG, et al. NF-kappaB antiapoptosis: induction of TRAF1 and TRAF2 and c-IAP1 and c-IAP2 to suppress caspase-8 activation. Science 1998;281:1680–3.

248. Lee R, Collins T. Nuclear factor-kappaB and cell survival: IAPs call for support. Circ Res 2001;88:262–4.

249. Liston P, Fong WG, Korneluk RG. The inhibitors of apoptosis: there is more to life than Bcl2. Oncogene 2003;22:8568–80.

250. Wright CW, Duckett CS. Reawakening the cellular death program in neoplasia through the therapeutic blockade of IAP function. J Clin Invest 2005;115:2673–8.

251. Burstein E, Ganesh L, Dick RD, et al. A novel role for XIAP in copper homeostasis through regulation of MURR1. EMBO J 2004;23:244–54.

252. Kaur S, Wang F, Venkatraman M, et al. X-linked inhibitor of apoptosis (XIAP) inhibits c-Jun N-terminal kinase 1 (JNK1) activation by transforming growth factor beta1 (TGF-beta1) through ubiquitin-mediated proteosomal degradation of the TGF-beta1-activated kinase 1 (TAK1). J Biol Chem 2005;280:38599–608.

253. Tamm I, Wang Y, Sausville E, et al. IAP-family protein survivin inhibits caspase activity and apoptosis induced by Fas (CD95), Bax, caspases, and anticancer drugs. Cancer Res 1998;58:5315–20.

254. Lee HH, Dadgostar H, Cheng Q, et al. NF-kappaB-mediated up-regulation of Bcl-x and Bfl-1/A1 is required for CD40 survival signaling in B lymphocytes. Proc Natl Acad Sci U S A 1999;96:9136–41.

255. Tamatani M, Che YH, Matsuzaki H, et al. Tumor necrosis factor induces Bcl-2 and Bcl-x expression through NFkappaB activation in primary hippocampal neurons. J Biol Chem 1999;274:8531–8.

256. Wang CY, Guttridge DC, Mayo MW, et al. NF-kappaB induces expression of the Bcl-2 homologue A1/Bfl-1 to preferentially suppress chemotherapy-induced apoptosis. Mol Cell Biol 1999;19:5923–9.

257. Chen C, Edelstein LC, Gelinas C. The Rel/NF-kappaB family directly activates expression of the apoptosis inhibitor Bcl-x(L). Mol Cell Biol 2000;20:2687–95.

258. Sun XM, Bratton SB, Butterworth M, et al. Bcl-2 and Bcl-xL inhibit CD95-mediated apoptosis by preventing mitochondrial release of Smac/DIABLO and subsequent inactivation of X-linked inhibitor-of-apoptosis protein. J Biol Chem 2002;277:11345–51.

259. Wadgaonkar R, Phelps KM, Haque Z, et al. CREB-binding protein is a nuclear integrator of nuclear factor-kappaB and p53 signaling. J Biol Chem 1999;274: 1879–82.
260. Xu Y, Kiningham KK, Devalaraja MN, et al. An intronic NF-kappaB element is essential for induction of the human manganese superoxide dismutase gene by tumor necrosis factor-alpha and interleukin-1beta. DNA Cell Biol 1999;18: 709–22.
261. Pham CG, Bubici C, Zazzeroni F, et al. Ferritin heavy chain upregulation by NF-kappaB inhibits TNFalpha-induced apoptosis by suppressing reactive oxygen species. Cell 2004;119:529–42.
262. Feuerhake F, Kutok JL, Monti S, et al. NFkappaB activity, function, and target-gene signatures in primary mediastinal large B-cell lymphoma and diffuse large B-cell lymphoma subtypes. Blood 2005;106:1392–9.
263. Stoffel A, Chaurushiya M, Singh B, et al. Activation of NF-kappaB and inhibition of p53-mediated apoptosis by API2/mucosa-associated lymphoid tissue 1 fusions promote oncogenesis. Proc Natl Acad Sci U S A 2004;101:9079–84.
264. Ohno H, Doi S, Yabumoto K, et al. Molecular characterization of the t(14;19)(q32;q13) translocation in chronic lymphocytic leukemia. Leukemia 1993;7:2057–63.
265. Cabannes E, Khan G, Aillet F, et al. Mutations in the IkBa gene in Hodgkin's disease suggest a tumour suppressor role for IkappaBalpha. Oncogene 1999;18: 3063–70.
266. Annunziata CM, Davis RE, Demchenko Y, et al. Frequent engagement of the classical and alternative NF-kappaB pathways by diverse genetic abnormalities in multiple myeloma. Cancer Cell 2007;12:115–30.
267. Keats JJ, Fonseca R, Chesi M, et al. Promiscuous mutations activate the noncanonical NF-kappaB pathway in multiple myeloma. Cancer Cell 2007;12:131–44.
268. Migliazza A, Lombardi L, Rocchi M, et al. Heterogeneous chromosomal aberrations generate 3' truncations of the NFKB2/lyt-10 gene in lymphoid malignancies. Blood 1994;84:3850–60.
269. Boehm JS, Zhao JJ, Yao J, et al. Integrative genomic approaches identify IKBKE as a breast cancer oncogene. Cell 2007;129:1065–79.
270. Hutti JE, Shen RR, Abbott DW, et al. Phosphorylation of the tumor suppressor CYLD by the breast cancer oncogene IKKepsilon promotes cell transformation. Mol Cell 2009;34:461–72.
271. Hamdane M, David-Cordonnier MH, D'Halluin JC. Activation of p65 NF-kappaB protein by p210BCR-ABL in a myeloid cell line (P210BCR-ABL activates p65 NF-kappaB). Oncogene 1997;15:2267–75.
272. Stirewalt DL, Meshinchi S, Radich JP. Molecular targets in acute myelogenous leukemia. Blood Rev 2003;17:15–23.
273. Garkavtsev I, Kozin SV, Chernova O, et al. The candidate tumour suppressor protein ING4 regulates brain tumour growth and angiogenesis. Nature 2004; 428:328–32.
274. Vitale-Cross L, Amornphimoltham P, Fisher G, et al. Conditional expression of K-ras in an epithelial compartment that includes the stem cells is sufficient to promote squamous cell carcinogenesis. Cancer Res 2004;64:8804–7.
275. Lu SL, Herrington H, Reh D, et al. Loss of transforming growth factor-beta type II receptor promotes metastatic head-and-neck squamous cell carcinoma. Genes Dev 2006;20:1331–42.
276. Molinolo AA, Amornphimoltham P, Squarize CH, et al. Dysregulated molecular networks in head and neck carcinogenesis. Oral Oncol 2009;45:324–34.

277. Patel V, Rosenfeldt HM, Lyons R, et al. Persistent activation of Rac1 in squamous carcinomas of the head and neck: evidence for an EGFR/Vav2 signaling axis involved in cell invasion. Carcinogenesis 2007;28:1145–52.

278. Romieu-Mourez R, Kim DW, Shin SM, et al. Mouse mammary tumor virus c-rel transgenic mice develop mammary tumors. Mol Cell Biol 2003;23:5738–54.

279. Benezra M, Chevallier N, Morrison DJ, et al. BRCA1 augments transcription by the NF-kappaB transcription factor by binding to the Rel domain of the p65/RelA subunit. J Biol Chem 2003;278:26333–41.

280. Pianetti S, Arsura M, Romieu-Mourez R, et al. Her-2/neu overexpression induces NF-kappaB via a PI3-kinase/Akt pathway involving calpain-mediated degradation of IkappaB-alpha that can be inhibited by the tumor suppressor PTEN. Oncogene 2001;20:1287–99.

281. Brose MS, Volpe P, Feldman M, et al. BRAF and RAS mutations in human lung cancer and melanoma. Cancer Res 2002;62:6997–7000.

282. Paez JG, Janne PA, Lee JC, et al. EGFR mutations in lung cancer: correlation with clinical response to gefitinib therapy. Science 2004;304:1497–500.

283. Stephens P, Hunter C, Bignell G, et al. Lung cancer: intragenic ERBB2 kinase mutations in tumours. Nature 2004;431:525–6.

284. Davies H, Hunter C, Smith R, et al. Somatic mutations of the protein kinase gene family in human lung cancer. Cancer Res 2005;65:7591–5.

285. Sher T, Dy GK, Adjei AA. Small cell lung cancer. Mayo Clin Proc 2008;83:355–67.

286. Chow JY, Ban M, Wu HL, et al. TGF-beta downregulates PTEN via activation of NF-kappaB in pancreatic cancer cells. Am J Physiol Gastrointest Liver Physiol 2010;298:G275–82.

287. Wilson W 3rd, Baldwin AS. Maintenance of constitutive IkappaB kinase activity by glycogen synthase kinase-3alpha/beta in pancreatic cancer. Cancer Res 2008;68:8156–63.

288. Evertsson S, Sun XF. Protein expression of NF-kappaB in human colorectal adenocarcinoma. Int J Mol Med 2002;10:547–50.

289. Koumakpayi IH, Le Page C, Mes-Masson AM, et al. Hierarchical clustering of immunohistochemical analysis of the activated ErbB/PI3K/Akt/NF-kappaB signalling pathway and prognostic significance in prostate cancer. Br J Cancer 2010;102:1163–73.

290. Dan HC, Cooper MJ, Cogswell PC, et al. Akt-dependent regulation of NF-{kappa}B is controlled by mTOR and raptor in association with IKK. Genes Dev 2008;22:1490–500.

291. Yang J, Splittgerber R, Yull FE, et al. Conditional ablation of Ikkb inhibits melanoma tumor development in mice. J Clin Invest 2010;120:2563–74.

292. Dhawan P, Su Y, Thu YM, et al. The lymphotoxin-beta receptor is an upstream activator of NF-kappaB-mediated transcription in melanoma cells. J Biol Chem 2008;283:15399–408.

293. Schwartz L, Guais A, Israel M, et al. Tumor regression with a combination of drugs interfering with the tumor metabolism: efficacy of hydroxycitrate, lipoic acid and capsaicin. Invest New Drugs 2013;31(2):256–64.

294. Kang JH, Kim CS, Han IS, et al. Capsaicin, a spicy component of hot peppers, modulates adipokine gene expression and protein release from obese-mouse adipose tissues and isolated adipocytes, and suppresses the inflammatory responses of adipose tissue macrophages. FEBS Lett 2007;581:4389–96.

295. Han SS, Keum YS, Chun KS, et al. Suppression of phorbol ester-induced NF-kappaB activation by capsaicin in cultured human promyelocytic leukemia cells. Arch Pharm Res 2002;25:475–9.

296. Singh S, Natarajan K, Aggarwal BB. Capsaicin (8-methyl-N-vanillyl-6-nonena-mide) is a potent inhibitor of nuclear transcription factor-kappa B activation by diverse agents. J Immunol 1996;157:4412–20.

297. Joung EJ, Li MH, Lee HG, et al. Capsaicin induces heme oxygenase-1 expression in HepG2 cells via activation of PI3K-Nrf2 signaling: NAD(P)H:quinone oxidoreductase as a potential target. Antioxid Redox Signal 2007;9:2087–98.

298. Mukhopadhyay A, Basu N, Ghatak N, et al. Anti-inflammatory and irritant activities of curcumin analogues in rats. Agents Actions 1982;12:508–15.

299. Sharma OP. Antioxidant activity of curcumin and related compounds. Biochem Pharmacol 1976;25:1811–2.

300. Lim GP, Chu T, Yang F, et al. The curry spice curcumin reduces oxidative damage and amyloid pathology in an Alzheimer transgenic mouse. J Neurosci 2001; 21:8370–7.

301. Arbiser JL, Klauber N, Rohan R, et al. Curcumin is an in vivo inhibitor of angiogenesis. Mol Med 1998;4:376–83.

302. Ray S, Chattopadhyay N, Mitra A, et al. Curcumin exhibits antimetastatic properties by modulating integrin receptors, collagenase activity, and expression of Nm23 and E-cadherin. J Environ Pathol Toxicol Oncol 2003;22:49–58.

303. Rao CV, Rivenson A, Simi B, et al. Chemoprevention of colon carcinogenesis by dietary curcumin, a naturally occurring plant phenolic compound. Cancer Res 1995;55:259–66.

304. Tian F, Zhang C, Tian W, et al. Comparison of the effect of p65 siRNA and curcumin in promoting apoptosis in esophageal squamous cell carcinoma cells and in nude mice. Oncol Rep 2012;28:232–40.

305. Chan MM. Inhibition of tumor necrosis factor by curcumin, a phytochemical. Biochem Pharmacol 1995;49:1551–6.

306. Lee KW, Kim JH, Lee HJ, et al. Curcumin inhibits phorbol ester-induced upregulation of cyclooxygenase-2 and matrix metalloproteinase-9 by blocking ERK1/2 phosphorylation and NF-kappaB transcriptional activity in MCF10A human breast epithelial cells. Antioxid Redox Signal 2005;7:1612–20.

307. Hatcher H, Planalp R, Cho J, et al. Curcumin: from ancient medicine to current clinical trials. Cell Mol Life Sci 2008;65:1631–52.

308. Ren J, Fan C, Chen N, et al. Resveratrol pretreatment attenuates cerebral ischemic injury by upregulating expression of transcription factor Nrf2 and HO-1 in rats. Neurochem Res 2011;36:2352–62.

309. Zhong M, Cheng GF, Wang WJ, et al. Inhibitory effect of resveratrol on interleukin 6 release by stimulated peritoneal macrophages of mice. Phytomedicine 1999;6:79–84.

310. Zhang Q, Tang X, Lu QY, et al. Resveratrol inhibits hypoxia-induced accumulation of hypoxia-inducible factor-1alpha and VEGF expression in human tongue squamous cell carcinoma and hepatoma cells. Mol Cancer Ther 2005;4: 1465–74.

311. Huderson AC, Myers JN, Niaz MS, et al. Chemoprevention of benzo(a)pyrene-induced colon polyps in Apc(Min) mice by resveratrol. J Nutr Biochem 2013; 24(4):713–24.

312. Liao PC, Ng LT, Lin LT, et al. Resveratrol arrests cell cycle and induces apoptosis in human hepatocellular carcinoma Huh-7 cells. J Med Food 2010; 13:1415–23.

313. Casanova F, Quarti J, da Costa DC, et al. Resveratrol chemosensitizes breast cancer cells to melphalan by cell cycle arrest. J Cell Biochem 2012;113: 2586–96.

314. Qureshi AA, Guan XQ, Reis JC, et al. Inhibition of nitric oxide and inflammatory cytokines in LPS-stimulated murine macrophages by resveratrol, a potent proteasome inhibitor. Lipids Health Dis 2012;11:76.

315. Yeung F, Hoberg JE, Ramsey CS, et al. Modulation of NF-kappaB-dependent transcription and cell survival by the SIRT1 deacetylase. EMBO J 2004;23: 2369–80.

316. Chen CY, Jang JH, Li MH, et al. Resveratrol upregulates heme oxygenase-1 expression via activation of NF-E2-related factor 2 in PC12 cells. Biochem Biophys Res Commun 2005;331:993–1000.

Targeting the p53 Pathway

Vita M. Golubovskaya, PhD[a,b], William G. Cance, MD[a,b,c],*

KEYWORDS

- p53 • Mdm-2 • FAK • Survival • Apoptosis

KEY POINTS

- The p53 gene is a tumor-suppressor gene whose genomic sequence contains 11 exons and spans 20 kilobases.
- p53 is the most commonly mutated gene in tumors, with up to 50% mutations in different types of cancers and 75% mutations in invasive cancers.
- Focal Adhesion Kinase (FAK) can suppress the transcriptional activity of p53 through its interaction.
- Understanding FAK biology during tumorigenesis, the mechanisms of its upregulation in different tumors, its role in stem cell biology, angiogenesis, and motility, and the mechanisms of its direct physical interaction with p53 protein and their downstream signaling pathways will be critical in developing targeted therapeutics.

INTRODUCTION

p53 is a guardian of the genome, and a tumor-suppressor gene that controls genetic stability and prevents cancer. p53 is highly mutated in different types of tumors or is inactivated by different mechanisms such as interacting with Mdm-2, Mdmx, Focal Adhesion Kinase (FAK), and other proteins. This review discusses different approaches to reactivate the p53 pathway either through targeting its inhibiting protein interactions with Mdm-2 and FAK proteins, through changing protein conformations with small-molecule inhibitors, through the introduction of wild-type p53, or through

Funding Source: This research was supported by the grant CA65910, from the National Cancer Institute.

Conflicts of Interest: Dr Golubovskaya and Dr Cance: Cofounders and stock holders of CureFAKtor Pharmaceuticals, Buffalo, NY.

During preparation of this review the below report was published, which demonstrated new approach of p53 reactivation by targeting FAK and p53 interaction with Roslin 2, R2 compound.[117]

[a] Department of Surgical Oncology, Roswell Park Cancer Institute, Elm & Carlton Streets, Buffalo, NY 14127, USA; [b] CureFAKtor Pharmaceuticals, 14 Rock Dove Lane, Orchard Park, Buffalo, NY 1427, USA; [c] Department of Surgery, University of Buffalo, 100 High Street, Buffalo, NY, USA

* Corresponding author. Department of Surgical Oncology, Roswell Park Cancer Institute, Elm & Carlton Streets, Buffalo, NY 14127.

E-mail addresses: William.Cance@roswellpark.org; wcance@curefaktor.com other pathways, focusing on future directions and perspectives in translational research on developing p53-targeting therapeutics. There are several homologous proteins to p53, such as p63 and p73, with similar and unique functions that are not discussed in this article.

P53 PROTEIN STRUCTURE AND FUNCTION

p53 is a tumor-suppressor gene whose genomic sequence contains 11 exons and spans 20 kilobases; it is located at the short arm of the chromosome 17p13.1 region and encodes p53 protein.[1] The p53 protein is a transcription factor that binds as a tetramer to the DNA consensus sequence 5'Pu-Pu-Pu-C-A/T-T/A-G-Py-Py-Py3' (Pu, purine; Py, pyrimidine) in the promoters of the several genes, such as p21, Bax, Mdm-2, and PUMA, and activates their transcription.[2] It has also been shown that p53 can repress transcription of several important genes such as survivin, Bcl-2, FAK, and others.[3] The promoter of p53 does not contain a TATA box and consists of various binding sites for known transcription factors, such as NF-κB, Sp1, or c-Jun.[4] The p53 gene encodes a 393-amino-acid tumor-suppressor protein, which contains several functional domains: 2 N-terminal transcriptional activating domains, TAD1 (amino acids [aa] 1–42) and TAD2 (aa 43–65); a proline-rich domain (aa 64–92); a central DNA-binding domain (aa 102–292); and a C-terminal tetramerization domain (aa 325–393) and basic region (aa 364–393) (**Fig. 1**).[5] The nuclear localization signal is located after the DNA-binding domain (aa 305–322) (see **Fig. 1**).

N-Terminal Transactivation Domain of p53

The 17 to 28 amino acids of the first N-terminal transactivation domain interact with Mdm-2 protein, double minute-2 homologue, which plays a major role in p53 degradation via the ubiquitin-proteasome pathway.[1] p53 activates Mdm-2 transcription through binding to its promoter, and upregulates Mdm-2 expression. In turn, Mdm-2 binds to p53 and negatively regulates its stability and activity. Thus, Mdm-2 regulates p53 via an autoregulatory feedback loop in which both proteins control its cellular expression. Amino acids 22 to 26 are involved in the binding of histone acetyltransferase P300 (reviewed in Ref.[6]). The second transactivation domain (aa 43–63) activates transcription of several p53 transcriptional targets.

Proline-Rich Domain of p53

A proline-rich domain (aa 64–92) contains 5 PXXP motifs, is important for interaction with various proteins, and regulates apoptosis.[6] The PXXP motifs of this domain

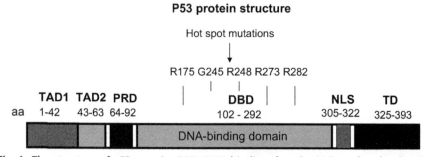

Fig. 1. The structure of p53 protein. DBD, DNA-binding domain; NLS, nuclear localization sequence; TAD, transactivating domain; TD, tetramerization domain.

were shown to create a binding site for Src-homology SH3 domains.[7] A mutant deleted for the proline-rich domain in human p53 (Δ62–91) was not able to cause apoptosis but was able to maintain cell-cycle arrest.[8] A polymorphism at the amino acid 72 of either proline or arginine could cause differences in binding of transcription factors, survival/apoptotic signaling, and response to chemotherapy agents.[9]

Central DNA-Binding Domain

The core central region of p53 is highly conserved, homologous to the regions of other p53 family members (p63 and p73). The DNA-binding domain binds to promoter binding sites 5'Pu-Pu-Pu-C-A/T-T/A-G-Py-Py-Py3'.[1] Several p53 mutation hot spots are located in this domain, such as: Arg175, Gly245, Arg248, Arg273, and Arg282 (see **Fig. 1**).

C-terminal Tetramerization Domain

This domain is involved in protein tetramerization and regulation of p53 activity. It contains the tetramerization region (aa 323–356) and a negative regulatory region (aa 363–393) (see Ref.[6] for a review).

P53 MUTATIONS IN CANCER CELLS

p53 is the most commonly mutated gene in tumors, with up to 50% mutations in different types of cancers and 75% mutations in invasive cancers. Most mutations are missense mutations, with 4 of 5 mutations in the DNA-binding domain, only 1% in the N-terminal domain, and 4% in the C-terminal tetramerization domain (reviewed in Ref.[10]). The most frequent hot-spot mutations are: 175 Arg → His (breaks bond between L2 and L3 loop); 248 Arg → Gln (Trp) (breaks contact with DNA in minor groove); 273 Arg → His (Cys) (breaks contact with DNA in major groove); and 282 Arg → Trp (destabilizes H2 helix and DNA binding in the major groove and breaks contacts on the β-hairpin) (reviewed in Ref.[10]) Arginines 248 and 273 are involved in interaction of p53 with DNA, and arginines 175 and 282 stabilize the DNA-binding sequence of p53.[4] Wild-type p53 binds to gene promoters with different affinity; for example, p53 activates p21 promoter with a higher affinity than the Bax promoter.[4]

P53 FUNCTION

p53 was discovered in 1979 and was first thought to play the role of oncogene, but was then revisited and found to be a tumor-suppressor gene. The model of the main functions of p53 is shown in **Fig. 2** and is discussed in a recent review summarizing the first 30 years of p53 research.[11] It is known that p53 is mutated in almost 50% of all tumors.[12] Inactivation of the p53 gene is a critical step in tumorigenesis.[13] Following induction by a variety of cell stresses, such as DNA damage, hypoxia, or the presence of activated oncogenes, p53 upregulates a set of genes that can promote either cell death, apoptosis, senescence, or growth arrest, such as *p21*, *GADD45*, *cyclin G*, and *Bax*, reviewed in Ref.[14] Recently it was shown that p53 can repress promoter activities of several antiapoptotic genes and cell cycle genes (survivin,[15] cyclin B1, cdc2,[16,17] cdc25 c,[18] stathmin,[19] Map4,[20] and bcl-2[16]). Overexpression of p53-induced apoptosis[21,22] and p53 inactivation caused a decrease in radiation-induced apoptosis.[23–25] More recently, new functions of p53, such as metabolism and antioxidant defense, have been reported and reviewed (see **Fig. 2**).[11]

p53 Binds Focal Adhesion Kinase Promoter and Represses its Activity

FAK is a 125-kDa nonreceptor kinase that plays an important role in survival signaling, adhesion, motility, invasion, angiogenesis, and proliferation.[26,27] FAK was shown to be

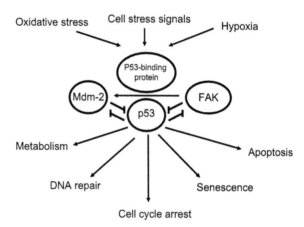

Fig. 2. FAK, p53, and Mdm-2 interaction and downstream signaling. FAK binds to p53 and blocks its functions; FAK binds to Mdm-2 to facilitate p53 proteosomal degradation, as shown in Ref.[46]; Mdm-2 binds to p53 and causes its degradation. p53 activates Mdm-2 and inhibits FAK.

overexpressed in many types of tumors and has been proposed as a therapeutic target.[28–30]

The first report on the indirect link of FAK and p53 signaling in apoptosis was reported by Ilic and colleagues,[31] who demonstrated that FAK suppressed a p53-regulated apoptotic pathway in anchorage-dependent cells such as fibroblasts and endothelial cells. These investigators showed that in the absence of FAK function, p53-regulated apoptosis was activated by protein kinase C and phospholipase A_2 and that this process was inhibited by dominant-negative p53 and Bcl-2. However, these processes were not studied in tumors and cancer cell lines.[31,32] In addition, immunohistochemical analysis of 115 endometrial carcinoma samples demonstrated a correlation between FAK and p53 overexpression.[33]

The authors' group[34] cloned the FAK promoter and found 2 p53 binding sites in this area, and showed that p53 binds to the FAK promoter and inhibits its transcriptional activity. Moreover, mutant p53 with hot-spot mutations did not inhibit FAK promoter activity, whereas the wild type did. The global analysis of p53 transcription factor binding sites demonstrated that induction of HCT116 colon cancer cells with 5-fluorouracil downregulated FAK.[35] It was therefore suggested that p53 can suppress metastasis through downregulation of metastasis-linked genes such as FAK. Because p53 is often mutated in cancer, the authors performed a population-based study on 600 tumors from patients with breast cancer, and found that p53 mutations highly correlated with FAK overexpression.[36] Recently, another group found a high correlation between high FAK expression and low levels of p53 in oral squamous cell carcinoma,[37] which may be explained by the absence of a repressive function on FAK promoter in p53-negative samples.

Direct p53 and FAK Protein Binding and Their Feedback Regulation

After finding that p53 regulates FAK promoter activity,[34] the authors demonstrated that the N-terminal transactivation domain of p53 is physically and directly associated with the N-terminal domain of FAK.[38] There have been several reports on the localization and function of the N-terminal part of FAK in the nucleus.[39–42] The N-terminal domain of FAK caused apoptosis in breast-cancer cell lines,[40] and its nuclear localization was regulated by caspase inhibitors in endothelial cells.[42] p53 was also reported to be localized in the cytoplasm.[43] p53 directly activated Bax and released proapoptotic molecules, activating multidomain protein complexes in the cytoplasm. This mechanism required the 62- to 91-amono acid proline-rich domain N-terminal domain of p53.[43] The authors also showed that FAK binds the 7 amino acids (aa 65–71) in the proline region of p53.[44] In addition, through computer modeling it was found that p53 peptides containing the amino acids 65 to 71 reactivated p53. This p53 peptide was modeled into the 3-dimensional structure of FAK, and small molecules that docked into this site of interaction were screened. In this way the authors identified novel small molecules targeting the FAK and p53 interaction that were able to activate p53 (see later discussion).

The authors have shown that FAK can suppress the transcriptional activity of p53 through its interaction, as p53-mediated activation of the p53 targets p21, Mdm-2, and Bax was blocked by overexpression of FAK, but not by ΔFAK-NT with a deleted N-terminal domain that binds p53.[38] Thus, p53 regulates FAK and, in turn, FAK regulates p53. Thus FAK and p53 can be regulated through a feedback mechanism.[27,45]

The binding of FAK and p53 was also studied by another group,[46] who showed interaction of FAK with p53 and also with Mdm-2 proteins whereby binding of FAK to Mdm-2 facilitated p53 ubiquitination and degradation.[46] The link between FAK and p53 was supported by a report on the FAK-interacting protein, FIP200.[47] FIP200 overexpression resulted in increased p21 levels and caused growth arrest, and FIP200 interacted with FAK and p53.[47] The investigators proposed a model of FAK-p53-FIP200 interaction, whereby FIP200/FAK and FIP200/p53 binding had competition and when FAK had low expression, FIP200 could bind p53 and increase its expression.[48]

Recently, the authors[49] showed that the stem-cell marker and transcription factor Nanog, which maintains stem-cell renewal and differentiation, was able to bind FAK promoter and upregulate its expression. In addition, FAK phosphorylated Nanog.[49] Of note, Nanog is repressed by p53 that induced differentiation of embryonic stem cells.[50] FAK is also repressed by p53, whereas it is activated is by Nanog. The mechanism of Nanog and FAK regulation and its cross-talk with p53 in cancer and stem cells requires further study. The novel mechanisms of FAK, p53, and Nanog survival function during carcinogenesis remain to be discovered.

P53-TARGETED THERAPY

This section discusses therapeutic approaches to target p53 function, beginning with p53-targeted therapy. The discussion then focuses on FAK-p53-targeted therapy based on data on FAK and p53 interaction.

Translational approaches that target p53 for cancer treatment include therapies targeting mutant p53 and therapies targeting wild-type p53 (reviewed in Ref.[51]), and are shown in **Fig. 3**.

Mutant p53–Targeted Therapy

To target mutant type p53, 2 therapeutic approaches are used: (1) deliver wild-type p53 with viruses (retroviruses or adenoviruses); and (2) use oncolytic therapy to destroy tumor cells with deleted or mutated p53 by lysis.

Exogenous expression of wild-type p53

Viral p53 delivery Retroviruses are attractive agents for cancer gene therapy, as they integrate in the stable form into the genome and require cell division for transduction. The second strategy is to use adenoviruses, which are double-stranded DNA viruses.

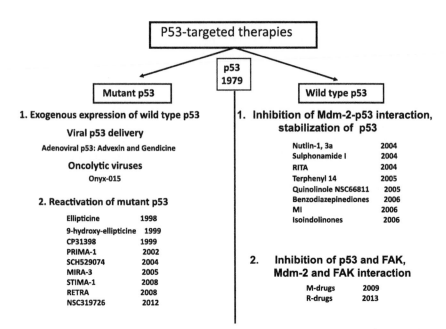

Fig. 3. p53-targeted therapies. p53 therapies target either mutant p53 (*left*) or wild-type p53 (*right*). Different therapeutic agents are shown with the year of their first report.

In contrast to retroviruses, their effect is not limited to highly proliferating cells and there is no risk of insertional mutagenesis or tumorigenesis.

Advexin One of the adenoviral drugs is Ad5CMV-p53 or (Advexin, developed by *Introgen Therapeutics Inc*; or Gendicine, *Shenzden SiBiono Gene Tech*), which is a recombinant E1-deleted serotype 5 adenoviral vector encoding p53. *In vitro* and *in vivo* studies confirmed the therapeutic effect of Ad5CMVp53. This therapeutic approach was used effectively in phase I and II clinical trials, although some cases of tumor resistance were also demonstrated (reviewed in Ref.[4]). The drug was not approved by the Food and Drug Administration (FDA), although Gendicine (adenoviral p53) is used for the treatment of head and neck cancer in China[52] and is effective in the treatment of hepatocellular carcinoma.[53]

Oncolytic viruses The second viral approach is to apply oncolytic viruses to kill p53-defective tumor cells, including the use of E1B-defective adenoviruses, which is a major approach.

Onyx-015 The delta 1520 virus (dl1520; ONYX-015), developed by Onyx Phramaceuticals, is an adenovirus that contains a deletion in the E1B region. ONYX-015 can be used as a selective drug against tumors with mutant p53. The problem of this and other adenoviral vectors is hepatotoxicity, and the FDA did not approve Onyx-015 after its use in numerous clinical trials.

Reactivation of mutant p53 with small molecules
To reactivate mutant p53, compounds were developed that targeted mutant p53 and reactivated wild-type p53 based on structural studies of p53 conformation, function, and regulation (see **Fig. 3**). The structures of all compounds are shown in review,[51]

and the compounds are presented here in chronologic order, according to when they were first reported (see **Fig. 3**).

Ellipticine (1998) One of the first compounds that targeted mutant p53 was ellipticine, an alkaloid that had cytotoxic and antiproliferative activity in a panel of cell lines with mutant p53.[54] Its derivative, 9-hydroxy-ellipticine (9HE), was developed in 1999.[55] Later studies showed the off-target effects of ellipticine, such as targeting topoisomerase II, FOX, and other mechanisms.

CP31398 (1999) In 1999, compound CP31398 (styrylquinazoline), which stabilized the DNA-binding domain of p53, was identified by high-throughput screening of a library of more than 100,000 synthetic small-molecule compounds by scientists from Pfizer Inc.[56] The compound increased conformationally active p53 in cells with mutant p53, increased p53 transcriptional activity with p21 target in cells with mutant p53, and decreased tumor growth.[56] CP31398 caused apoptosis in different cancer cell lines and stabilized wild-type p53 protein independently from Mdm-2.[57,58] However, different quantitative biophysical methods under a wide range of conditions did not detect the interaction of CP31398 and p53 core domain, but detected intercalation of CP31398 with DNA and destabilization of DNA-p53 complex.[59,60] The compound had several p53-independent functions, such as increase of apoptotic Bax protein.[59] CP31398 did not affect binding of wild-type p53 with DNA and did not affect p63 and p73 homologues binding to DNA, but increased the amount and affinity (K_d) of mutant p53 with DNA.[61] CP31398 restored the functions of mutant p53 to suppress ultraviolet B–induced skin carcinogenesis in mice, which was associated with increased p53, p21, and BclXs.[62,63] CP31398 was shown to have a chemopreventive effect on the development of intestinal adenoma in an animal model of familial adenomatous polyposis.[64] The compound suppressed development of tumors by 36% and 75% at low and high doses, respectively, and increased expression of p53, p21, cleaved caspase-3, and PARP-1.[64] The chemopreventive effect of CP31398 was observed in combination with celecoxib on azoxymethane-induced aberrant crypt foci and colon adenocarcinomas in F344 rats.[65] The combination of CP31398 and celecoxib reduced the incidence of adenocarcinoma by 78% and its multiplicity by 90%.[65] Rats fed with a combination of these drugs had increased p21 expression and apoptosis, and reduced tumor-cell proliferation.[65]

PRIMA-1 (2002) Another p53-reactivating compound was found in 2002 and named PRIMA (p53 Reactivation and Induction of Massive Apoptosis).[66] PRIMA had antitumor activity *in vivo* in a mutant p53–dependent manner.[66] It restored the p53-binding activity of R273H mutant and also other p53 mutants in the DNA-binding domain.[66] A methylated form of PRIMA-1 was more active than the parent compound and synergized with cisplatin to induce tumor-cell apoptosis, and induced apoptotic Bax and PUMA p53 targets.[67] PRIMA-1MET had suppressive effects in different mutant p53–carrying mouse tumors: mouse sarcomas, mammary carcinoma, and chemically induced fibrosarcoma.[68] PRIMA-1 entered into phase I clinical trials based on its high efficacy in the animal models.

SCH529074 (2004) Another small-molecule compound was discovered in 2004 and named SCH529074.[69] This compound was able to bind the DNA-binding domain of p53, restore the growth-suppressive functions of mutant p53, and interrupt the HDM2-regulated ubiquitination of wild-type p53.[69]

MIRA-3 (2005) The MIRA-1 derivative, MIRA-3, was also able to reactivate mutant p53 and to express antitumor activity in tumor xenografts with human mutant p53 *in vivo*.[70]

STIMA-1 (2008) The compound STIMA-1 had structural similarities with CP-31398 and was able to reactivate mutant p53.[71]

RETRA (2008) Screening of a small-molecule library to induce p53-dependent reporter activity in A431 cells with R273H mutation identified another compound, RETRA-1 (REactivation of Transcriptional Reporter Activity).[72] RETRA-1 showed antitumor activity in mouse xenografts, and also targeted homologous p53 protein p73.[72] RETRA was suggested to sequester and release p73 from its inhibitory complex with mutant p53. Thus, targeting homologous to p53 proteins, such as p63 and p73, is a potential approach that can be used in therapy.

NSC319726 (2012) In 2012 3 new compounds, NSC319725, NSC319726, and NSC328784, were found by *in silico* modeling screening of an National Cancer Institute (NCI) library of small-molecule compounds in a panel of 60 cancer cell lines carrying p53 mutations, and were reported to selectively kill cancer cells while not affecting normal cells.[73] After compound validation, NSC319726 had the best and most specific killing effects on cancer cells, changing the conformation of p53 and restoring wild-type function of p53R175 mutant. The compound killed R172Hp53 knock-in mice, caused apoptosis, and activated p21 (p53 target) in mice xenograft tumors in a 175-allele–specific mutant p53–dependent manner.[73] The activity of the compound was dependent on the zinc-chelating properties as well as redox changes. It was concluded that the *in silico* method on a panel of cancer cell lines promises to be a future strategy in searching for p53-reactivating compounds.

Wild-Type p53–Targeted Therapy

The small-molecule compounds were described to mostly target the p53 and Mdm-2 interaction, and are described herein (see **Fig. 3**). Also described are the FAK-p53 pathway small-molecule inhibitors developed by the authors, along with analysis of the structural data of these complexes and the small molecules targeting these complexes.

p53 and Mdm-2 interaction

The p53–Mdm-2 complex does not involve large protein areas, as many protein-protein interactions make it suitable for the development of targeted drug therapy. Of the 6 p53 amino acids from the p53 N-terminal transactivation domain, [18]TFSDLW[23] specifically binds to the pocket in the Mdm-2 protein.[74] The cocrystallization of p53 peptide and Mdm-2 protein identified the 109-amino-acid region of the amino-terminal domain of Mdm-2 bound to p53 peptide and detected that Phe19, Trp23, and Leu26 were deeply inserted inside the hydrophobic Mdm-2 cleft.[75] Two hybrid genetic analyses identified amino acids of Mdm-2 involved in interaction with p53, and included G58, D68, V75, and C77 amino acids of the N-terminal domain of Mdm-2.[76] A later study identified additional sites in the N-terminal transactivation domain of p53, residues 40 to 45 and residues 49 to 54, which are involved in binding with Mdm-2.[77] This binding is weaker than at the main site of p53–Mdm-2 interaction, but can provide additional approaches to drug development. The first drugs developed to target p53-Mdm-2 interaction were peptides, which were superseded by small-molecule compounds, owing to their higher stability, bioavailability, and other pharmacologic and pharmacokinetic properties (see later discussion).

Sulfonamide (2004) Sulfonamide I was identified by computational screening using a 3-dimensional pharmacophore model and small molecules from the National Center for Biotechnology Information database, and this compound effectively inhibited p53–Mdm-2 interaction and activated p53.[78] In the binding assay IC_{50} was 32 µM, which was higher than that of p53 peptide, which caused 100% inhibition of p53–Mdm-2 binding at 100 µM. The functional efficacy was demonstrated in a reporter luciferase assay, whereby sulfonamide increased p53-transcriptional activity in Mdm-2-overexpressing cell line.

Nutlins (2004) The small-molecule drugs that target p53 and Mdm-2 interaction were developed by La Roche in Nutley, New Jersey and were named Nutlins. These compounds bind Mdm-2 in the p53-binding pocket with a nanomolar range of binding affinity. The first 3 compounds, Nutlin-1, -2, and -3, share a common structure.[79,80] The binding of Nutlin with Mdm-2 was confirmed by cocrystallization studies. The compounds activated the p53 pathway in cancer cells, activated the p21 target, caused apoptosis, and led to inhibition of tumor xenograft growth. The Nutlin-3 antitumor activity was shown in different types of cancer, including acute myeloid leukemia, neuroblastoma, osteosarcoma, and prostate cancer.[81–85] The effect of Nutlins was p53 dependent. An oral Nutlin-3 entered clinical trials recently for the treatment of patients with solid tumors and hematologic cancers.

RITA (2004) RITA (Reactivation of p53 and Induction of Tumor Apoptosis) was identified by screening a chemical library from the NCI set of compounds.[86] RITA inhibited growth of colon cancer cell HCT116 more efficiently than p53−/− cells and caused a p53-dependent decrease of xenograft tumor growth *in vivo*. RITA prevented interaction of p53 and Mdm-2 *in vitro*, owing to p53 conformational change.[86] RITA reactivated p53 and induced apoptosis in multiple myeloma cancer and leukemia cells.[87,88] RITA synergized with Nutlin to induce apoptosis in melanoma.[89] RITA reactivated p53 and also activated the JNK-1 pathway in multiple myeloma cancer cells.[90] RITA caused a decrease of cervical carcinoma xenograft growth *in vivo*, associated with reactivation with p53 transcriptional targets: Bax, Noxa-1, and PUMA-1.[91]

Terphenyl 14 (2005) The computational screening of a small terphenyl library identified terphenyl 14, which was able to bind to the hydrophobic groove of Mdm-2 protein, to mimic the α-helical region of p53, and to disrupt p53–Mdm-2 protein interaction.[92]

Benzodiazepinediones (2005) High-throughput screening of chemical libraries using the assay that detected the effect of compounds on protein stability identified the benzodiazepinedione family of compounds, and the lead compound I stabilized p53 and induced p21 expression.[93] The optimization of compound I resulted in TDP521252 and TD665759, which both inhibited Mdm-2.[94] TDP521252 and TDP665759 inhibited the proliferation of wild-type p53 cell lines with an IC_{48} of 14 and 0.7 µM, respectively, and disrupted the complex of Mdm-2 and p53.[94] Administration of TD665759 to mice increased p21 in liver samples. The compound synergized with doxorubicin in an A375 xenograft model, and decreased tumor growth.[94]

Quinolinole (NSC66811) (2006) The computational screening of small molecules identified 354 Mdm-2 potential candidates to disrupt interaction with p53. The binding assay demonstrated that quinolinole (7-[anilino(phenyl)methyl]-2-methyl-8-quinolinol) (NSC66811) is the best to inhibit Mdm-2 in nanomolar concentrations, with a K_i (120 nM), was lower than that of p53 peptide.[95] The compound mimicked 3 amino acids of p53 that were involved in interaction with Mdm-2, and disrupted interaction with Mdm-2.

MI (2006) The MI compounds were generated by the University of Michigan and Ascenta, and belong to the family of potent tryptophan-based inhibitors, which bind to Mdm-2 with high affinity, mimicking the binding of Trp23 from the p53 peptide, and disrupt the interaction of Mdm-2 with p53. At first oxindole was found to mimic the interaction of Trp23. The subsequent chemical modifications and optimizations resulted in a series of MI compounds.[96] One of the most potent inhibitors was MI-63, with a K_i of 3 nM, IC_{50} of 280 nM, and induced p53 and p21 expression.[96] The MI-43 was designed to target 4 amino acids of p53 peptide: Phe19, Trp23, Leu22, and Leu26.[97] MI-43 inhibited cell growth and survival of colon cancer cells with wild-type p53.[97] The MI-43 compound induced cell-cycle arrest that required p53 and p21. The optimization of MI-63 resulted in MI-219, inhibiting tumor growth *in vivo*.[97] The next derivative of MI-219 was MI-319, which demonstrated efficient tumor growth suppression of lymphoma cells.[98] MI-319 synergized with cisplatin and decreased cell growth in pancreatic cancer.[99]

Isoindolinones (2006) Isoindolinones were identified as scaffold Mdm-2 inhibitors, blocking the pocket of interaction with p53.[100] The IC_{50} values of these inhibitors are 5 to 16 μM in growth inhibition assays and reporter assays, and they inhibit the binding of Mdm-2 to p53. The most potent inhibitor was (+)-*R*-3-(4-chlorophenyl)-3-(1-hydroxymethylcyclopropylmethoxy)-2-(4-nitrobenzyl)-2,3-dihydroisoindol-1-one or isoindolinone compound 74a, which effectively disrupted interaction of Mdm-2 and p53 and activated p53, p21, and Mdm-2 transcription.[101] The IC_{50} of 74a was 170 nM, versus 61 nM of Nutlin, in an Mdm-2 binding assay, and was similar in viability assays.[101] The cellular activity of 74a was p53 dependent.

FOCAL ADHESION KINASE AS A THERAPEUTIC TARGET
FAK Inhibition with Antisense Oligonucleotides, siRNA, and Dominant-Negative FAK

Recently, FAK has been proposed as a new therapeutic target.[102] Several *in vitro* approaches were used to downregulate FAK, such as adenoviral FAK-CD (dominant-negative FAK),[103] antisense oligonucleotides,[104] and siRNA for FAK.[105] The authors[106] linked FAK expression to apoptosis by treating FAK-positive tumor cell lines with different antisense oligonucleotides to FAK that specifically inhibited p125 FAK expression. The cells treated with antisense oligonucleotides lost their attachment and underwent apoptosis.[106] The authors[105] also analyzed the FAK siRNA effect on tumor growth, and found that silencing of FAK expression significantly decreased tumor growth in an MCF-7 xenograft model. FAK siRNA directly affected important genes involved in survival/apoptotic, cell cycle pathways.[105]

Small-Molecule Inhibitors Targeting FAK Functions

Small molecules targeting FAK adenosine triphosphate–binding site
Several pharmaceutical companies such as Novartis, Pfizer, and Glaxo developed several FAK inhibitors that targeted the adenosine triphosphate (ATP)-binding site of FAK. The Novartis inhibitor, TAE-226, did not enter clinical trials owing to its toxicity and nonspecifity. Of the Pfizer inhibitors, PF-573,228 did not enter clinical study[107] and PF-562271 did enter clinical study phase I, but has been reported to inhibit FAK homologue Pyk-1[108]; another Pfizer inhibitor, PF-04554878, was also entered the first clinical studies. Another group from Poniard developed a PND-1186 FAK inhibitor that also had nonspecific effects by inhibiting different proteins at 1 μM, such as Aurora, Flt-3, Lck1, and others.[109] Thus, these FAK inhibitors targeting the FAK ATP were nonspecific because of the highly conservative nature of kinase domains with the ATP-binding site that limited their clinical use.

Allosteric FAK inhibitors

Another approach to FAK inhibition involves the allosteric FAK inhibitors that target the FAK kinase–dependent and kinase-independent (scaffolding) functions of FAK. The inhibitors targeting kinase function but not the active ATP-binding site (K454) were named allosteric inhibitors, and targeted other sites of FAK phosphorylation such as the main Y397 autophosphorylation site. Small-molecule drugs were found through computer modeling and database screening using 3-dimensional target protein crystal structures and libraries of small-molecule compounds. By using computer modeling and screening of more than 200,000 small molecules from the NCI database and docking compounds into the structural functional pockets of FAK, the authors found 40 different potential FAK inhibitors. Using this method, a FAK inhibitor targeting the Y397 site of FAK was identified,[110] called Y15 or FAK inhibitor 14, which blocked breast,[110] pancreatic,[111] and neuroblastoma tumor growth.[112] The Y15 inhibitor also had antitumor activity in glioblastoma[113] and colon cancer xenograft models.[114] The similar allosteric FAK inhibitor, named Y11, also targeted the Y397 FAK site and inhibited growth of colon cancer tumors.[115]

Small-Molecule Inhibitors Targeting FAK-Scaffolding Function

One of the approaches to inhibit FAK kinase–independent scaffolding function was targeting its protein-protein interaction with its binding partners, such VEGFR-3 or other p53 and Mdm-2. One of the lead FAK inhibitors, the FAK inhibitor C4, targeted the FAK–VEGFR-3 interaction and inhibited tumor growth in different types of tumor xenografts.[116]

Small-molecule drug inhibitors are effectively used to target p53 protein-protein interactions, particularly with Mdm-2 protein.[117] The first potent inhibitors targeting p53–Mdm-2 interaction have been identified by high-throughput screening followed by structure-based optimization.[117] The screening identified Nutlins, which represent a class of *cis*-imidazole analogues that bind to the p53 pocket interacting with Mdm-2. The same strategy was used to target interaction with Mdm-2 and FAK (M drugs)[118] and p53 and FAK (Roslin drugs or R drugs).[119] The authors also found the lead FAK and Mdm-2 targeting compound, M13, which reactivated p53 and inhibited tumor growth.[118] In addition, the authors developed FAK-p53 targeting compounds (R drugs) (see **Fig. 3**) that reactivated p53 and its transcriptional targets in p53+/+ HCT116 colon cancer cells but not in p53−/− cells.[119] These drugs reactivated p53 transcription *in vitro* and *in vivo*, and effectively decreased viability, clonogenicity, and tumor growth.

PERSPECTIVES

Understanding FAK biology during tumorigenesis, the mechanisms of its upregulation in different tumors, its role in stem-cell biology, angiogenesis, and motility, and, especially, the mechanisms of its direct physical interaction with p53 protein and their downstream signaling pathways, will be critical in developing targeted therapeutics. Studies with peptide inhibitors already have indicated that the blockade of specific protein-protein interactions has therapeutic promise for treating a variety of diseases, including cancer.[120–123] Small-molecule drugs are particularly attractive as inhibitors of intracellular protein-protein interactions because of their ability to modify their structures to achieve optimal target binding. As the mechanisms of FAK signaling in cancer cells are further defined, the optimal sites for targeting this protein and disrupting its signaling to cause apoptosis in human tumors will be identified. Thus, targeting of the FAK and p53 interaction, as well as other binding partners, can be important therapeutic targets in cancer treatment programs.[124]

The review of Levine and Oren,[11] summarizing the first 30 years of p53 research, proposed that the next decade of research will bring novel and important p53-targeted therapies. The authors hope that the approaches to p53 therapy discussed in this review will create new ideas and help in developing novel therapies targeting p53 signaling pathways in cancer cells.

REFERENCES

1. Levine AJ. p53, the cellular gatekeeper for growth and division. Cell 1997;88: 323–31.
2. Farmer G, Bargonetti J, Zhu H, et al. Wild-type p53 activates transcription in vitro. Nature 1992;358:83–6.
3. Golubovskaya VM, Cance WG. Focal adhesion kinase and p53 signaling in cancer cells. Int Rev Cytol 2007;263:103–53.
4. Bouchet BP, de Fromentel CC, Puisieux A, et al. p53 as a target for anti-cancer drug development. Crit Rev Oncol Hematol 2006;58:190–207.
5. Khoury MP, Bourdon JC. The isoforms of the p53 protein. Cold Spring Harb Perspect Biol 2010;2:a000927.
6. Lacroix M, Toillon RA, Leclercq G. p53 and breast cancer, an update. Endocr Relat Cancer 2006;13:293–325.
7. Yu H, Chen JK, Feng S, et al. Structural basis for the binding of proline-rich peptides to SH3 domains. Cell 1994;76:933–45.
8. Edwards SJ, Hananeia L, Eccles MR, et al. The proline-rich region of mouse p53 influences transactivation and apoptosis but is largely dispensable for these functions. Oncogene 2003;22:4517–23.
9. Bergamaschi D, Gasco M, Hiller L, et al. p53 polymorphism influences response in cancer chemotherapy via modulation of p73-dependent apoptosis. Cancer Cell 2003;3:387–402.
10. Stoklsa T, Golab J. Prospects for p53-based cancer therapy. Acta Biochim Pol 2005;52:321–8.
11. Levine AJ, Oren M. The first 30 years of p53: growing ever more complex. Nat Rev Cancer 2009;9:749–58.
12. Baker SJ, Preisinger AC, Jessup JM, et al. p53 gene mutations occur in combination with 17p allelic deletions as late events in colorectal tumorigenesis. Cancer Res 1990;50:7717–22.
13. Fearon ER, Vogelstein B. A genetic model for colorectal tumorigenesis. Cell 1990;61:759–67.
14. Giaccia AJ, Kastan MB. The complexity of p53 modulation: emerging patterns from divergent signals. Genes Dev 1998;12:2973–83.
15. Hoffman WH, Biade S, Zilfou JT, et al. Transcriptional repression of the anti-apoptotic survivin gene by wild type p53. J Biol Chem 2002;277: 3247–57.
16. Wu Y, Mehew JW, Heckman CA, et al. Negative regulation of bcl-2 expression by p53 in hematopoietic cells. Oncogene 2001;20:240–51.
17. Taylor WR, Stark GR. Regulation of the G2/M transition by p53. Oncogene 2001; 20:1803–15.
18. Krause K, Wasner M, Reinhard W, et al. The tumour suppressor protein p53 can repress transcription of cyclin B. Nucleic Acids Res 2000;28: 4410–8.

19. Johnsen JI, Aurelio ON, Kwaja Z, et al. p53-mediated negative regulation of stathmin/Op18 expression is associated with G(2)/M cell-cycle arrest. Int J Cancer 2000;88:685–91.

20. Murphy M, Hinman A, Levine AJ. Wild-type p53 negatively regulates the expression of a microtubule-associated protein. Genes Dev 1996;10:2971–80.

21. Yonish-Rouach E, Resnitzky D, Lotem J, et al. Wild-type p53 induces apoptosis of myeloid leukaemic cells that is inhibited by interleukin-6. Nature 1991;352:345–7.

22. Oren M. Decision making by p53: life, death and cancer. Cell Death Differ 2003;10:431–42.

23. Lowe SW, Ruley HE, Jacks T, et al. p53-dependent apoptosis modulates the cytotoxicity of anticancer agents. Cell 1993;74:957–67.

24. Lowe SW, Jacks T, Housman DE, et al. Abrogation of oncogene-associated apoptosis allows transformation of p53-deficient cells. Proc Natl Acad Sci U S A 1994;91:2026–30.

25. Fridman JS, Lowe SW. Control of apoptosis by p53. Oncogene 2003;22:9030–40.

26. Owens LV, Xu L, Craven RJ, et al. Overexpression of the focal adhesion kinase (p125FAK) in invasive human tumors. Cancer Res 1995;55:2752–5.

27. Cance WG, Golubovskaya VM. Focal adhesion kinase versus p53: apoptosis or survival? Sci Signal 2008;1:pe22.

28. Cance WG, Harris JE, Iacocca MV, et al. Immunohistochemical analyses of focal adhesion kinase expression in benign and malignant human breast and colon tissues: correlation with preinvasive and invasive phenotypes. Clin Cancer Res 2000;6:2417–23.

29. Owens LV, Xu L, Dent GA, et al. Focal adhesion kinase as a marker of invasive potential in differentiated human thyroid cancer. Ann Surg Oncol 1996;3:100–5.

30. Golubovskaya VM. Targeting focal adhesion kinase in cancer—part I. Anticancer Agents Med Chem 2010;10:713.

31. Ilic D, Almeida EA, Schlaepfer DD, et al. Extracellular matrix survival signals transduced by focal adhesion kinase suppress p53-mediated apoptosis. J Cell Biol 1998;143:547–60.

32. Zhang Y, Lu H, Dazin P, et al. Squamous cell carcinoma cell aggregates escape suspension-induced, p53-mediated anoikis: Fibronectin and integrin {alpha} mediate survival signals through focal adhesion kinase. J Biol Chem 2004;279:48342–9.

33. Livasy CA, Moore D, Cance WG, et al. Focal adhesion kinase overexpression in endometrial neoplasia. Appl Immunohistochem Mol Morphol 2004;12:342–5.

34. Golubovskaya V, Kaur A, Cance W. Cloning and characterization of the promoter region of human focal adhesion kinase gene: nuclear factor kappa B and p53 binding sites. Biochim Biophys Acta 2004;1678:111–25.

35. Wei CL, Wu Q, Vega VB, et al. A global map of p53 transcription-factor binding sites in the human genome. Cell 2006;124:207–19.

36. Golubovskaya VM, Conway-Dorsey K, Edmiston SN, et al. FAK overexpression and p53 mutations are highly correlated in human breast cancer. Int J Cancer 2009;125:1735–8.

37. Rosado P, Lequerica-Fernandez P, Pena I, et al. In oral squamous cell carcinoma, high FAK expression is correlated with low P53 expression. Virchows Arch 2012;461:163–8.

38. Golubovskaya VM, Finch R, Cance WG. Direct Interaction of the N-terminal domain of focal adhesion kinase with the N-terminal transactivation domain of p53. J Biol Chem 2005;280:25008–21.

39. Stewart A, Ham C, Zachary I. The focal adhesion kinase amino-terminal domain localises to nuclei and intercellular junctions in HEK 293 and MDCK cells independently of tyrosine 397 and the carboxy-terminal domain. Biochem Biophys Res Commun 2002;299:62–73.

40. Beviglia L, Golubovskaya V, Xu L, et al. Focal adhesion kinase N-terminus in breast carcinoma cells induces rounding, detachment and apoptosis. Biochem J 2003;373:201–10.

41. Jones G, Stewart G. Nuclear import of N-terminal FAK by activation of the FcepsilonRI receptor in RBL-2H3 cells. Biochem Biophys Res Commun 2004;314: 39–45.

42. Lobo M, Zachary I. Nuclear localization and apoptotic regulation of an amino-terminal domain focal adhesion kinase fragment in endothelial cells. Biochem Biophys Res Commun 2000;276:1068–74.

43. Chipuk JE, Green DR. Cytoplasmic p53: bax and forward. Cell Cycle 2004;3: 429–31.

44. Golubovskaya VM, Finch R, Zheng M, et al. The 7-amino-acid site in the proline-rich region of the N-terminal domain of p53 is involved in the interaction with FAK and is critical for p53 functioning. Biochem J 2008;411:151–60.

45. Golubovskaya VM, Cance W. Focal adhesion kinase and p53 signal transduction pathways in cancer. Front Biosci 2010;15:901–12.

46. Lim ST, Chen XL, Lim Y, et al. Nuclear FAK promotes cell proliferation and survival through FERM-enhanced p53 degradation. Mol Cell 2008;29:9–22.

47. Melkoumian ZK, Peng X, Gan B, et al. Mechanism of cell cycle regulation by FIP200 in human breast cancer cells. Cancer Res 2005;65:6676–84.

48. Mitra SK, Schlaepfer DD. Integrin-regulated FAK-Src signaling in normal and cancer cells. Curr Opin Cell Biol 2006;18:516–23.

49. Ho B, Olson G, Figel S, et al. Nanog increases Focal Adhesion Kinase (FAK) promoter activity and expression and directly binds to FAK protein to be phosphorylated. J Biol Chem 2012;287:18656–73.

50. Lin T, Chao C, Saito S, et al. p53 induces differentiation of mouse embryonic stem cells by suppressing Nanog expression. Nat Cell Biol 2005;7: 165–71.

51. Essmann F, Schulze-Osthoff K. Translational approaches targeting the p53 pathway for anti-cancer therapy. Br J Pharmacol 2012;165:328–44.

52. Shi J, Zheng D. An update on gene therapy in China. Curr Opin Mol Ther 2009; 11:547–53.

53. Yang ZX, Wang D, Wang G, et al. Clinical study of recombinant adenovirus-p53 combined with fractionated stereotactic radiotherapy for hepatocellular carcinoma. J Cancer Res Clin Oncol 2010;136:625–30.

54. Shi LM, Myers TG, Fan Y, et al. Mining the National Cancer Institute Anticancer Drug Discovery Database: cluster analysis of ellipticine analogs with p53-inverse and central nervous system-selective patterns of activity. Mol Pharmacol 1998;53:241–51.

55. Sugikawa E, Hosoi T, Yazaki N, et al. Mutant p53 mediated induction of cell cycle arrest and apoptosis at G1 phase by 9-hydroxyellipticine. Anticancer Res 1999; 19:3099–108.

56. Foster BA, Coffey HA, Morin MJ, et al. Pharmacological rescue of mutant p53 conformation and function. Science 1999;286:2507–10.

57. Wang W, Takimoto R, Rastinejad F, et al. Stabilization of p53 by CP-31398 inhibits ubiquitination without altering phosphorylation at serine 15 or 20 or MDM2 binding. Mol Cell Biol 2003;23:2171–81.

58. Takimoto R, Wang W, Dicker DT, et al. The mutant p53-conformation modifying drug, CP-31398, can induce apoptosis of human cancer cells and can stabilize wild-type p53 protein. Cancer Biol Ther 2002;1:47–55.

59. Rippin TM, Bykov VJ, Freund SM, et al. Characterization of the p53-rescue drug CP-31398 in vitro and in living cells. Oncogene 2002;21:2119–29.

60. Rippin TM, Freund SM, Veprintsev DB, et al. Recognition of DNA by p53 core domain and location of intermolecular contacts of cooperative binding. J Mol Biol 2002;319:351–8.

61. Demma MJ, Wong S, Maxwell E, et al. CP-31398 restores DNA-binding activity to mutant p53 in vitro but does not affect p53 homologs p63 and p73. J Biol Chem 2004;279:45887–96.

62. Tang X, Zhu Y, Han L, et al. CP-31398 restores mutant p53 tumor suppressor function and inhibits UVB-induced skin carcinogenesis in mice. J Clin Invest 2007;117:3753–64.

63. El-Deiry WS. Targeting mutant p53 shows promise for sunscreens and skin cancer. J Clin Invest 2007;117:3658–60.

64. Rao CV, Swamy MV, Patlolla JM, et al. Suppression of familial adenomatous polyposis by CP-31398, a TP53 modulator, in APCmin/+ mice. Cancer Res 2008;68:7670–5.

65. Rao CV, Steele VE, Swamy MV, et al. Inhibition of azoxymethane-induced colorectal cancer by CP-31398, a TP53 modulator, alone or in combination with low doses of celecoxib in male F344 rats. Cancer Res 2009;69:8175–82.

66. Bykov VJ, Issaeva N, Selivanova G, et al. Mutant p53-dependent growth suppression distinguishes PRIMA-1 from known anticancer drugs: a statistical analysis of information in the National Cancer Institute database. Carcinogenesis 2002;23:2011–8.

67. Bykov VJ, Zache N, Stridh H, et al. PRIMA-1(MET) synergizes with cisplatin to induce tumor cell apoptosis. Oncogene 2005;24:3484–91.

68. Zache N, Lambert JM, Wiman KG, et al. PRIMA-1MET inhibits growth of mouse tumors carrying mutant p53. Cell Oncol 2008;30:411–8.

69. Demma M, Maxwell E, Ramos R, et al. SCH529074, a small molecule activator of mutant p53, which binds p53 DNA binding domain (DBD), restores growth-suppressive function to mutant p53 and interrupts HDM2-mediated ubiquitination of wild type p53. J Biol Chem 2010;285:10198–212.

70. Bykov VJ, Issaeva N, Zache N, et al. Reactivation of mutant p53 and induction of apoptosis in human tumor cells by maleimide analogs. J Biol Chem 2005;280:30384–91.

71. Zache N, Lambert JM, Rokaeus N, et al. Mutant p53 targeting by the low molecular weight compound STIMA-1. Mol Oncol 2008;2:70–80.

72. Kravchenko JE, Ilyinskaya GV, Komarov PG, et al. Small-molecule RETRA suppresses mutant p53-bearing cancer cells through a p73-dependent salvage pathway. Proc Natl Acad Sci U S A 2008;105:6302–7.

73. Yu X, Vazquez A, Levine AJ, et al. Allele-specific p53 mutant reactivation. Cancer Cell 2012;21:614–25.

74. Picksley SM, Vojtesek B, Sparks A, et al. Immunochemical analysis of the interaction of p53 with MDM2; fine mapping of the MDM2 binding site on p53 using synthetic peptides. Oncogene 1994;9:2523–9.

75. Kussie PH, Gorina S, Marechal V, et al. Structure of the MDM2 oncoprotein bound to the p53 tumor suppressor transactivation domain. Science 1996;274:948–53.

76. Freedman DA, Epstein CB, Roth JC, et al. A genetic approach to mapping the p53 binding site in the MDM2 protein. Mol Med 1997;3:248–59.

77. Chi SW, Lee SH, Kim DH, et al. Structural details on mdm2-p53 interaction. J Biol Chem 2005;280:38795–802.
78. Galatin PS, Abraham DJ. A nonpeptidic sulfonamide inhibits the p53-mdm2 interaction and activates p53-dependent transcription in mdm2-overexpressing cells. J Med Chem 2004;47:4163–5.
79. Vassilev LT, Vu BT, Graves B, et al. In vivo activation of the p53 pathway by small-molecule antagonists of MDM2. Science 2004;303:844–8.
80. Vassilev LT. Small-molecule antagonists of p53-MDM2 binding: research tools and potential therapeutics. Cell Cycle 2004;3:419–21.
81. Tovar C, Rosinski J, Filipovic Z, et al. Small-molecule MDM2 antagonists reveal aberrant p53 signaling in cancer: implications for therapy. Proc Natl Acad Sci U S A 2006;103:1888–93.
82. Tovar C, Higgins B, Kolinsky K, et al. MDM2 antagonists boost antitumor effect of androgen withdrawal: implications for therapy of prostate cancer. Mol Cancer 2011;10:49.
83. Barbarotto E, Corallini F, Rimondi E, et al. Differential effects of chemotherapeutic drugs versus the MDM-2 antagonist nutlin-3 on cell cycle progression and induction of apoptosis in SKW6.4 lymphoblastoid B-cells. J Cell Biochem 2008;104:595–605.
84. Secchiero P, Zerbinati C, Melloni E, et al. The MDM-2 antagonist nutlin-3 promotes the maturation of acute myeloid leukemic blasts. Neoplasia 2007;9: 853–61.
85. Van Maerken T, Ferdinande L, Taildeman J, et al. Antitumor activity of the selective MDM2 antagonist nutlin-3 against chemoresistant neuroblastoma with wild-type p53. J Natl Cancer Inst 2009;101:1562–74.
86. Issaeva N, Bozko P, Enge M, et al. Small molecule RITA binds to p53, blocks p53-HDM-2 interaction and activates p53 function in tumors. Nat Med 2004; 10:1321–8.
87. Saha MN, Jiang H, Mukai A, et al. RITA inhibits multiple myeloma cell growth through induction of p53-mediated caspase-dependent apoptosis and synergistically enhances nutlin-induced cytotoxic responses. Mol Cancer Ther 2010;9:3041–51.
88. Kazemi A, Safa M, Shahbazi A. RITA enhances chemosensivity of pre-B ALL cells to doxorubicin by inducing p53-dependent apoptosis. Hematology 2011; 16:225–31.
89. de Lange J, Ly LV, Lodder K, et al. Synergistic growth inhibition based on small-molecule p53 activation as treatment for intraocular melanoma. Oncogene 2012;31:1105–16.
90. Saha MN, Jiang H, Yang Y, et al. Targeting p53 via JNK pathway: a novel role of RITA for apoptotic signaling in multiple myeloma. PLoS One 2012;7:e30215.
91. Zhao CY, Szekely L, Bao W, et al. Rescue of p53 function by small-molecule RITA in cervical carcinoma by blocking E6-mediated degradation. Cancer Res 2010;70:3372–81.
92. Yin H, Lee GI, Park HS, et al. Terphenyl-based helical mimetics that disrupt the p53/HDM2 interaction. Angew Chem Int Ed Engl 2005;44:2704–7.
93. Grasberger BL, Lu T, Schubert C, et al. Discovery and cocrystal structure of benzodiazepinedione HDM2 antagonists that activate p53 in cells. J Med Chem 2005;48:909–12.
94. Koblish HK, Zhao S, Franks CF, et al. Benzodiazepinedione inhibitors of the Hdm2:p53 complex suppress human tumor cell proliferation in vitro and sensitize tumors to doxorubicin in vivo. Mol Cancer Ther 2006;5:160–9.

95. Lu Y, Nikolovska-Coleska Z, Fang X, et al. Discovery of a nanomolar inhibitor of the human murine double minute 2 (MDM2)-p53 interaction through an integrated, virtual database screening strategy. J Med Chem 2006;49:3759–62.

96. Ding K, Lu Y, Nikolovska-Coleska Z, et al. Structure-based design of spiro-oxindoles as potent, specific small-molecule inhibitors of the MDM2-p53 interaction. J Med Chem 2006;49:3432–5.

97. Shangary S, Ding K, Qiu S, et al. Reactivation of p53 by a specific MDM2 antagonist (MI-43) leads to p21-mediated cell cycle arrest and selective cell death in colon cancer. Mol Cancer Ther 2008;7:1533–42.

98. Mohammad RM, Wu J, Azmi AS, et al. An MDM2 antagonist (MI-319) restores p53 functions and increases the life span of orally treated follicular lymphoma bearing animals. Mol Cancer 2009;8:115.

99. Azmi AS, Aboukameel A, Banerjee S, et al. MDM2 inhibitor MI-319 in combination with cisplatin is an effective treatment for pancreatic cancer independent of p53 function. Eur J Cancer 2010;46:1122–31.

100. Hardcastle IR, Ahmed SU, Atkins H, et al. Small-molecule inhibitors of the MDM2-p53 protein-protein interaction based on an isoindolinone scaffold. J Med Chem 2006;49:6209–21.

101. Hardcastle IR, Liu J, Valeur E, et al. Isoindolinone inhibitors of the murine double minute 2 (MDM2)-p53 protein-protein interaction: structure-activity studies leading to improved potency. J Med Chem 2011;54:1233–43.

102. McLean GW, Carragher NO, Avizienyte E, et al. The role of focal-adhesion kinase in cancer—a new therapeutic opportunity. Nat Rev Cancer 2005;5: 505–15.

103. Xu LH, Yang X, Craven RJ, et al. The COOH-terminal domain of the focal adhesion kinase induces loss of adhesion and cell death in human tumor cells. Cell Growth Differ 1998;9:999–1005.

104. Smith CS, Golubovskaya VM, Peck E, et al. Effect of focal adhesion kinase (FAK) downregulation with FAK antisense oligonucleotides and 5-fluorouracil on the viability of melanoma cell lines. Melanoma Res 2005;15:357–62.

105. Golubovskaya VM, Zheng M, Zhang L, et al. The direct effect of focal adhesion kinase (FAK), dominant-negative FAK, FAK-CD and FAK siRNA on gene expression and human MCF-7 breast cancer cell tumorigenesis. BMC Cancer 2009;9: 280.

106. Xu LH, Owens LV, Sturge GC, et al. Attenuation of the expression of the focal adhesion kinase induces apoptosis in tumor cells. Cell Growth Differ 1996;7: 413–8.

107. Slack-Davis JK, Martin KH, Tilghman RW, et al. Cellular characterization of a novel focal adhesion kinase inhibitor. J Biol Chem 2007;282:14845–52.

108. Roberts WG, Ung E, Whalen P, et al. Antitumor activity and pharmacology of a selective focal adhesion kinase inhibitor, PF-562,271. Cancer Res 2008;68: 1935–44.

109. Tanjoni I, Walsh C, Uryu S, et al. PND-1186 FAK inhibitor selectively promotes tumor cell apoptosis in three-dimensional environments. Cancer Biol Ther 2010;9:764–77.

110. Golubovskaya VM, Nyberg C, Zheng M, et al. A small molecule inhibitor, 1,2,4,5-benzenetetraamine tetrahydrochloride, targeting the y397 site of focal adhesion kinase decreases tumor growth. J Med Chem 2008;51:7405–16.

111. Hochwald SN, Nyberg C, Zheng M, et al. A novel small molecule inhibitor of FAK decreases growth of human pancreatic cancer. Cell Cycle 2009;8: 2435–43.

112. Beierle EA, Ma X, Stewart J, et al. Inhibition of focal adhesion kinase decreases tumor growth in human neuroblastoma. Cell Cycle 2010;9:1005–15.

113. Golubovskaya VM, Huang G, Ho B, et al. Pharmacologic blockade of FAK auto-phosphorylation decreases human glioblastoma tumor growth and synergizes with temozolomide. Mol Cancer Ther 2013;12:162–72.

114. Heffler M, Golubovskaya VM, Dunn KM, et al. Focal Adhesion kinase autophos-phorylation inhibition decreases colon cancer cell growth and enhances the efficacy of chemotherapy. Cancer Biol Ther 2013. [Epub ahead of print].

115. Golubovskaya VM, Figel S, Ho BT, et al. A small molecule focal adhesion kinase (FAK) inhibitor, targeting Y397 site: 1-(2-hydroxyethyl)-3, 5, 7-triaza-1-azoniatri-cyclo [3.3.1.1(3,7)]decane; bromide effectively inhibits FAK autophosphoryla-tion activity and decreases cancer cell viability, clonogenicity and tumor growth in vivo. Carcinogenesis 2012;33:1004–13.

116. Kurenova EV, Hunt DL, He D, et al. Small molecule chloropyramine hydrochlo-ride (C4) targets the binding site of focal adhesion kinase and vascular endothe-lial growth factor receptor 3 and suppresses breast cancer growth in vivo. J Med Chem 2009;52:4716–24.

117. Vassilev LT. p53 Activation by small molecules: application in oncology. J Med Chem 2005;48:4491–9.

118. Golubovskaya V, Palma NL, Zheng M, et al. A small-molecule inhibitor, 5′-o-tritylthymidine, targets FAK And Mdm-2 interaction, and blocks breast and colon tumorigenesis in vivo. Anticancer Agents Med Chem 2013;13:532–45.

119. Golubovskaya VM, Ho B, Zheng M, et al. Disruption of focal adhesion kinase and p53 interaction with small molecule compound R2 reactivated p53 and blocked tumor growth. BMC Cancer 2013;13(1):342.

120. Akhter SA, Luttrell LM, Rockman HA, et al. Targeting the receptor-Gq interface to inhibit in vivo pressure overload myocardial hypertrophy. Science 1998;280: 574–7.

121. Aramburu J, Yaffe MB, Lopez-Rodriguez C, et al. Affinity-driven peptide selec-tion of an NFAT inhibitor more selective than cyclosporin A. Science 1999;285: 2129–33.

122. May MJ, D'Acquisto F, Madge LA, et al. Selective inhibition of NF-kappaB acti-vation by a peptide that blocks the interaction of NEMO with the IkappaB kinase complex. Science 2000;289:1550–4.

123. van Rooij E, Doevendans PA, de Theije CC, et al. Requirement of nuclear factor of activated T-cells in calcineurin-mediated cardiomyocyte hypertrophy. J Biol Chem 2002;277:48617–26.

124. Cance WG, Kurenova E, Marlowe T, et al. Disrupting the scaffold to improve focal adhesion kinase-targeting therapeutics. Sci Signaling 2013;6:pe10.

Cancer Immunotherapy
Current Status and Future Directions

Fumito Ito, MD, PhD[a], Alfred E. Chang, MD[b],*

KEYWORDS

- Cancer immunotherapy • Cancer vaccine • Immune-modulating antibodies
- Immune checkpoints • Adoptive cell therapy

KEY POINTS

- Despite recognition of durable therapeutic responses in some patients with cancer historically, immunotherapeutic agents have provided limited evidence of clinical success until recently.
- Recent discoveries by which tumors evade immune T-cell recognition have led to a variety of clinically effective cancer immunotherapies.
- Understanding the pivotal role of the tumor microenvironment in suppressing antitumor immunity and the exploration of combinatorial treatment regimens will further enhance the efficacy of cancer immunotherapies.

HISTORY OF CANCER IMMUNOTHERAPY

The first systematic study of immunotherapy for the treatment of malignant tumors was conducted by a New York bone sarcoma surgeon, William B. Coley (1862–1936), whose line of clinical research began in the 1890s. Coley's interest in immunotherapy stemmed from the loss of a young patient with a soft tissue sarcoma of the arm, who developed metastatic disease and died shortly after Coley's radical excision of the tumor. Coley investigated the medical records of the hospital and found a patient with a four-time recurrent inoperable sarcoma of the neck, which regressed after a postoperative infection of erysipelas (a superficial, streptococcal infection of the skin).[1] This incident stimulated Coley's clinical research, and he started to infect patients with cancer with various bacterial isolates. He developed "Coley's toxin," the combination of heat-killed *Streptococcus pyogenes* and *Serratia marcescens*.[2] He started intratumoral injections of Coley's toxin in 1891, and treated hundreds of

Conflict of Interest: None.

[a] Department of Surgery, University of Michigan Health System, 3410 Cancer Center/5932, 1500 East Medical Center Drive, Ann Arbor, MI 48109–5932, USA; [b] Department of Surgery, University of Michigan Health System, 3303 Cancer Center/5932, 1500 East Medical Center Drive, Ann Arbor, MI 48109–5932, USA
* Corresponding author.
E-mail address: aechang@umich.edu

patients with inoperable bone and soft tissue sarcomas using immunotherapy over the ensuing 40 years.[3] Despite a remarkable result of durable response (5-year survival rate >44%) in selected patients with inoperable soft tissue sarcoma,[4] his strategy gradually fell out of favor because of poorly controlled and documented patient follow-up and many different preparations and administration of the toxins making it difficult for others to reproduce his results. In addition, Coley's successes lacked a solid theoretical foundation. Clinical interest in cancer immunotherapy diminished in preference to the more broadly applicable chemotherapy and radiation treatment. However, Coley's intriguing observations and encouraging clinical results led to the understanding that the immunologic host response may affect the biologic behavior of malignant tumors and that manipulation of the immune system might cause recognition of the tumor, initiation of tumor-specific immunity, and eventually tumor destruction.

CLASSIFICATION OF CANCER IMMUNOTHERAPY

Cancer immunotherapy can be classified into two types: active and passive (**Fig. 1**). Active immunotherapies stimulate the endogenous immune system, and are further

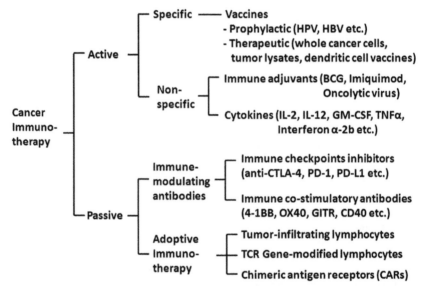

Fig. 1. Classification of cancer immunotherapy. Cancer immunotherapy can be classified into two types: active and passive. Active immunotherapies stimulate the endogenous immune system, and are further divided into two systems: specific and nonspecific immunotherapy. Active specific immunotherapy includes either prophylactic or therapeutic vaccines. Active nonspecific immunotherapy uses the components of the nonspecific immune system of the body, such as immune adjuvants and cytokines. Passive immunotherapies do not stimulate the immune system and bypass the requirement to activate endogenous immunity. The passive transfers of monoclonal antibodies can augment antitumor immunity by either blockade of immune checkpoints or enhancement of stimulatory signals. Adoptive cell therapy involves infusion of tumor-reactive cells that are autologous tumor-infiltrating lymphocytes, T-cell receptor gene-modified lymphocytes, or chimeric antigen receptors that are recombinant receptors providing antigen-binding and T-cell activation functions. BCG, bacillus Calmette-Guérin; CTLA, cytotoxic T-lymphocyte–associated antigen; GITR, glucocorticoid-induced tumor necrosis factor receptor; GM-CSF, granulocyte-macrophage colony–stimulating factor; HBV, hepatitis B virus; HPV, human papillomavirus; IL, interleukin; PD, programmed death; TNF, tumor necrosis factor.

divided into two systems: specific and nonspecific immunotherapy. Active specific immunotherapy includes either prophylactic or therapeutic approaches. Prophylactic vaccines target infectious agents that cause or contribute to the development of cancer, which include hepatitis B virus (HBV) vaccine and human papillomavirus (HPV) vaccine. Therapeutic vaccines are designed to treat existing cancers and may use attenuated whole cancer cells, tumor lysates, or purified tumor antigens, with or without adjuvants, to stimulate the patient's immune system. Active nonspecific immunotherapy uses the components of the nonspecific immune system of the body. These components include immune adjuvants, such as bacillus Calmette-Guérin (BCG), and cytokines including interleukin (IL)-2, IL-12, granulocyte-macrophage colony–stimulating factor (GM-CSF), tumor necrosis factor (TNF)-α, and interferon (IFN)-α-2b.

Passive immunotherapies do not stimulate the immune system and bypass the requirement to activate endogenous immunity. These therapies are comprised of antibodies or cells that are made or modified in the laboratory and administered to patients to provide or enhance immunity against cancer. The passive transfer of monoclonal antibodies (mAbs) and cells to augment antitumor immunity are effective treatments for a variety of hematologic and solid malignancies.[5]

Examples of mAbs used to enhance the immune system include anti–cytotoxic T-lymphocyte antigen (CTLA)-4, anti–programmed death (PD)-1, anti-PD ligand 1 (PD-L1), and anti-4-1BB. Adoptive cell therapy (ACT) is another form of passive immunotherapy that involves identification, isolation, activation, and reinfusion of autologous lymphocytes reactive to the tumor into patients.

PROPHYLACTIC AND THERAPEUTIC CANCER VACCINES

Prophylactic vaccines have been used with considerable success for the prevention of cancers attributable to infectious agents, such as HBV and HPV. HBV vaccines protect against HBV infection, and the potentially subsequent severe and deadly sequelae, such as cirrhosis and hepatocellular carcinoma.[6] The quadrivalent HPV vaccine is efficacious in preventing persistent cervical infection with HPV-6, -11, -16, or -18 and high-grade cervical intraepithelial neoplasia associated with these infections.[7,8] Recently, the quadrivalent HPV vaccine has been shown to also prevent vaginal, vulvar, and anal precancers.[9,10]

In contrast, the development of therapeutic vaccines to treat established tumor has been problematic. Therapeutic cancer vaccines directly target not the tumor, but the immune system, which in turn targets the tumor and its microenvironment to recalibrate the existing host-tumor interaction, skewing the balance from tumor tolerance toward tumor control. Although therapeutic cancer vaccines, when used as monotherapy, have minimal toxicity compared with conventional chemotherapy, the efficacy of ex vivo derived therapeutic vaccines has still to be proved for human cancers, and the limited success has been attributed to a variety of factors regarding the preparation and administration of the vaccine, the disease stage of patients in clinical trials, or the heterogeneous nature of malignant tumors.[11,12]

The first therapeutic cancer vaccine approved by the US Food and Drug Administration is sipuleucel-T to treat minimally symptomatic or asymptomatic metastatic castration-resistant prostate cancer. Sipuleucel-T is a cellular product comprised of autologous dendritic cells pulsed ex vivo with a recombinant fusion protein (PA2024) consisting of GM-CSF and prostatic acid phosphatase.[13] Dendritic cells are potent antigen-presenting cells that are responsible for inducing T and B immune responses. After processing, the dendritic cells are reinfused into the patient, with the goal of generating an immune response against prostatic acid phosphatase. A phase III randomized placebo-controlled double-blind multicenter study enrolled 512 men with minimally symptomatic or asymptomatic metastatic castration-resistant prostate cancer and randomized them 2:1 to receive sipuleucel-T or placebo every 2 weeks for three treatments. Sipuleucel-T was found to be well tolerated and prolonged median overall survival by 4.1 months compared with placebo (25.8 vs 21.7 months, respectively) but failed to show benefit in progression-free survival, and tumor regressions were rare.[14]

IMMUNE ADJUVANTS

Cancer cells often express a variety of abnormal proteins (tumor antigens) as targets for an immune response. Because tumors are poorly immunogenic, spontaneous immune responses to these antigens are weak and rarely sufficient to cause tumor regression. However, the local administration of immune-activating agents (immune adjuvants) can increase the strength of the immune response and induce protective immunity. In general, immune adjuvant-based therapies have only proved effective against early stage tumors.

In 1908, Albert Calmette and Camille Guérin of the Pasteur Institute in Lille, France began to investigate a vaccine for human tuberculosis and developed the attenuated form of bovine tuberculosis, *Mycobacterium bovis*, or BCG. The use of BCG as a cancer therapy was started when an autopsy series by Raymond Pearl in 1929 showed a lower frequency of cancer in patients with tuberculosis.[15] Since the first report on successful treatment of superficial bladder cancer with intravesical BCG in 1976,[16] it remains a clinically accepted and approved therapy for bladder cancer. Combination therapy with surgery and BCG was associated with progression-free survival in 62% of patients, compared with 37% of patients who underwent surgery alone.[17] Although the mechanism in BCG immunotherapy is not fully understood, the degree of local inflammatory reaction correlates with efficacy, suggesting an immune response elicited by BCG rather than a direct antitumor effect.[18]

Invasion of microbial pathogens triggers immune responses by activating evolutionarily conserved pattern-recognition receptors, such as members of the Toll-like receptor (TLR) family. TLRs comprise the main class of cell-surface pattern-recognition receptors that are expressed on antigen-presenting cells, such as macrophages and dendritic cells.[19] TLR ligation was found to activate the innate and adaptive immune systems, and plays an important role in antitumor immunity.[20] A significant amount of effort has been devoted to exploit the therapeutic potential of TLR agonists. Imiquimod is a low-molecular-weight immune-response modifier that can activate TLR-7 on dendritic cells and induce secretion of various cytokines, such as IFN-α, IFN-γ, TNF-α, IL-1, IL-6, IL-8, IL-10, and IL-12.[21] Imiquimod was initially approved in 1997 for the treatment of external anogenital and perianal warts caused by HPV infection. Because Imiquimod was also found to demonstrate efficacy against low-grade epithelial tumors and precancerous lesions, it is now approved for the treatment of superficial basal cell carcinoma and actinic keratosis, the precursor lesion of squamous cell carcinoma, and is being tested for melanoma and vulvar intraepithelial neoplasia.[22–26]

Another attractive approach is the use of oncolytic viruses that can exert a direct cytotoxic effect and promote immune-mediated tumor rejection. These features have prompted investigators to further explore oncolytic viruses for cancer immunotherapy. Herpes simplex virus-1 vectors have shown promising efficacy against a wide variety of malignancies including colorectal, head and neck, breast, prostate cancer, melanoma, and glioblastoma.[27] A phase II clinical trial with intratumoral injection of attenuated herpes simplex virus-1 engineered to secrete GM-CSF (OncovexGM-CSF) for the treatment of patients with stage IIIc or IV metastatic melanoma has shown 26% objective response rate including uninjected regional and distant soft tissue and visceral metastatic sites.[28]

CYTOKINES

Cytokines are proteins secreted by cells of the immune system and can be delivered systemically to activate antitumor immunity. IL-2 was first identified as a T-cell growth factor in 1976, and has been found to be an important mediator of immune function through its effects on the growth, development, and activity of T and B lymphocytes, and natural killer cells.[29] Based on potent, dose-dependent immunomodulatory and antitumor activity shown in preclinical models,[30] clinical studies were conducted. Treatment with high-dose, single-agent IL-2 in patients with metastatic melanoma and renal cell carcinoma demonstrated 15% to 20% objective responses and 7% complete remission in metastatic melanoma or renal cell carcinoma.[31]

Subsequent publications of retrospective analysis with extended follow-up of 270 patients treated with high-dose IL-2 conducted at the National Cancer Institute between 1985 and 1993 showed 16% objective response including 17 (6%) complete responses, and 59% of complete responders remained progression-free at 7 years.[32–34] Phase II studies evaluating the efficacy of high-dose IL-2 for 259 patients with metastatic renal cell carcinoma treated at the National Cancer Institute showed 20% objective responses including 23 (8.9%) complete responders, of which 19 (83%) remained free of recurrence at follow-up between 24 and 221 months.[35] Although immunotherapy with high-dose IL-2 carries significant risk of serious systemic toxicities, which requires administration as an in-patient, these durable complete responses led to the approval of high-dose IL-2 for clinical use in 1992 for metastatic renal cell carcinoma and in 1998 for metastatic melanoma.

IFNs are pleiotropic cytokines and were first discovered as an antiviral agent during studies on virus interference.[36] IFN-mediated signaling and transcriptional activation of cellular gene expression are best understood in the context of JAK-STAT pathway proteins, which is a major signaling system that cells use to transmit extracellular information from many cytokines and growth factors to the nucleus.[37,38] Although the antitumor mechanism of action for IFN-α-2b therapy in patients with melanoma has not been universal, preclinical and clinical models suggest that the effects of IFN-α-2b are mediated by host cells rather than direct effects on tumor cells.[39,40] The use of IFN-α-2b has been studied as an adjuvant treatment in patients with melanoma. High-dose IFN-α-2b demonstrated increased disease-free survival and in some studies, overall survival in high-risk patients with melanoma in randomized clinical trials.[41–44] A meta-analysis analyzing data from 14 randomized trials including 8122 patients showed adjuvant immunotherapy with IFN-α-2b has been found to prolong disease-free and overall survival in selected patients with melanoma at increased risk for disease dissemination.[45] IFN-α-2b has a large variety of possible side effects in virtually all organ systems, which often hamper the attainment of optimal dose intensity and sometimes even necessitates premature cessation of therapy. Pegylated IFN-α-2b has been developed to decrease the frequency with which IFN-α-2b is administered while maintaining a high level of exposure. A randomized clinical trial that enrolled 1256 patients with resected stage III melanoma showed significantly increased 7-year relapse-free ($P = .06$), distant metastasis-free ($P = .02$), and overall survival (P = .006) with pegylated IFN-α-2b in patients with sentinel lymph node involvement and ulcerated melanoma compared with observation.[46]

IMMUNE-MODULATING ANTIBODIES

The capacity of mAbs to induce tumor-directed T-cell responses is intriguing. Intratumoral T-cell composition and distribution have been associated with clinical outcomes,[47] suggesting the relevance of T cells in antitumor immunity. Moreover, T cells can target intracellular antigens that are thought to be inaccessible to antibody therapies. The ultimate amplitude and quality of the response of T cells is regulated by a balance between costimulatory and inhibitory signals (immune checkpoints). After activation, T cells upregulate the expression of inhibitory receptors, which protects against deleterious autoimmunity. The importance of these pathways was highlighted by studies showing that total blockade by genetic disruption led to massive T-cell hyperproliferation and protracted multiorgan autoimmunity.[48,49] Thus, under normal physiologic conditions, immune checkpoints are crucial for the maintenance of self-tolerance to prevent overactivation. Cancer takes advantage of this ability to hide from the immune system by exploiting a series of immune escape mechanisms that were developed to avoid autoimmunity.

Recently, preclinical and clinical data showed that blockade of these immune checkpoints can significantly enhance antitumor immunity. Blockade of one of these checkpoints, CTLA-4, provided the first evidence of improvement in overall survival for the treatment of patients with metastatic melanoma.[50,51] CTLA-4 is a key negative regulator, expressed exclusively on T cells, and counteracts the activity of the T-cell costimulatory receptor, CD28 (**Fig. 2**). After antigen is engaged by T-cell receptor (TCR), CD28 signaling amplifies TCR signaling to activate T cells.

CD28 and CTLA-4 share B7 family of accessory molecules (CD80, CD86) expressed by antigen-presenting cells.[52] Because CTLA-4 has a much higher affinity for CD80 and CD86, ligation to CTLA-4 inhibits further activation and expansion, thereby controlling the progress of an immune response.[53-55] CTLA-4 ligation is not only through the activated CD4 and CD8 T cells, but also associated with enhancement of regulatory T-cell immunosuppressive activity.[56] In a placebo-controlled phase III trial, 676 patients with relapsed-refractory metastatic melanoma were randomly assigned in a 3:1:1 ratio to ipilimumab plus glycoprotein 100 (gp100) peptide vaccine, ipilimumab alone, or gp100 alone. Overall survival was significantly increased in patients given ipilimumab (22%, 24%, and 14% at 24 months, respectively). Of note, 18% of the ipilimumab-treated patients survived beyond 2 years compared with 5% of patients receiving the gp100 peptide vaccine alone.[50] In another randomized trial involving 502 patients with previously untreated metastatic melanoma, the addition of ipilimumab to standard dacarbazine alone was shown to improve overall survival compared with dacarbazine alone (11.2 months vs 9.1 months; P<.001).[51] Immune-related toxicity involving various tissue sites, such as enterocolitis, hepatitis, dermatitis, and endocrinopathy, were also observed in 25% to 30% of patients. PD-1 is another T-cell coinhibitory receptor with a structure similar to that of CTLA-4 but with a distinct biologic function and ligand specificity.[57,58] PD-1 predominantly regulates effector T-cell activity within tissue and tumors (effector phase), whereas CTLA-4 predominantly regulates T-cell activation (priming phase) (see **Fig. 2**).[59] PD-1 is more broadly expressed than CTLA-4: it is induced on non–T lymphocytes subsets, including B cells and natural killer cells.[60,61] PD-1 has two principal ligands, PD-L1 and PD-L2. PD-L1 is not only expressed on many tumors,[62-64] but also on myeloid cells in the tumor microenvironment.[65-67]

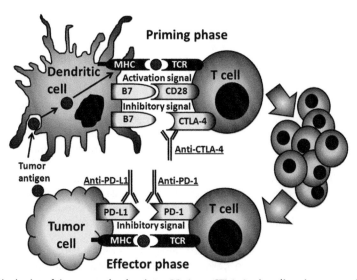

Fig. 2. Blockade of immune checkpoints, PD-1 or CTLA-4, signaling in cancer immunotherapy. Tumor antigen is picked up, processed, and presented on the major histocompatibility complex (MHC) by antigen-presenting cells, such as dendritic cells. T cells recognize MHC-antigen complex through their T-cell receptor (TCR). Antigen-specific T cells are activated by a second signal delivered by the B7 costimulatory molecules B7-1 (or CD80) and B7-2 (or CD86), which bind to CD28 on T cells. Cytotoxic T-lymphocyte–associated antigen 4 (CTLA-4), which has a higher affinity for B7 costimulatory molecules, is upregulated shortly after T-cell activation and initiates inhibitory signal on T cells. The interaction between CTLA-4 and the costimulatory molecules happens primarily in the priming phase of a T-cell response within lymph nodes. Programmed death 1 (PD-1) inhibitory receptor is expressed by T cells during long-term antigen exposure and results in negative regulation on T cells during ligation with PD-L1, which is expressed within the tumor microenvironment. The PD-1 interaction happens in the effector phase of a T-cell response in peripheral tissues. Its blockade with antibodies to PD-1 or PD-L1 results in the preferential activation of T cells with specificity for the cancer.

PD-L2 is expressed on antigen-presenting cells and various tumors, such as B-cell lymphoma and Hodgkin disease.[68] Expression of PD-L1 is correlated with unfavorable prognosis in cancers of lung, kidney, pancreas, and ovaries.[69–72] Ligation of PD-1, which is expressed on a large proportion of tumor-infiltrating lymphocytes (TILs) from many different tumor types,[73,74] renders these cells unresponsive or exhausted as has been suggested by decreased cytokine production by PD-1$^+$ compared with PD-1$^-$ TILs from melanomas.[74] Blockade of this interaction by PD-1/PD-L1 axis is expected to revitalize these exhausted tumor-specific T cells. Recently, two large clinical trials of anti–PD-1 therapy or anti–PD-L1 therapy reported impressive durable response rates.[75,76] Nivolumab is a humanized mAb that targets the PD-1 protein. This mAb was evaluated in a phase I/II study in 296 patients with a variety of heavily pretreated malignancies including melanoma (104 patients); renal cell cancer (34 patients); and non–small cell lung cancer (122 patients). Cumulative response rates were 28% among patients with melanoma, 27% among patients with renal cell cancer, and 18% among patients with non–small cell lung cancer. Of note, none of the patients with PD-L1$^-$ tumors had an objective response, whereas 36% of patients with PD-L1$^+$ tumors had and objective response ($P = .006$).[75] BMS-936559 is a mAb that binds to PD-L1, and has been tested in a dose escalation phase I/II study in

207 patients with a variety of malignancies including melanoma (55 patients); renal cell cancer (17 patients); non–small cell lung cancer (75 patients); and ovarian cancer (17 patients). Objective response rate was 17% in melanoma, 11% in renal cell cancer, 10% in non–small-cell lung cancer, and 6% in ovarian cancer. Responses lasted for 1 year or more in 50% of patients with at least 1 year of follow-up.[76] Autoimmune phenomena have been reported with blockade of PD-1/PD-L1 axis, albeit less frequently than with CTLA-4–specific antibodies, which is consistent with the generally milder autoimmune phenotype seen in PD-1$^{-/-}$ mice compared with CTLA-4$^{-/-}$ mice.[48,49,77,78]

Another strategy to augmenting T cell–specific immunity against tumor cells aims to activate costimulatory receptors including glucocorticoid-induced TNF receptor, 4-1BB, OX40, and CD40. Glucocorticoid-induced TNF receptor, OX40, and 4-1BB are members of TNF receptor family expressed on T cells, and ligation of these receptors augments effector T-cell function.[79] Agonistic antibodies directed against each of these proteins were found to increase the efficacy of antitumor immunity in preclinical model.[80–84]

CD40 is a member of the TNF super family and costimulatory molecule that is expressed by various immune cells and by cancer cells of different histologies. CD40 expression on immune cells has been implicated in the regulation of humoral and cellular immunity, whereas CD40 expression on certain tumor cell types has been implicated in proapoptotic and antiproliferative activity.[85–87] CD40 is also broadly expressed on dendritic cells and its activation by CD40 ligand, found on activated T cells, seems to "license" the antigen-presenting cell for T-cell activation.[88] Consistent with these findings, a recent phase I trial of the anti-CD40 antibody showed encouraging preliminary results in patients with advanced melanoma.[89]

To achieve the desired antitumor immunity while maintaining immunologic tolerance to self-antigens expressed on normal tissue cells to avoid autoimmune response is a major challenge. Despite some encouraging results with anti–CTLA-4 or anti–PD-1/PD-L1 mAb, clinicians need to be aware that targeting the immunologic synapse can backfire. Early clinical trial of an agonist antibody against the costimulatory receptor CD28 caused a massive cytokine storm and multiorgan failure in six healthy volunteers.[90] One of the clinical trials with agonists of another costimulatory receptor, 4-1BB, which are expressed on activated T cells and natural killer cells, was recently suspended because a considerable degree of liver toxicity was observed with higher doses of the antibody.[91] These findings emphasize that the balance between antitumor effects and autoimmune side effects must be considered in clinical targeting of the immunologic synapse.

ADOPTIVE CELL THERAPY

Adoptive T-cell therapy involves the transfer of ex vivo expanded effector cells as a means of augmenting the antitumor immune response. Tumor-specific T cells can be derived from the patient's peripheral blood, the tumor environment (TILs), or they can be genetically modified to express a high-affinity antitumor TCR.[92,93] There are several advantages to the use of lymphocyte transfer as an immune-based approach to treat cancer. T cells are potent effectors of adaptive immunity because of their ability to initiate killing after their receptor-mediated engagement of antigens expressed on the surface of tumor cells. T-cell cytotoxicity requires direct contact with target cells, thereby limiting any possible damage to bystander cells. The attractiveness of target-specific approaches lies in avoidance of the serious side effects of other conventional treatments, such as chemotherapy and radiation, which have relatively nonspecific mechanisms of action. A unique feature of the immune response, unlike conventional cancer therapies, is that it can elicit long-term protection from recurring disease. Another significant advantage of T cell-based immunotherapies is that they do not depend on knowledge of tumor location. T cells, through the expression of trafficking molecules, are equipped to search out and destroy widely disseminated heterogeneous tumor cell targets.

In ACT, T cells can be selected in vitro for high reactivity against tumor antigens and grown under conditions that overcome the tolerizing influences in tumor microenvironment. Recently, ACT with TILs has emerged as one of the most effective treatments in patients with metastatic melanoma. TILs from resected melanoma deposits can be grown to large numbers in IL-2 while retaining reactivity against endogenous tumor-associated antigens. This approach was first described in 1988 by Rosenberg and colleagues,[94] but significant improvement in efficacy came in 2002 with the introduction of a nonmyeloablative lymphodepleting chemotherapy preparative regimen given before the adoptive transfer,[95] which could improve enhanced persistence of the transferred T cells. This regimen can be accomplished using chemotherapy alone or in combination with total-body irradiation for the temporary ablation of the immune system in a patient with cancer. Two potential mechanisms enhancing in vivo clonal expansion of administered autologous TILs have been proposed based on studies in preclinical models: the elimination of suppressor T cells[96]; or the decreased competition by endogenous lymphocytes for homeostatic regulatory cytokines, such as IL-7 or IL-15.[97–99] In their most recent report, they treated 93 patients with metastatic melanoma refractory to all other treatments with the adoptive transfer of autologous TILs administered in conjunction with systemic IL-2 administration after a lymphodepleting regimens (chemotherapy alone or with 2 or 12 Gy total body irradiation). Objective tumor regression was observed in 49% to 72% of patients (including 20 patients [22%] of complete regression) with the greater the degree of host lymphodepletion, the more effective was the treatment. Responses were durable (>5 years) and 19 of 20 patients have ongoing complete regressions with a minimum follow-up of 57 months.[92,100]

There are some drawbacks of this approach in addition to the costs and labor intensity of the treatment. First, not all patients have preexisting tumor-reactive lymphocytes that can be expanded ex vivo: only approximately half of melanomas give rise to antitumor TILs and other types of tumor only rarely contain identifiable tumor-reactive lymphocytes.[101,102] Isolation and expansion of TILs can take 5 to 6 weeks making this treatment difficult for patients with progressive disease. It involves a rather toxic regimen that entails systemic IL-2 administration and preparative lymphodepleting protocol with chemotherapy with or without total body irradiation, making only patients with good performance status eligible for this treatment.[103,104]

Genetic engineering of circulating autologous lymphocytes from patients with cancer by using genes that encode receptors capable of recognizing cancer antigens to generate high-affinity T cells with specificity for tumors is used to overcome these limitations. These high-affinity T cells can be equipped with conventional TCRs expressing a heterodimeric αβ receptor, which recognize processed antigenic peptides presented by major histocompatibility complex (MHC) proteins or with chimeric antigen receptors (CARs), which recognize tumor-associated antigen through single-chain variable fragments that are isolated from antigen-specific mAbs. Gene encoding TCRs can be obtained from high-affinity T cells isolated from a patient who had an excellent response to ACT and cloned into a retrovirus or lentivirus, which can then be used to transduce autologous T cells from other patients with matching HLA restriction elements.[102] Morgan and colleagues[105] reported the first successful application of gene-modified T cells to treat 15 patients with melanoma with a TCR that targeted the MART-1 melanocyte/melanoma differentiation antigen and achieved an objective response in 2 of 15 patients including one complete response. Since then, this approach has been applied with a variety of antigens including MART-1 and gp100 (melanoma); NY-ESO-1 (epithelial tumor and sarcomas); CEA (colorectal cancer); and 2G-1 (renal cell carcinoma).[102,106–108] However, this approach is complicated by potential "on-target, off-organ" adverse effects caused by recognition of low-level expression of tumor-associated antigen on healthy tissues, which can be recognized by high-affinity TCRs. These side effects include vitiligo, uveitis, and auditory toxicity (MART-1 and gp100)[102] and inflammatory colitis (CEA).[106] The major challenge for immunotherapy using gene-modified T cells remains the identification of antigens that can be targeted to destroy the cancer without causing toxicity to normal tissues. The use of CARs that recognize non–MHC-restricted structures on the surface of target cells is highly attractive because tumors can frequently lose tumor antigen expression through the downregulation of MHC expression.[109] In addition, CAR-modified T cells can specifically traffic to tumor sites and persist as memory cells in vivo, compared with mAbs. Currently, the most successful use of CARs has been reported in the treatment of B-cell lymphoma to target the CD19 molecule, which is expressed on most B-cell malignancies and normal B cells. An intriguing report showed regression in a patient with heavily pretreated B-cell lymphoma with anti–CD19-CAR-transduced T cells,[110] and subsequent reports from the same group and others have shown encouraging results.[111–113] The use of CARs now has broadened the application of ACT to a variety of cancers including renal cell carcinoma, neuroblastoma, colorectal cancer, and ovarian cancer.[114–117]

COMBINING IMMUNOTHERAPY WITH OTHER THERAPEUTIC MODALITIES

Cytotoxic chemotherapy has been considered to cause immunosuppression because of its toxicity for dividing cells in the bone marrow and peripheral lymphoid tissue, and therefore to negate the benefits of immunotherapy. However, as early as the 1970s, a preclinical model demonstrated that intratumoral injection of chemotherapeutic agents, such as actinomycin D, adriamycin, and mitomycin C, not only cured intradermal tumors but also caused systemic immune response resistant to tumor rechallenge.[118] Certain chemotherapeutic agents were found to enhance vaccine-mediated T-cell killing by several distinct mechanisms. Oxaliplatin and anthracyclines induce immunogenic tumor cell death, which results in enhanced crosspriming of tumor-associated antigen by dendritic cells and subsequent activation of T cells.[119,120] Docetaxel was found to suppress myeloid-derived suppressor cells (MDSC) and enhance IFN production by CD8+ T cells.[121,122] Low-dose cyclophosphamide treatment not only decreases the number of regulatory T cells but also inhibits their suppressive function.[123,124] Synergic effect of chemotherapy and immunotherapy was described in preclinical mouse model with administration of gemcitabine and agonistic–anti-CD40 antibody, demonstrating enhanced T-cell infiltration at the tumor site and CD8 T cell dependent synergistic antitumor immunity.[125] Several phase I/II clinical studies have shown encouraging results with chemoimmunotherapy.[126–128]

Immunomodulatory antibodies may enhance antitumor immune responses elicited by other treatment, such as radiotherapy and in some instances mediate promising abscopal effects. Abscopal effect is the bystander effect of radiotherapy observed at a site distant to that irradiated within the same subject. Recently, an abscopal effect in a patient with metastatic melanoma treated with ipilimumab and radiotherapy was reported. A female patient with metastatic melanoma to spleen, hilar lymph nodes who had been on maintenance ipilimumab underwent palliative radiotherapy to paraspinal mass. The patient showed significant response not only at the primary irradiated site but also in areas not targeted by radiotherapy.[129]

A clinical trial combining ipilimumab and radiotherapy in patients with metastatic melanoma is currently under way.

FUTURE DIRECTIONS

An important biologic and clinical question is whether the effector function of tumor reactive T cells expressing multiple inhibitory receptors can be fully recovered by targeting a single receptor, or whether combinational checkpoint blockade is required for sustained tumor protection. Preclinical mouse models of cancer have shown that dual blockade of coordinately expressed receptors can produce additive or synergistic antitumor immunity.[130–132] Because the rationale for blocking immune checkpoint inhibitors is based on the assumption that tumor protective T cells exist in the patient before therapy and that these cells exert antitumor activity if immune checkpoint receptors are blocked, combining blockade of immune checkpoint inhibitors and ACT with activated TILs might potentially have additive or synergistic effects.

The concept of "immunoediting" relates to the manner in which tumors manipulate their microenvironment through tumor-derived cytokines, chemokines, and other soluble factors.[133] By the time tumors have become clinically detectable, they have already developed mechanisms to evade the host immune response. Immune suppression is a common feature of the tumor microenvironment and a substantial barrier to cancer immunotherapy. Myeloid-derived suppressor cells (MDSCs), tumor-associated macrophages (TAMs), and regulatory T cells are major components of the immune suppressive tumor microenvironment. MDSCs are a heterogeneous cell population composed mainly of myeloid progenitor cells that do not completely differentiate into mature macrophages, dendritic cells, or granulocytes. Increased circulating MDSCs have been correlated with tumor stage and metastatic tumor burden in different types of tumors.[134,135] These findings suggest a potential use for those cells in immune monitoring of patients with cancer.

TAMs are derived from circulating monocytes, differentiate within the tumor microenvironment, and are different from immature myeloid cells because of their high expression of MHC class II.[136,137] Preclinical studies demonstrated that TAMs play an important role in tumor growth, angiogenesis, metastasis, matrix remodeling, and immune evasion in various human and animal tumors.[136–139] Regulatory T cells infiltrate many tumors and increased frequency of regulatory T cells is associated with poor outcome for several cancer types.[140–142]

Tumor-infiltrating regulatory T cells directly promote malignant cell proliferation and dissemination through the secretion of receptor activator of nuclear factor-κB ligand.[143] Regulatory T cells also suppress immune responses through the secretion of suppressive cytokines, transforming growth factor-β, and IL-10, and express negative costimulatory molecule, CTLA-4. Regulatory T cells pose a significant barrier to the success of immunotherapy and they represent an attractive target for enhancing antitumor immunity. The future of immunotherapy will likely involve agents to manipulate the suppressive tumor microenvironment to improve trafficking of immune cells to the tumor site in combinations with vaccines, ACT, or immunomodulatory antibodies. The careful evaluation of immune responses to tumors and normal tissue during combined application of immunotherapy is critical to achieve optimal benefits to patients with cancer.

REFERENCES

1. Coley WB. II. Contribution to the knowledge of sarcoma. Ann Surg 1891;14(3): 199–220.
2. Coley WB. The treatment of inoperable sarcoma by bacterial toxins (the mixed toxins of the streptococcus erysipelas and the bacillus prodigiosus). Proc R Soc Med 1910;3(Surg Sect):1–48.
3. Coley WB. End results in Hodgkin's disease and lymphosarcoma treated by the mixed toxins of erysipelas and bacillus prodigiosus, alone or combined with radiation. Ann Surg 1928;88(4):641–67.
4. Wiemann B, Starnes CO. Coley's toxins, tumor necrosis factor and cancer research: a historical perspective. Pharmacol Ther 1994;64(3):529–64.
5. Dougan M, Dranoff G. Immune therapy for cancer. Annu Rev Immunol 2009;27: 83–117.
6. McMahon BJ, Bruden DL, Petersen KM, et al. Antibody levels and protection after hepatitis B vaccination: results of a 15-year follow-up. Ann Intern Med 2005; 142(5):333–41.
7. FUTURE II Study Group. Quadrivalent vaccine against human papillomavirus to prevent high-grade cervical lesions. N Engl J Med 2007;356(19):1915–27.
8. Garland SM, Hernandez-Avila M, Wheeler CM, et al. Quadrivalent vaccine against human papillomavirus to prevent anogenital diseases. N Engl J Med 2007;356(19):1928–43.
9. Joura EA, Leodolter S, Hernandez-Avila M, et al. Efficacy of a quadrivalent prophylactic human papillomavirus (types 6, 11, 16, and 18) L1 virus-like-particle vaccine against high-grade vulval and vaginal lesions: a combined analysis of three randomised clinical trials. Lancet 2007;369(9574):1693–702.
10. Palefsky JM, Giuliano AR, Goldstone S, et al. HPV vaccine against anal HPV infection and anal intraepithelial neoplasia. N Engl J Med 2011;365(17): 1576–85.
11. Soruri A, Zwirner J. Dendritic cells: limited potential in immunotherapy. Int J Biochem Cell Biol 2005;37(2):241–5.
12. Figdor CG, de Vries IJ, Lesterhuis WJ, et al. Dendritic cell immunotherapy: mapping the way. Nat Med 2004;10(5):475–80.
13. So-Rosillo R, Small EJ. Sipuleucel-T (APC8015) for prostate cancer. Expert Rev Anticancer Ther 2006;6(9):1163–7.
14. Kantoff PW, Higano CS, Shore ND, et al. Sipuleucel-T immunotherapy for castration resistant prostate cancer. N Engl J Med 2010;363(5):411–22.
15. Meyer JP, Persad R, Gillatt DA. Use of bacille Calmette-Guerin in superficial bladder cancer. Postgrad Med J 2002;78(922):449–54.
16. Morales A, Eidinger D, Bruce AW. Intracavitary bacillus Calmette-Guerin in the treatment of superficial bladder tumors. J Urol 1976;116(2):180–3.
17. Herr HW, Schwalb DM, Zhang ZF, et al. Intravesical bacillus Calmette-Guerin therapy prevents tumor progression and death from superficial bladder cancer: ten-year followup of a prospective randomized trial. J Clin Oncol 1995;13(6): 1404–8.
18. Bohle A, Brandau S. Immune mechanisms in bacillus Calmette-Guerin immunotherapy for superficial bladder cancer. J Urol 2003;170(3):964–9.
19. Medzhitov R, Janeway CA Jr. Decoding the patterns of self and nonself by the innate immune system. Science 2002;296(5566):298–300.
20. Bendelac A, Medzhitov R. Adjuvants of immunity: harnessing innate immunity to promote adaptive immunity. J Exp Med 2002;195(5):F19–23.

21. Zuany-Amorim C, Hastewell J, Walker C. Toll-like receptors as potential therapeutic targets for multiple diseases. Nat Rev Drug Discov 2002;1(10):797–807.
22. van Seters M, van Beurden M, ten Kate FJ, et al. Treatment of vulvar intraepithelial neoplasia with topical imiquimod. N Engl J Med 2008;358(14):1465–73.
23. Geisse J, Caro I, Lindholm J, et al. Imiquimod 5% cream for the treatment of superficial basal cell carcinoma: results from two phase III, randomized, vehicle-controlled studies. J Am Acad Dermatol 2004;50(5):722–33.
24. Hadley G, Derry S, Moore RA. Imiquimod for actinic keratosis: systematic review and meta-analysis. J Invest Dermatol 2006;126(6):1251–5.
25. Turza K, Dengel LT, Harris RC, et al. Effectiveness of imiquimod limited to dermal melanoma metastases, with simultaneous resistance of subcutaneous metastasis. J Cutan Pathol 2010;37(1):94–8.
26. Daayana S, Elkord E, Winters U, et al. Phase II trial of imiquimod and HPV therapeutic vaccination in patients with vulval intraepithelial neoplasia. Br J Cancer 2010;102(7):1129–36.
27. Kasuya H, Takeda S, Nomoto S, et al. The potential of oncolytic virus therapy for pancreatic cancer. Cancer Gene Ther 2005;12(9):725–36.
28. Senzer NN, Kaufman HL, Amatruda T, et al. Phase II clinical trial of a granulocytemacrophage colony-stimulating factor-encoding, second-generation oncolytic herpesvirus in patients with unresectable metastatic melanoma. J Clin Oncol 2009;27(34):5763–71.
29. Morgan DA, Ruscetti FW, Gallo R. Selective in vitro growth of T lymphocytes from normal human bone marrows. Science 1976;193(4257):1007–8.
30. Rosenberg SA, Mule JJ, Spiess PJ, et al. Regression of established pulmonary metastases and subcutaneous tumor mediated by the systemic administration of highdose recombinant interleukin 2. J Exp Med 1985;161(5):1169–88.
31. Rosenberg SA, Yang JC, Topalian SL, et al. Treatment of 283 consecutive patients with metastatic melanoma or renal cell cancer using high-dose bolus interleukin 2. JAMA 1994;271(12):907–13.
32. Rosenberg SA, Lotze MT, Muul LM, et al. Observations on the systemic administration of autologous lymphokine-activated killer cells and recombinant interleukin-2 to patients with metastatic cancer. N Engl J Med 1985;313(23):1485–92.
33. Atkins MB, Kunkel L, Sznol M, et al. High-dose recombinant interleukin-2 therapy in patients with metastatic melanoma: long-term survival update. Cancer J Sci Am 2000;6(Suppl 1):S11–4.
34. Atkins MB, Lotze MT, Dutcher JP, et al. High-dose recombinant interleukin 2 therapy for patients with metastatic melanoma: analysis of 270 patients treated between 1985 and 1993. J Clin Oncol 1999;17(7):2105–16.
35. Klapper JA, Downey SG, Smith FO, et al. High-dose interleukin-2 for the treatment of metastatic renal cell carcinoma: a retrospective analysis of response and survival in patients treated in the surgery branch at the National Cancer Institute between 1986 and 2006. Cancer 2008;113(2):293–301.
36. Isaacs A, Lindenmann J. Virus interference. I. The interferon. Proc R Soc Lond B Biol Sci 1957;147(927):258–67.
37. Sen GC. Viruses and interferons. Annu Rev Microbiol 2001;55:255–81.
38. Darnell JE Jr, Kerr IM, Stark GR. Jak-STAT pathways and transcriptional activation in response to IFNs and other extracellular signaling proteins. Science 1994;264(5164):1415–21.
39. Lesinski GB, Anghelina M, Zimmerer J, et al. The antitumor effects of IFN-alpha are abrogated in a STAT1-deficient mouse. J Clin Invest 2003;112(2):170–80.

40. Moschos SJ, Edington HD, Land SR, et al. Neoadjuvant treatment of regional stage IIIB melanoma with high-dose interferon alfa-2b induces objective tumor regression in association with modulation of tumor infiltrating host cellular immune responses. J Clin Oncol 2006;24(19):3164–71.

41. Kirkwood JM, Strawderman MH, Ernstoff MS, et al. Interferon alfa-2b adjuvant therapy of high-risk resected cutaneous melanoma: the Eastern Cooperative Oncology Group Trial EST 1684. J Clin Oncol 1996;14(1):7–17.

42. Kirkwood JM, Ibrahim JG, Sondak VK, et al. High- and low-dose interferon alfa-2b in high-risk melanoma: first analysis of intergroup trial E1690/S9111/C9190. J Clin Oncol 2000;18(12):2444–58.

43. Kirkwood JM, Ibrahim JG, Sosman JA, et al. High-dose interferon alfa-2b significantly prolongs relapse-free and overall survival compared with the GM2-KLH/QS-21 vaccine in patients with resected stage IIB-III melanoma: results of intergroup trial E1694/S9512/C509801. J Clin Oncol 2001;19(9):2370–80.

44. Pehamberger H, Soyer HP, Steiner A, et al. Adjuvant interferon alfa-2a treatment in resected primary stage II cutaneous melanoma. Austrian Malignant Melanoma Cooperative Group. J Clin Oncol 1998;16(4):1425–9.

45. Sabel MS, Sondak VK. Point: interferon-alpha for adjuvant therapy for melanoma patients. J Natl Compr Canc Netw 2004;2(1):61–8.

46. Eggermont AM, Suciu S, Testori A, et al. Long-term results of the randomized phase III trial EORTC 18991 of adjuvant therapy with pegylated interferon alfa-2b versus observation in resected stage III melanoma. J Clin Oncol 2012; 30(31):3810–8.

47. Galon J, Costes A, Sanchez-Cabo F, et al. Type, density, and location of immune cells within human colorectal tumors predict clinical outcome. Science 2006; 313(5795):1960–4.

48. Tivol EA, Borriello F, Schweitzer AN, et al. Loss of CTLA-4 leads to massive lymphoproliferation and fatal multiorgan tissue destruction, revealing a critical negative regulatory role of CTLA-4. Immunity 1995;3(5):541–7.

49. Waterhouse P, Penninger JM, Timms E, et al. Lymphoproliferative disorders with early lethality in mice deficient in CTLA-4. Science 1995;270(5238): 985–8.

50. Hodi FS, O'Day SJ, McDermott DF, et al. Improved survival with ipilimumab in patients with metastatic melanoma. N Engl J Med 2010;363(8):711–23.

51. Robert C, Thomas L, Bondarenko I, et al. Ipilimumab plus dacarbazine for previously untreated metastatic melanoma. N Engl J Med 2011;364(26):2517–26.

52. Leach DR, Krummel MF, Allison JP. Enhancement of antitumor immunity by CTLA-4 blockade. Science 1996;271(5256):1734–6.

53. Linsley PS, Greene JL, Brady W, et al. Human B7-1 (CD80) and B7-2 (CD86) bind with similar avidities but distinct kinetics to CD28 and CTLA-4 receptors. Immunity 1994;1(9):793–801.

54. Riley JL, Mao M, Kobayashi S, et al. Modulation of TCR-induced transcriptional profiles by ligation of CD28, ICOS, and CTLA-4 receptors. Proc Natl Acad Sci U S A 2002;99(18):11790–5.

55. Schneider H, Downey J, Smith A, et al. Reversal of the TCR stop signal by CTLA-4. Science 2006;313(5795):1972–5.

56. Wing K, Onishi Y, Prieto-Martin P, et al. CTLA-4 control over Foxp3+ regulatory T cell function. Science 2008;322(5899):271–5.

57. Ishida Y, Agata Y, Shibahara K, et al. Induced expression of PD-1, a novel member of the immunoglobulin gene superfamily, upon programmed cell death. EMBO J 1992;11(11):3887–95.

58. Okazaki T, Honjo T. PD-1 and PD-1 ligands: from discovery to clinical application. Int Immunol 2007;19(7):813–24.
59. Ribas A. Tumor immunotherapy directed at PD-1. N Engl J Med 2012;366(26): 2517–9.
60. Fanoni D, Tavecchio S, Recalcati S, et al. New monoclonal antibodies against B-cell antigens: possible new strategies for diagnosis of primary cutaneous B-cell lymphomas. Immunol Lett 2011;134(2):157–60.
61. Terme M, Ullrich E, Aymeric L, et al. IL-18 induces PD-1-dependent immunosuppression in cancer. Cancer Res 2011;71(16):5393–9.
62. Blank C, Brown I, Peterson AC, et al. PD-L1/B7H-1 inhibits the effector phase of tumor rejection by T cell receptor (TCR) transgenic CD8+ T cells. Cancer Res 2004;64(3):1140–5.
63. Dong H, Strome SE, Salomao DR, et al. Tumor-associated B7-H1 promotes T-cell apoptosis: a potential mechanism of immune evasion. Nat Med 2002;8(8): 793–800.
64. Iwai Y, Ishida M, Tanaka Y, et al. Involvement of PD-L1 on tumor cells in the escape from host immune system and tumor immunotherapy by PD-L1 blockade. Proc Natl Acad Sci U S A 2002;99(19):12293–7.
65. Curiel TJ, Wei S, Dong H, et al. Blockade of B7-H1 improves myeloid dendritic cell mediated antitumor immunity. Nat Med 2003;9(5):562–7.
66. Kuang DM, Zhao Q, Peng C, et al. Activated monocytes in peritumoral stroma of hepatocellular carcinoma foster immune privilege and disease progression through PDL1. J Exp Med 2009;206(6):1327–37.
67. Liu Y, Zeng B, Zhang Z, et al. B7-H1 on myeloid-derived suppressor cells in immune suppression by a mouse model of ovarian cancer. Clin Immunol 2008; 129(3):471–81.
68. Rosenwald A, Wright G, Leroy K, et al. Molecular diagnosis of primary mediastinal B cell lymphoma identifies a clinically favorable subgroup of diffuse large B cell lymphoma related to Hodgkin lymphoma. J Exp Med 2003;198(6): 851–62.
69. Thompson RH, Gillett MD, Cheville JC, et al. Costimulatory B7-H1 in renal cell carcinoma patients: indicator of tumor aggressiveness and potential therapeutic target. Proc Natl Acad Sci U S A 2004;101(49):17174–9.
70. Hamanishi J, Mandai M, Iwasaki M, et al. Programmed cell death 1 ligand 1 and tumorinfiltrating CD8+ T lymphocytes are prognostic factors of human ovarian cancer. Proc Natl Acad Sci U S A 2007;104(9):3360–5.
71. Konishi J, Yamazaki K, Azuma M, et al. B7-H1 expression on non-small cell lung cancer cells and its relationship with tumor-infiltrating lymphocytes and their PD-1 expression. Clin Cancer Res 2004;10(15):5094–100.
72. Nomi T, Sho M, Akahori T, et al. Clinical significance and therapeutic potential of the programmed death-1 ligand/programmed death-1 pathway in human pancreatic cancer. Clin Cancer Res 2007;13(7):2151–7.
73. Sfanos KS, Bruno TC, Meeker AK, et al. Human prostate-infiltrating CD8+ T lymphocytes are oligoclonal and PD-1+. Prostate 2009;69(15):1694–703.
74. Ahmadzadeh M, Johnson LA, Heemskerk B, et al. Tumor antigen-specific CD8 T cells infiltrating the tumor express high levels of PD-1 and are functionally impaired. Blood 2009;114(8):1537–44.
75. Topalian SL, Hodi FS, Brahmer JR, et al. Safety, activity, and immune correlates of anti-PD-1 antibody in cancer. N Engl J Med 2012;366(26):2443–54.
76. Brahmer JR, Tykodi SS, Chow LQ, et al. Safety and activity of anti-PD-L1 antibody in patients with advanced cancer. N Engl J Med 2012;366(26):2455–65.

77. Keir ME, Butte MJ, Freeman GJ, et al. PD-1 and its ligands in tolerance and immunity. Annu Rev Immunol 2008;26:677–704.

78. Nishimura H, Nose M, Hiai H, et al. Development of lupus-like autoimmune diseases by disruption of the PD-1 gene encoding an ITIM motif-carrying immunoreceptor. Immunity 1999;11(2):141–51.

79. Watts TH. TNF/TNFR family members in costimulation of T cell responses. Annu Rev Immunol 2005;23:23–68.

80. Cohen AD, Diab A, Perales MA, et al. Agonist anti-GITR antibody enhances vaccine induced CD8(+) T-cell responses and tumor immunity. Cancer Res 2006; 66(9):4904–12.

81. Lynch DH. The promise of 4-1BB (CD137)-mediated immunomodulation and the immunotherapy of cancer. Immunol Rev 2008;222:277–86.

82. Piconese S, Valzasina B, Colombo MP. OX40 triggering blocks suppression by regulatory T cells and facilitates tumor rejection. J Exp Med 2008;205(4): 825–39.

83. Ramirez-Montagut T, Chow A, Hirschhorn-Cymerman D, et al. Glucocorticoid-induced TNF receptor family related gene activation overcomes tolerance/ignorance to melanoma differentiation antigens and enhances antitumor immunity. J Immunol 2006;176(11):6434–42.

84. Sugamura K, Ishii N, Weinberg AD. Therapeutic targeting of the effector T-cell costimulatory molecule OX40. Nat Rev Immunol 2004;4(6):420–31.

85. Diehl L, den Boer AT, Schoenberger SP, et al. CD40 activation in vivo overcomes peptide-induced peripheral cytotoxic T-lymphocyte tolerance and augments anti-tumor vaccine efficacy. Nat Med 1999;5(7):774–9.

86. Pan PY, Ma G, Weber KJ, et al. Immune stimulatory receptor CD40 is required for T-cell suppression and T regulatory cell activation mediated by myeloid-derived suppressor cells in cancer. Cancer Res 2010;70(1):99–108.

87. Sotomayor EM, Borrello I, Tubb E, et al. Conversion of tumor-specific CD4+ T-cell tolerance to T-cell priming through in vivo ligation of CD40. Nat Med 1999;5(7):780–7.

88. van Mierlo GJ, Boonman ZF, Dumortier HM, et al. Activation of dendritic cells that crosspresent tumor-derived antigen licenses CD8+ CTL to cause tumor eradication. J Immunol 2004;173(11):6753–9.

89. Vonderheide RH, Flaherty KT, Khalil M, et al. Clinical activity and immune modulation in cancer patients treated with CP-870,893, a novel CD40 agonist monoclonal antibody. J Clin Oncol 2007;25(7):876–83.

90. Suntharalingam G, Perry MR, Ward S, et al. Cytokine storm in a phase 1 trial of the anti-CD28 monoclonal antibody TGN1412. N Engl J Med 2006;355(10):1018–28.

91. Croft M, Benedict CA, Ware CF. Clinical targeting of the TNF and TNFR superfamilies. Nat Rev Drug Discov 2013;12(2):147–68.

92. Restifo NP, Dudley ME, Rosenberg SA. Adoptive immunotherapy for cancer: harnessing the T cell response. Nat Rev Immunol 2012;12(4):269–81.

93. Rosenberg SA. Raising the bar: the curative potential of human cancer immunotherapy. Sci Transl Med 2012;4(127):127ps8.

94. Rosenberg SA, Packard BS, Aebersold PM, et al. Use of tumor-infiltrating lymphocytes and interleukin-2 in the immunotherapy of patients with metastatic melanoma. A preliminary report. N Engl J Med 1988;319(25):1676–80.

95. Dudley ME, Wunderlich JR, Yang JC, et al. Adoptive cell transfer therapy following nonmyeloablative but lymphodepleting chemotherapy for the treatment of patients with refractory metastatic melanoma. J Clin Oncol 2005;23(10): 2346–57.

96. Antony PA, Piccirillo CA, Akpinarli A, et al. CD8+ T cell immunity against a tumor/selfantigen is augmented by CD4+ T helper cells and hindered by naturally occurring T regulatory cells. J Immunol 2005;174(5):2591–601.
97. Ma J, Urba WJ, Si L, et al. Anti-tumor T cell response and protective immunity in mice that received sublethal irradiation and immune reconstitution. Eur J Immunol 2003;33(8):2123–32.
98. Klebanoff CA, Finkelstein SE, Surman DR, et al. IL-15 enhances the in vivo antitumor activity of tumor-reactive CD8+ T cells. Proc Natl Acad Sci U S A 2004; 101(7):1969–74.
99. Gattinoni L, Finkelstein SE, Klebanoff CA, et al. Removal of homeostatic cytokine sinks by lymphodepletion enhances the efficacy of adoptively transferred tumor-specific CD8+ T cells. J Exp Med 2005;202(7):907–12.
100. Rosenberg SA, Yang JC, Sherry RM, et al. Durable complete responses in heavily pretreated patients with metastatic melanoma using T-cell transfer immunotherapy. Clin Cancer Res 2011;17(13):4550–7.
101. Dudley ME, Wunderlich JR, Shelton TE, et al. Generation of tumor-infiltrating lymphocyte cultures for use in adoptive transfer therapy for melanoma patients. J Immunother 2003;26(4):332–42.
102. Johnson LA, Morgan RA, Dudley ME, et al. Gene therapy with human and mouse T-cell receptors mediates cancer regression and targets normal tissues expressing cognate antigen. Blood 2009;114(3):535–46.
103. Yee C. Adoptive T cell therapy: addressing challenges in cancer immunotherapy. J Transl Med 2005;3(1):17.
104. Weber J, Atkins M, Hwu P, et al. White paper on adoptive cell therapy for cancer with tumor-infiltrating lymphocytes: a report of the CTEP subcommittee on adoptive cell therapy. Clin Cancer Res 2011;17(7):1664–73.
105. Morgan RA, Dudley ME, Wunderlich JR, et al. Cancer regression in patients after transfer of genetically engineered lymphocytes. Science 2006;314(5796):126–9.
106. Parkhurst MR, Yang JC, Langan RC, et al. T cells targeting carcinoembryonic antigen can mediate regression of metastatic colorectal cancer but induce severe transient colitis. Mol Ther 2011;19(3):620–6.
107. Robbins PF, Morgan RA, Feldman SA, et al. Tumor regression in patients with metastatic synovial cell sarcoma and melanoma using genetically engineered lymphocytes reactive with NY-ESO-1. J Clin Oncol 2011;29(7):917–24.
108. Hanada K, Wang QJ, Inozume T, et al. Molecular identification of an MHC-independent ligand recognized by a human {alpha}/{beta} T-cell receptor. Blood 2011;117(18):4816–25.
109. Garrido F, Ruiz-Cabello F, Cabrera T, et al. Implications for immunosurveillance of altered HLA class I phenotypes in human tumours. Immunol Today 1997; 18(2):89–95.
110. Kochenderfer JN, Wilson WH, Janik JE, et al. Eradication of B-lineage cells and regression of lymphoma in a patient treated with autologous T cells genetically engineered to recognize CD19. Blood 2010;116(20):4099–102.
111. Kochenderfer JN, Dudley ME, Feldman SA, et al. B-cell depletion and remissions of malignancy along with cytokine-associated toxicity in a clinical trial of anti-CD19 chimeric-antigen-receptor-transduced T cells. Blood 2012;119(12):2709–20.
112. Porter DL, Levine BL, Kalos M, et al. Chimeric antigen receptor-modified T cells in chronic lymphoid leukemia. N Engl J Med 2011;365(8):725–33.
113. Kalos M, Levine BL, Porter DL, et al. T cells with chimeric antigen receptors have potent antitumor effects and can establish memory in patients with advanced leukemia. Sci Transl Med 2011;3(95):95ra73.

114. Lamers CH, Sleijfer S, Vulto AG, et al. Treatment of metastatic renal cell carcinoma with autologous T-lymphocytes genetically retargeted against carbonic anhydrase IX: first clinical experience. J Clin Oncol 2006;24(13):e20–2.

115. Park JR, Digiusto DL, Slovak M, et al. Adoptive transfer of chimeric antigen receptor redirected cytolytic T lymphocyte clones in patients with neuroblastoma. Mol Ther 2007;15(4):825–33.

116. Kershaw MH, Westwood JA, Parker LL, et al. A phase I study on adoptive immunotherapy using gene-modified T cells for ovarian cancer. Clin Cancer Res 2006;12(20 Pt 1):6106–15.

117. Morgan RA, Yang JC, Kitano M, et al. Case report of a serious adverse event following the administration of T cells transduced with a chimeric antigen receptor recognizing ERBB2. Mol Ther 2010;18(4):843–51.

118. Bast RC Jr, Segerling M, Ohanian SH, et al. Regression of established tumors and induction of tumor immunity by intratumor chemotherapy. J Natl Cancer Inst 1976;56(4):829–32.

119. Tesniere A, Schlemmer F, Boige V, et al. Immunogenic death of colon cancer cells treated with oxaliplatin. Oncogene 2010;29(4):482–91.

120. Obeid M, Tesniere A, Ghiringhelli F, et al. Calreticulin exposure dictates the immunogenicity of cancer cell death. Nat Med 2007;13(1):54–61.

121. Garnett CT, Schlom J, Hodge JW. Combination of docetaxel and recombinant vaccine enhances T-cell responses and antitumor activity: effects of docetaxel on immune enhancement. Clin Cancer Res 2008;14(11):3536–44.

122. Kodumudi KN, Woan K, Gilvary DL, et al. A novel chemoimmunomodulating property of docetaxel: suppression of myeloid-derived suppressor cells in tumor bearers. Clin Cancer Res 2010;16(18):4583–94.

123. Lutsiak ME, Semnani RT, De Pascalis R, et al. Inhibition of CD4(+)25+ T regulatory cell function implicated in enhanced immune response by low-dose cyclophosphamide. Blood 2005;105(7):2862–8.

124. Ghiringhelli F, Menard C, Puig PE, et al. Metronomic cyclophosphamide regimen selectively depletes CD4+CD25+ regulatory T cells and restores T and NK effector functions in end stage cancer patients. Cancer Immunol Immunother 2007;56(5):641–8.

125. Nowak AK, Robinson BW, Lake RA. Synergy between chemotherapy and immunotherapy in the treatment of established murine solid tumors. Cancer Res 2003;63(15):4490–6.

126. Antonia SJ, Mirza N, Fricke I, et al. Combination of p53 cancer vaccine with chemotherapy in patients with extensive stage small cell lung cancer. Clin Cancer Res 2006;12(3 Pt 1):878–87.

127. Arlen PM, Gulley JL, Parker C, et al. A randomized phase II study of concurrent docetaxel plus vaccine versus vaccine alone in metastatic androgen-independent prostate cancer. Clin Cancer Res 2006;12(4):1260–9.

128. Wheeler CJ, Das A, Liu G, et al. Clinical responsiveness of glioblastoma multiforme to chemotherapy after vaccination. Clin Cancer Res 2004;10(16):5316–26.

129. Postow MA, Callahan MK, Barker CA, et al. Immunologic correlates of the abscopal effect in a patient with melanoma. N Engl J Med 2012;366(10):925–31.

130. Woo SR, Turnis ME, Goldberg MV, et al. Immune inhibitory molecules LAG-3 and PD-1 synergistically regulate T-cell function to promote tumoral immune escape. Cancer Res 2012;72(4):917–27.

131. Sakuishi K, Apetoh L, Sullivan JM, et al. Targeting Tim-3 and PD-1 pathways to reverse T cell exhaustion and restore anti-tumor immunity. J Exp Med 2010; 207(10):2187–94.

132. Curran MA, Montalvo W, Yagita H, et al. PD-1 and CTLA-4 combination blockade expands infiltrating T cells and reduces regulatory T and myeloid cells within B16 melanoma tumors. Proc Natl Acad Sci U S A 2010;107(9):4275–80.

133. Swann JB, Vesely MD, Silva A, et al. Demonstration of inflammation-induced cancer and cancer immunoediting during primary tumorigenesis. Proc Natl Acad Sci U S A 2008;105(2):652–6.

134. Diaz-Montero CM, Salem ML, Nishimura MI, et al. Increased circulating myeloid-derived suppressor cells correlate with clinical cancer stage, metastatic tumor burden, and doxorubicin-cyclophosphamide chemotherapy. Cancer Immunol Immunother 2009;58(1):49–59.

135. Serafini P, Mgebroff S, Noonan K, et al. Myeloid-derived suppressor cells promote cross-tolerance in B-cell lymphoma by expanding regulatory T cells. Cancer Res 2008;68(13):5439–49.

136. Sica A, Bronte V. Altered macrophage differentiation and immune dysfunction in tumor development. J Clin Invest 2007;117(5):1155–66.

137. Solinas G, Germano G, Mantovani A, et al. Tumor-associated macrophages (TAM) as major players of the cancer-related inflammation. J Leukoc Biol 2009;86(5):1065–73.

138. Qian BZ, Pollard JW. Macrophage diversity enhances tumor progression and metastasis. Cell 2010;141(1):39–51.

139. Sica A, Larghi P, Mancino A, et al. Macrophage polarization in tumour progression. Semin Cancer Biol 2008;18(5):349–55.

140. Sasada T, Kimura M, Yoshida Y, et al. CD4+CD25+ regulatory T cells in patients with gastrointestinal malignancies: possible involvement of regulatory T cells in disease progression. Cancer 2003;98(5):1089–99.

141. Curiel TJ, Coukos G, Zou L, et al. Specific recruitment of regulatory T cells in ovarian carcinoma fosters immune privilege and predicts reduced survival. Nat Med 2004;10(9):942–9.

142. Bates GJ, Fox SB, Han C, et al. Quantification of regulatory T cells enables the identification of high-risk breast cancer patients and those at risk of late relapse. J Clin Oncol 2006;24(34):5373–80.

143. Tan W, Zhang W, Strasner A, et al. Tumour-infiltrating regulatory T cells stimulate mammary cancer metastasis through RANKL-RANK signalling. Nature 2011; 470(7335):548–53.

Clinical Applications of Translational Research

Translational Research in Melanoma

Madhury Ray, MD[a], Jeffrey M. Farma, MD[b], Cary Hsu, MD[c],*

KEYWORDS

- Melanoma • Translational research • Immunotherapy • Targeted therapy

KEY POINTS

- Recent advances in systemic therapy for melanoma have altered the outlook for patients afflicted with advanced stages of the disease.
- Effective immunotherapy is associated with infrequent and slowly developing responses, which may result in durable remission of disease at the expense of significant autoimmune toxicities.
- Targeted therapies are associated with high response rates and rapid tumor regression, however drug resistance almost invariably develops.
- Robust biomarkers need to be identified in order to increase the probability that the individual patient is likely to benefit from a specific therapeutic strategy.

Melanoma is the fifth most common malignancy in the United States, representing a remarkable increase in incidence, as noted in population studies.[1,2] It follows that melanoma also carries one of the fastest increasing death rates.[3] Surgery has long been the cornerstone of melanoma therapy, with only limited efficacy reported from an array of adjuvant strategies and therapies for unresectable disease. Although survival for patients with localized disease is excellent, survival declines precipitously for those with metastatic disease, who have an expected 2-year survival rate of 10% to 20%.[4,5] Until 2011, only 3 drugs had been approved as treatment options for patients with metastatic melanoma: dacarbazine (DTIC), fotemustine, and interleukin 2 (IL-2). Standard chemotherapy regimens have response rates of approximately 15%, and duration of response tends to be on the order of months, although durable, complete responses (CRs) have been reported. Combinations of cytotoxic agents have been investigated and have not substantially improved survival outcomes compared with

Disclosures: The authors have nothing to disclose.
a Division of General Surgery, Department of Surgery, David Geffen School of Medicine at the University of California, Los Angeles, 10833 Le Conte Avenue, Los Angeles, CA 90095, USA; b Fox Chase Cancer Center, 333 Cottman Avenue, Philadelphia, PA 19111, USA; c Division of Surgical Oncology, Department of Surgery, David Geffen School of Medicine at the University of California, Los Angeles, 10833 Le Conte Avenue, Los Angeles, CA 90095, USA
* Corresponding author. 1304 15th Street, Suite 102, Santa Monica, CA 90404.
E-mail address: caryhsu@mednet.ucla.edu

Surg Oncol Clin N Am 22 (2013) 785–804
http://dx.doi.org/10.1016/j.soc.2013.06.009
1055-3207/13/$ – see front matter © 2013 Elsevier Inc. All rights reserved.

DTIC alone.[6] Despite vigorous efforts to bring new therapies from the bench to bedside, approval by the US Food and Drug Administration (FDA) of the cytokine IL-2 in 1998 was the only new therapy to arise in more than 30 years after standard cytotoxic chemotherapy regimens had been established.[6,7] Effective therapies for unresectable melanoma have long represented an unmet need based on the rapidly increasing incidence and poor prognosis of advanced disease states.

During the past 2 years, there has been renewed optimism as the translation of basic scientific findings into positive clinical trial data has resulted in the approval of efficacious new agents. In addition, several promising new therapies are in the final stages of clinical testing. These advances have evolved through 2 seemingly unrelated approaches: immunotherapy and targeted therapy. This review highlights important recent translational research findings and their impact on the care of patients with melanoma (**Table 1**).

IMMUNOTHERAPY

The foundation for modern cancer immunotherapy for melanoma was the development of the cytokine IL-2 as a therapeutic agent during the 1980s. IL-2 is a common γ-chain cytokine required for T-cell growth and activation. It has no direct tumoricidal activity; rather, its antitumor activity derives from its influence on the cytotoxic activity of T lymphocytes, which recognize and destroy the tumor.[8] Although objective responses occur in only approximately 15% of patients with melanoma, nearly half of responding patients have a CR. With long-term follow-up, complete responders frequently (>80%) have durable remission, with many of these patients believed to be cured.[9] The sustainability of responses and potential for cure clearly distinguish immunotherapy from other available systemic therapies.

Most of the work in the immunotherapy for melanoma has focused on T-cell–mediated responses. Dendritic cells (DCs) are professional antigen-presenting cells (APCs) that capture antigens and present them to naive T cells in the context of activating costimulatory signals, thereby initiating the immune response.[10] In the absence of costimulation, T cells are induced into a state of unresponsiveness, or anergy.[11] Tumor-associated antigens (TAA) are bound to major histocompatibility complex (MHC) class I molecules and presented on the surface of tumor cells. When activated CD8+ T cells with the appropriate receptor encounter a tumor cell showing the TAA, they are able to perform their cytolytic killing functions on the tumor target and release inflammatory cytokines to activate neighboring immune cells. This summary is inadequate to encompass all of the complexities involved in the regulation of cellular immune responses against tumors, but it provides the framework to understand the work to be discussed.

Vaccines

Melanoma vaccines have been investigated as adjuvant therapy in resected patients with high risk of recurrence as well as in the therapy for metastatic disease. Generically, vaccines consist of tumor antigen(s) in a formulation designed to activate the cellular arm of the immune system. A common approach has been the use of peptide vaccines of variable length containing the sequence of the target TAAs. These peptides are typically administered with an adjuvant, such as incomplete Freund's adjuvant or bacterial derivatives like bacillus Calmette-Guérin, which stimulate immune responses nonspecifically. Vaccination strategies using viruses or naked DNA encoding TAAs have been investigated. A spectrum of strategies with DC vaccines have been explored.[10] Irradiated autologous or allogeneic tumor preparations have been

Table 1
Selected clinical trials for advanced melanoma

Reference	Classification	Patients (n)	Treatment	Response Rate (%)	Duration of Response (mo)	Median PFS (mo)	Overall Survival (%)
Schwartzentruber et al,[14] 2011	Immunotherapy (vaccine) phase 3	94 91	gp100 + IL-2 IL-2	16 6	NR NR	2.2 1.6	NR NR
Bedikian et al,[16] 2010	Immunotherapy (vaccine) phase 2	127	Allovectin-7	11.8	13.8	1.6	NR
Senzer et al,[22] 2009	Immunotherapy (vaccine) phase 2	50	OncoVEX GM-CSF	26	NR	NR	58 at 1 y 52 at 2 y
Hodi et al,[49] 2010	Immunotherapy (checkpoint blockade) phase 3	137 136	Ipilimumab ± gp100 gp100	10.9 1.5	NR NR	2.8 2.8	45.6 at 1 y 23.5 at 2 y 25.3 at 1 y 13.7 at 2 y
Robert et al,[50] 2011	Immunotherapy (checkpoint blockade) phase 3	250 252	Ipilimumab + DTIC DTIC	15.2 10.3	NR NR	2.8 2.8	47.3 at 1 y 28.5 at 2 y 36.3 at 1 y 17.9 at 2 y
Topalian et al,[57] 2012	Immunotherapy (checkpoint blockade) phase 1	94	Anti-PD-1 Ab	28	NR	NR	NR
Brahmer et al,[56] 2012	Immunotherapy (checkpoint blockade) phase 1	52	Anti-PD-L1 Ab	17.3	NR	NR	NR
Chapman et al,[67] 2011	Targeted therapy (BRAF inhibition) phase 3	337 338	Vemurafenib DTIC	48.4 5.4	6.7 NR	5.3 1.6	84 at 6 mo 56 at 1 y 66 at 6 mo 44 at 1 y
Hauschild et al,[77] 2012	Targeted therapy (BRAF inhibition) phase 3	187 63	Dabrafenib DTIC	49.7 6.3	5.6 (estimated) NR	5.1 2.7	NR NR
Flaherty et al,[89] 2012	Targeted therapy (MEK inhibition) phase 3	214 108	Trametinib DTIC or paclitaxel	22 8.3	5.5 NR	4.8 1.5	81 at 6 mo 67 at 6 mo
Flaherty et al,[92] 2012	Targeted therapy (combined BRAF/MEK inhibition) phase 1/2	54 54	Dabrafenib plus trametinib Dabrafenib	75.9 53.7	10.5 6.1	9.4 5.8	79 at 1 y 70 at 1 y

Abbreviations: Ab, antibody; NR, not reported.
Data from Refs.[14,16,22,30,36,37,49,67,77,89,92]

used as vaccines. Vaccines have been administered in conjunction with immunostimulatory cytokines such as IL-2, IL-12, and granulocyte-macrophage colony-stimulating factor (GM-CSF).

There are several conceptually appealing features of vaccine strategies: vaccines are most often administered in the outpatient setting, with minimal need for specialized care; they are typically associated with minimal side effects; and, if successful, they may lead to lasting tumor immunity. Investigations in this area have been disappointing in their failure to consistently and clearly show clinical efficacy.[7,12] Klebanoff and colleagues[13] recently examined notable contemporary cancer vaccine trials reported since 2004; overall, only 12 of 309 (3.9%) patients with melanoma had objective responses. In retrospect, this entire body of work highlights our incomplete understanding of the mechanisms required to trigger antitumor immunity. Through these early failures, there have been substantial gains in fundamental knowledge and promise for a path to improving on immunization strategies.

The lack of efficacy in vaccine trials has been attributed to a variety of shortcomings. First, the central role of DCs in successful immunization was not recognized as cancer vaccines were first being developed, and this point has only recently been addressed in newer vaccine studies. It has been recognized that adjuvant agents are crucial for the initiation of immune responses, yet the array of approved adjuvants remains woefully limited and their function poorly understood. Despite the identification of hundreds of TAAs, it remains unclear which are the best targets to reach the end point of clinical efficacy. Also, antigen expression within any given tumor is heterogeneous and the ability of the tumor to show these antigens is often compromised. Another previously underappreciated component of vaccine strategies is the need to overcome mechanisms of immunosuppression mediated by the tumor or present in the tumor microenvironment. Each successive generation of studies of cancer vaccines has incorporated strategies based in the continuously expanding knowledge of immunobiology.

We have only recently reached the important benchmark of a positive phase 3 study of melanoma vaccines, with 2 promising unrelated studies soon to be reported. Schwartzentruber and colleagues[14] recently published the findings of a multicenter, phase 3 study evaluating the combination of the peptide vaccine gp100 with high-dose IL-2 compared with IL-2 alone. The addition of the peptide vaccine significantly improved response rates (16% vs 6%) and progression-free survival (PFS) (2.2 months vs 1.6 months). There was a trend toward improved median survival (17.8 months vs 11.1 months; $P = .06$). This monumental effort validates the potential of vaccine strategies in the treatment of established metastatic melanoma but also underscores the need for innovation to enhance efficacy.

Allovectin-7 is a novel vaccine for metastatic melanoma that has shown promise in early-phase clinical studies.[15–17] Downregulation or loss of expression of MHC class I and β_2 microglobulin molecules has been identified as 1 mechanism through which tumor cells may escape immune detection.[18,19] Allovectin-7 is a plasmid DNA encoding HLA-B7 and β_2 microglobulin. This vaccine is injected directly into tumors and results in the assembly of a complete MHC class I complex on the tumor surface. It is proposed that the vaccine may have activity through several mechanisms, including expression of a foreign antigen (in HLA-B7–negative patients), increased TAA presentation in the context of HLA-B7, and increased surface expression of MHC class I molecules on the tumor surface (because of the increased availability of β_2 microglobulin molecules). In addition, it is possible that unmethylated bacterial CpG motifs in the plasmid backbone may stimulate immune responses, as has been shown in animal models.[20] Objective response rates of 4% to 11% have been reported in phase 2 studies, with some patients undergoing CR. Antitumor responses have been reproducible in multiple phase 2 trials, and all studies document an extremely favorable toxicity profile. A phase 3 clinical trial comparing Allovectin-7 with DTIC or temozolomide has recently completed accrual.

Another promising vaccine is OncoVEX[GM-CSF], an oncolytic herpes simplex virus type 1 that has been genetically engineered for tumor-selective replication and enhanced tumoricidal activity.[21] In addition, the virus encodes the immunomodulatory cytokine GM-CSF, which stimulates the proliferation, maturation, and differentiation of DCs. The vaccine is injected intratumorally. Responses are seen both in the injected lesions and at distant sites. It is presumed that tumor lysis at the site of injection releases antigens, which are subsequently presented by DCs, initiating systemic antitumor effects. In a phase 2 study, the objective response rate was 26%, with more than half of patients achieving CR.[22] Subsequently, an eagerly anticipated phase 3 study has completed accrual, with results expected shortly.

Adoptive Cell Transfer Therapy

Adoptive cell transfer therapy (ACT) for patients with unresectable melanoma has evolved through elegant basic, translational, and clinical research.[23] ACT involves resection of a melanoma metastasis, isolation of tumor-infiltrating lymphocytes (TILs) from the tumor explant, expansion of the T-cell cultures in vitro, and reinfusion of autologous tumor reactive cells together with IL-2 into the patient, after a lymphodepleting preparation. Transgenic mouse models of ACT have played a major role in the optimization of human protocols. Murine studies have clarified desirable characteristics of transferred T cells, the importance of lymphodepletion, and the role of APCs.[24] The Surgery Branch of the National Cancer Institute[25] recently reported their extensive experience with ACT in the therapy for 93 heavily pretreated patients with metastatic melanoma. Objective response rates greater than 70% were achieved in the most recent series. Durable, complete tumor regression was achieved in 22% of patients, with an actuarial 5-year survival of 93% in patients with CR. No other therapy has matched these outcomes.

More recently, genetically modified peripheral blood lymphocytes have been used in ACT studies.[26] Antitumor activity has been reported in patients with melanoma treated with T cells retrovirally transduced with high-affinity T-cell receptors (TCRs) recognizing tumor antigens such as MART-1, NY-ESO-1, and MAGE-A3.[27–29] Chimeric antigen receptors (CARs) comprise the tumor antigen-binding domain of an antibody molecule fused to the intracellular signaling domain of a TCR. CARs specific for high-molecular-weight melanoma-associated antigen and ganglioside GD3 have shown promise in preclinical testing.[30,31] CARs have several theoretic advantages over TCR-based gene transfer. Effector cell engagement does not depend on peptide antigen expression and MHC-restricted presentation by the tumor, potential mechanisms by which tumors may escape immune detection. Because they function in an MHC-independent manner, there may be wider applicability to patients as an off-the-shelf reagent. In addition, there is the ability to engineer these CARs to express the intracellular signaling domains of a variety of costimulatory molecules to improve T-cell function and survival.

Immunomodulation

Clinical trials of IL-2 showed that the immune system could be activated nonspecifically to promote tumor regression in patients with melanoma.[9,32,33] One implication of these trials is that patients with melanoma frequently have endogenous lymphocytes capable of recognizing tumor antigens; it has also been established that lymphocytes that recognize the tumor frequently reside near the tumor.[34] Substantial evidence indicates that the tumor interacts with responding lymphocytes to subvert the immune response and permit tumor growth, a process referred to as immunoediting.[18]

According to the classic 2-signal model of T-cell activation, the first signal is provided through the interaction of the antigen-MHC complex with the TCR. Naive T cells encountering an antigen must also receive a second signal to initiate an immune response. This process occurs through the interaction of CD28 receptors on T cells with B7-1 (CD80) and B7-2 (CD86) molecules, which are present on APCs. In the absence of costimulation, T cells become anergic.[11,35] Subsequently, additional costimulatory pathways providing both activating (CD28, OX40, GITR, CD137, CD27, HVEM) and inhibiting (CTLA-4, PD-1, TIM-3, BTLA, VISTA, LAG-3) second signals have been identified.[36] The interplay of these costimulatory molecules serves to precisely control the intensity and duration of cellular immune responses. Elucidation of these diverse pathways has broadened the concept of costimulation, and these immunologic checkpoints represent new targets for therapeutic intervention.

Cytotoxic T Lymphocyte Antigen 4 Blockade

Cytotoxic T lymphocyte antigen 4 (CTLA-4) was identified as a homologue of CD28, which receives the second signal in T-cell activation.[37] In contrast to CD28, it is not present on the surface of naive T cells but is rapidly upregulated with T-cell activation.[37,38] CTLA-4 binds B7-1 and B7-2 with significantly higher affinity than CD28, and signaling through CTLA-4 engagement serves to attenuate T-cell activation and proliferation.[39,40] Its native function has been described a brake that prevents productive immune responses from progressing to autoimmune injury; CTLA-4–deficient mice die at 3 to 4 weeks of age from a fatal lymphoproliferative disorder.[41] CTLA-4 is overexpressed on chronically stimulated and exhausted T cells.[42,43] In addition, CTLA-4 is constitutively expressed on T-regulatory cells, which may be crucial for their suppressive function.[44] Blockade of CTLA-4 results in enhanced T-cell–mediated immune responses, and numerous animal models have shown that tumor immunity can be induced by interfering with CTLA-4 signaling.[41] Subsequently, ipilimumab, a fully human monoclonal antibody, was developed as a therapeutic agent to block CTLA-4. Early-phase clinical trials reported activity in patients with metastatic melanoma.[45–48]

Ipilimumab received FDA approval in 2011 after the publication of a phase 3 study in which patients with metastatic melanoma were treated with ipilimumab alone or in combination with the gp100 peptide vaccine. The control arm received only the gp100 vaccine. All patients had received previous therapy with other agents, including more than 20% of patients receiving IL-2. There were significant differences in survival with 1-year and 2-year overall survival of 45.6% and 23.5% in patients receiving ipilimumab compared with 25.3% and 13.7% in patients receiving gp100 alone. Overall survival was independent of previous IL-2 therapy, suggesting that these immunomodulating agents act through different mechanisms. Grade 3 or 4 toxicities were frequent (10% to 15%), and death attributed to immune-related adverse events occurred in approximately 1% of patients.[49] The gp100 vaccine did not enhance the efficacy of CTLA-4 blockade, as was seen when this vaccine was combined with IL-2.[14] This finding reinforces the concept that IL-2 and anti-CTLA-4 have inherently different mechanisms of action. This landmark study is the first randomized clinical trial showing a benefit in overall survival for patients metastatic with melanoma. Another pivotal phase 3 study examined the efficacy and safety of ipilimumab plus DTIC compared with DTIC alone in 502 patients with previously untreated metastatic melanoma.[50] The 1-year, 2-year, and 3-year survival were 47.3%, 28.5%, and 20.8% for patients receiving ipilimumab and DTIC compared with 36.3%, 17.9%, and 12.2% for patients receiving DTIC alone. Grade 3 or higher immune-mediated adverse events were documented in 38.1% of patients receiving ipilimumab; there were no deaths attributed to autoimmune phenomena.

Prieto and colleagues[51] recently reported the longest follow-up on patients with melanoma treated with ipilimumab in 3 consecutive trials conducted at the National Cancer Institute. With median follow-up of 71 to 92 months, this study reveals unique and important features of this therapy that are often not apparent in the randomized studies. First, objective responses frequently evolved slowly; in complete responders, the median time to CR was 30 months, with 1 patient achieving CR at 71 months. Reports with shorter follow-up may underestimate the true objective response rate. Second, CRs are remarkably durable, with only 1 of 15 patients recurring after CR; all of the other patients with CR were alive without evidence of disease with median follow-up of 83 months. This finding is reminiscent of the experience with IL-2, and it is tempting to speculate that some of these patients may be cured.

Programmed Death 1/Programmed Death Ligand 1 Blockade

Programmed death 1 (PD-1) and its ligands, PD-L1 and PD-L2, have recently attracted attention as another immunologic checkpoint that can be manipulated to achieve antitumor immune responses.[52] PD-1 was first identified in 1992 and its ligands nearly 10 years later. Signaling through the PD-1/PD-L1(-L2) axis serves to dampen T-cell–mediated immune responses and plays a critical role in central tolerance induction. Inflammation and cardiomyopathy have been observed in PD-1 knockout mice. This autoimmune phenotype is considerably milder than that seen in CTLA-4 knockout mice and does not manifest until 6 to 9 months after birth. PD-1 is not expressed on naive T cells but is induced quickly on activation. When antigen-specific T cells are chronically stimulated, PD-1 is upregulated, and the cells become functionally impaired; T-cell function can be restored with PD-1 blockade.[53] In TILs derived from patients with melanoma, increased PD-1 expression has been correlated with an exhausted phenotype and impaired effector function.[42] PD-L1 is constitutively expressed in hematopoietic cells and a wide variety of other tissues. Because of this distribution, it has been postulated that this pathway serves to protect normal peripheral tissues from activated T cells, thus limiting autoimmunity. PD-L1 is also expressed by many tumors, including melanoma. In solid tumors, PD-L1 can inhibit the cytolytic activity of tumor-infiltrating T cells.[54,55] Furthermore, PD-L1 expression has been correlated with an unfavorable prognosis in a variety of cancer histologies.[52] Expression of PD-L1 is believed to be a mechanism by which tumors may escape immune rejection.

Two concurrently published phase 1 clinical trials using monoclonal antibodies to disrupt the PD-1/PD-L1 axis have shown promising clinical efficacy across an array of histologies including non–small cell lung cancer, melanoma, and renal cell cancer.[56,57] In the study reported by Topalian and colleagues, anti-PD-1 antibody was administered in escalating doses to 296 patients. These individuals included 94 patients with melanoma, for whom the objective response rate was 28%. Most responding patients had durable responses of greater than 1 year. Pretreatment tumor specimens were available from a few study patients, and it was noted that objective responses were observed only in patients whose tumors expressed PD-L1, suggesting that this may be a potential biomarker for patient selection. Grade 3 or higher toxicities occurred in 14% of patients. Potential autoimmune toxicities included pneumonitis, vitiligo, colitis, hepatitis, hypophysitis, and thyroiditis. There were 3 cases of fatal pneumonitis. Brahmer and colleagues reported the companion trial, in which patients with a variety of histologies were treated with escalating does of anti-PD-L1 antibody. In the patients with melanoma, 9 of 52 patients had objective responses (17%), including 3 CRs. As reported with the anti-PD-1 antibody, responses tended to be durable, and stable disease (27%) was a frequent outcome in patients not classified as having an objective response. Grade 3 or 4 toxicities occurred in only 9% of study patients. Potentially immune-related toxicities included rash, hypothyroidism, hepatitis, sarcoidosis, endophthalmitis, diabetes mellitus, and myasthenia gravis. Taken together, these studies show that blockade of PD-1 or PD-L1 can result in tumor regression, with a pattern of response similar to that seen with CTLA-4 blockade. The immune-related toxicities attributed to anti-PD-1 and anti-PD-L1 are less infrequent and milder than those associated with anti-CTLA-4. Phase 2 and 3 trials will further define the efficacy and applicability of these therapies, and FDA approval of 1 or both agents seems imminent based on the dramatic results already reported.

TARGETED THERAPIES

Significant advances have come in our understanding of the molecular signaling pathways and the genetic mutations involved in the progression from normal melanocyte to melanoma.[58] Therapies directed toward specific melanoma driver mutations have subsequently evolved. Inhibitors of the mitogen-activated protein kinase (MAPK), AKT, and KIT pathways are discussed.

The MAPK Pathway and BRAF Mutations in Melanoma

The BRAF protein, a serine-threonine kinase, mediates an early step of the MAPK signaling pathway, which, in the normal cell, connects the activation of RAS (a membrane-bound G-protein) with the nuclear-mediated activities of angiogenesis, cell growth, and avoidance of apoptosis.[59] Specifically, activated RAS activates the RAF proteins (A-, B-, C-), which results in the phosphorylation of MEK, which in turn phosphorylates ERK, which translocates into the nucleus and acts as a progrowth and antiapoptotic agent (**Fig. 1**).[60]

In 2002, by sequencing the genomes of several different types of tumor cells, Davies and colleagues[61] described a single mutation in *BRAF* that occurred frequently in melanomas but also in colon and ovarian cancers. This V600 mutation was later confirmed to be present in approximately 50% of melanomas and 7% of all cancers. Additional work in the same study showed that cells with a V600E mutation show constitutive activation of the MAPK pathway independent of RAS activation. Because RAS did not seem to be relevant in V600E-mediated cancer, attention was focused on the RAF proteins. BRAF, 1 of the 3 RAF proteins, was already known to be the main activator of MEK.[62]

In 2007, Terai and colleagues[63] showed that, in the normal cell, after activation by RAS, BRAF homodimerizes (or occasionally heterodimerizes with CRAF) in order to become the primary activator of MEK. However, the V600E mutants express a constitutively active monomeric BRAF, which does not require catalytic activation by RAS to activate MEK, and subsequently active ERK. In addition to promoting tumor growth and resisting apoptosis, V600E mutants also alter the tumor microenvironment and allow cancerous cells to evade the immune system.[64]

The initial unsuccessful clinical efforts to target RAF used sorafenib, a nonselective RAF inhibitor that only weakly inhibited both mutant and wild-type BRAF.[65] In 2008, Tsai and colleagues published in vitro and animal data describing a selective BRAF inhibitor, which blocked mutant, but not wild-type, BRAF activity. By 2011, the

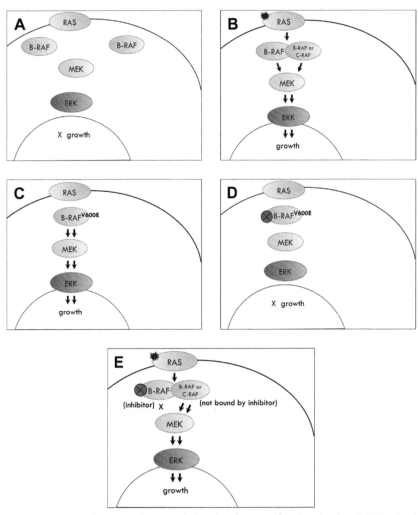

Fig. 1. RAS-RAF signaling in melanoma. (*A*) In the absence of RAS activation, BRAF exists in a monomeric form. The remainder of the pathway remains inactive. (*B*) On RAS activation, BRAF either homodimerizes or heterodimerizes with CRAF. Each dimer protein activates MEK, which in turn activates ERK, propagating downstream signaling. (*C*) Mutant BRAF is active as a monomer in the absence of RAS activation, and activates MEK constitutively. Activated MEK in turn activates ERK, leading to cell growth. (*D*) When selective BRAF inhibitors inactivate mutant BRAF, cell growth is arrested. (*E*) In the setting of RAS activation, selective BRAF inhibitors inactivate only 1 member of the BRAF dimer. The other protein in the dimer is transactivated and downstream signaling is paradoxically activated.

selective inhibitor PLX4032, now known as vemurafenib, was approved by the FDA for the treatment of metastatic melanoma.[66,67]

Selective BRAF Inhibitors: Vemurafenib and Dabrafenib

Vemurafenib is a synthetic small molecule that competitively binds the adenosine triphosphate (ATP)-binding site of both mutant and wild-type BRAF kinases. The selectivity of the drug is based on nuanced differences between the wild-type and mutant MAPK pathways at the level of BRAF.[68] At rest, in the wild-type cell, BRAF exists as a monomer with minimal phosphorylation of MEK. When growth factors cause RAS activation, BRAF dimerizes into an active form, and MEK is activated by phosphorylation. The V600E mutant BRAF exists in a constitutively active monomeric form that does not require dimerization, growth signals, or RAS activation to activate MEK.[69]

The ATP-binding site is conserved between wild-type and mutant BRAF. Direct binding of vemurafenib blocks ATP and inhibits kinase activity. However, in the wild-type cell, therapeutic doses of vemurafenib (960 mg orally twice a day), results in a conformational change that increases the activity of the unbound monomer. The net result is that the total activity of the BRAF dimer remains unchanged, and normal feedback loops regulate growth and activity of the cell. The mutant monomer does not have a second, hyperactive BRAF monomer to compensate for its inactivity, and its ability to activate MEK is compromised by vemurafenib.[64]

In 2010, this elegant model culminated in the BRIM 3 (BRAF Inhibitor in Melanoma 3) phase 3 clinical trial of vemurafenib in patients with metastatic melanoma bearing the V600E mutation. At 6 months, patients treated with vemurafenib had a survival of 84% (vs 64% in the standard melanoma therapy arm), and progression of the disease was delayed by nearly 4 months. Approximately half of patients (vs 5.5% with standard therapy) responded to treatment. This finding translated to a relative reduction of 63% in the risk of death and of 74% in the risk of either death or disease progression.[67] Cutaneous side effects and arthralgia are the most common adverse events encountered with vemurafenib and occur in 5% to 40% of cases.[67] Of the cutaneous side effects, the most striking has recently been labeled the RASopathy. This term refers to the development of secondary, RAS-driven (as opposed to RAS-independent, BRAF-driven) cancers such as keratoacanthomas and other squamous cell neoplasms, which occur in approximately 25% of patients.[70] In general, these de novo cancers are well differentiated, easy to diagnose with active surveillance, generally curable with local treatment, and regress on cessation of vemurafenib treatment.[71]

In 2010, preclinical studies elucidated a mechanism to explain these secondary malignancies. Although vemurafenib was developed based on the activation of MEK and ERK by BRAF monomers and homodimers, a minor pathway also exists in which BRAF and CRAF form an active heterodimer that can also activate MEK and ERK.[72] In RAS-primed cells, which already bear a RAS mutation, this BRAF-CRAF heterodimer pathway becomes more prevalent, but these cells are not oncogenic.[73] In the setting of inactivated BRAF, the situation changes. Similar to the way that an inhibited wild-type BRAF monomer transactivates its uninhibited partner BRAF in a homodimer during vemurafenib treatment, inactive BRAF transphosphorylates CRAF in the RAS-primed heterodimer and paradoxically renders it more active, resulting in excessive activation of MEK and ERK, which in turn results in malignant cellular growth.[74] Pathologic and dermatologic studies confirm that most of these cutaneous lesions bear RAS mutations.[75] New cutaneous neoplasms are not a contraindication to the treatment of melanoma with vemurafenib, but as the scope and duration of treatment expand, the significance of RAS-primed malignancies may increase.

Approximately a decade after the discovery of the role of V600E mutant BRAF in melanoma, elucidation of this key pathway was translated into a targeted therapy with efficacy and minor side effects. At 6 months, the phase 3 trial evaluation of vemurafenib was closed early because of the clear benefits of treatment, and the drug was granted FDA approval for treatment in metastatic melanoma. Despite impressive initial tumor shrinkage in responding patients, it quickly became apparent that responses are short-lived. In more than 90% of cases, the dramatic tumor responses of reverse course and disease progression are evident within 6 to 8 months after the initiation of treatment.[76]

In June, 2012, a phase 3 clinical trial was completed on dabrafenib, another selective BRAF inhibitor with a similar mechanism to vemurafenib, which may retain the efficacy of vemurafenib with a lower incidence of secondary cutaneous malignancies. Median PFS was 5.1 months in the dabrafenib arm compared with 2.7 months for DTIC.[77] In patients with metastatic melanoma, brain metastases are a frequent finding and are associated with a poor prognosis. Because of the size of vemurafenib (ie, >300 kDa), it was never expected to cross the blood-brain barrier. For this reason, all of the initial trials of vemurafenib excluded patients with brain metastases.[78] However, anecdotal reports and an open-label pilot study have shown some efficacy in the treatment of brain metastases.[79] Dabrafenib is a smaller molecule than vemurafenib, and thus may have better penetration of the blood-brain barrier. In a phase 1 dose escalation trial of dabrafenib, 9 of 10 V600 mutant patients with asymptomatic, untreated brain metastases showed a decrease in the size of the brain metastases, with complete resolution in 4. The median duration of response was 4.2 months.[80] As with metastases outside the brain, resistance seems to develop to both of these drugs.[81] However, as strategies to combat resistance are developed, selective BRAF inhibitors may prove to be a useful therapy for melanoma brain metastases.

The mechanisms of resistance seem to be multifactorial and complex. Mutations in the ATP-binding site of mutant BRAF kinase, the so-called gatekeeper mutations that cause resistance to other targeted therapies, do not seem to be the cause of resistance to vemurafenib.[82] Investigations have focused on MAPK-dependent and MAPK-independent mechanisms of resistance.[83]

MAPK-Dependent Resistance

An understanding of the MAPK pathway and the paradoxic transactivation of dimeric RAF kinases in mutant BRAF-inhibited cells explains both the selectivity of vemurafenib and some of its most significant side effects. Similarly, genetic studies of melanoma cells that have acquired resistance to vemurafenib show slightly overactive RAF dimers because of an activated RAS mutation.[84] In the setting of V600E BRAF mutant inhibition, cells with a mutation that allows them to be transactivated by vemurafenib are selected for and overcome MAPK pathway inhibition.[85]

One proposed method for treating resistance relies on the idea that these vemurafenib-resistant transactivated mutant melanoma cells may become dependent on the drug to activate them. Recent work by Das Thakur and colleagues[86] shows a significant delay in the development of resistance using a discontinuous dosing therapy, which interferes with the proliferation of vemurafenib-driven clones during breaks in therapy. In addition, a new class of paradox breaker BRAF inhibitors that do not paradoxically activate the downstream MAPK pathway are being investigated. These agents retain the selectivity of vemurafenib and have shown increased PFS.[87]

At the end of 2010, Johannessen and colleagues[88] described a mechanism of resistance that relied on MAPK pathway activation, but bypassed RAF entirely. Using genetic screening, the group used cell lines and biopsy samples from patients with vemurafenib resistance to identify COT, a MAP kinase and activator of MEK encoded by the MAPK38 gene, which acts independently of RAF and RAS kinases. These investigators found that COT protein expression is almost completely suppressed when V600E-mutant BRAF is expressed, but in the setting of mutant BRAF inhibition or knockdown, COT is overexpressed and thus overactivates the MAPK pathway at the level of MEK.

With RAF inhibition, the MAPK pathway can be activated by other kinases to cause side effects and resistance. Thus, there have been efforts to target the pathway downstream. Phase 3 trials were recently completed on trametinib, a reversible small molecule inhibitor of both MEK I and MEK II, the kinases immediately downstream to the RAF kinases. In metastatic patients with melanoma with a *V600* BRAF mutation who were naive to BRAF inhibitor therapy, 6-month survival rates were improved versus standard cytotoxic chemotherapy alone (81%), and although PFS was better than standard cytotoxic chemotherapy, it was shorter than PFS observed in studies of vemurafenib (4.8 vs 7 months). The side effect profile was also different, with rash (a different type of rash than that caused by BRAF inhibitors), edema, hypertension, and diarrhea being most common. Ocular side effects and a rare, reversible cardiomyopathy were also noted. The squamous cell carcinomas observed with BRAF inhibitor therapy were not seen with trametinib treatment.[89,90]

Based on its mechanism as a downstream inhibitor of the MAPK pathway, trametinib was also evaluated as a therapy in metastatic melanoma that had acquired resistance to the BRAF inhibitors. In 2013, phase 2 trials were completed comparing trametinib treatment in BRAF inhibitor–naive metastatic patients with melanoma with treatment in patients who were already BRAF inhibitor resistant. Trametinib therapy in the setting of BRAF resistance conferred no clinically objective advantage.[91] In vitro studies showed minimal response of COT kinase to trametinib.[88] Thus, trametinib does not show promise as a single agent over vemurafenib (or its successor dabrafenib), nor does it seem effective in combating BRAF inhibitor resistance. However, its role in combination therapy seems more promising.

Phase 3 trials are under way to evaluate combination therapy with dabrafenib and trametinib, based on promising phase 2 results. These results showed a response rate of 76% (vs 54% for dabrafenib alone) and an impressive PFS of 9.4 months and duration of response of 10.5 months. Furthermore, cutaneous neoplasms were less frequent with combination therapy compared with dabrafenib alone. Hypertension and diarrhea were decreased relative to trametinib alone.[92]

MAPK-Independent Resistance: the PI3/AKT Pathway

Another canonical pathway in oncogenesis is the PI3/AKT pathway. In this pathway, one of several membrane-bound receptors, such as RAS or insulinlike growth factor 1 receptor (IGF-1R), activates the PI3 kinase, which in turn activates the AKT kinase, which activates small molecules such as mammalian target of rapamycin (mTOR) and results in cell growth and evasion of apoptosis. The pathway is inhibited by the molecule PTEN.[93,94] In vitro studies have shown cross-talk between the 2 pathways in multiple cancers.[95]

In 2010, Villaneueva and colleagues[96] reported the increased presence of IGF-1R and activated AKT in biopsy samples from patients with melanoma who had developed vemurafenib resistance, and several other groups have noted a decrease in PTEN in BRAF-inhibitor–resistant cells.[95,97] In 2011, Atefi and colleagues[98] induced vemurafenib resistance in melanoma cell lines in vitro and showed the reversal of resistance with inhibition of AKT or mTOR; however, concomitant therapy with a MAPK pathway inhibitor was required to achieve cell death. Based on these in vitro results, several clinical trials exploring combination therapy for *V600E* mutant metastatic melanoma with inhibitors of BRAF and the PI3/AKT/mTOR pathway are under way.[99]

KIT Mutations in Melanoma

Curtin and colleagues[100] used comparative genomic hybridization to evaluate somatic activation of KIT in mucosal and acral melanomas as well as melanomas with and without chronic, sun-induced damage. They hypothesized that these melanomas may have alternative genetic aberrations, because these subtypes of melanoma infrequently harbor mutations related to BRAF and NRAS. Overall, KIT mutations were identified in 39% of mucosal, 36% of acral, 28% of melanomas in skin with chronic sun-induced damage (CSD), and 0% of melanomas in skin without CSD. In these same specimens, BRAF mutations were present in 3%, 21%, 6%, and 56%, respectively. Increased KIT protein expression based on immunohistochemistry staining was identified in 79% of melanomas in the vertical growth phase with a known KIT mutation. These investigators suggested that aberrant KIT signaling in melanoma may represent an activating mutation.

The study by Beadling and colleagues[101] was envisioned after a patient with anorectal melanoma was identified to harbor a KIT exon 11 mutation and responded to treatment with imatinib. Formalin-fixed, paraffin-embedded melanoma specimens were analyzed for KIT mutations. Screening was performed using a combination of polymerase chain reaction amplification and denaturing high-performance liquid chromatography. All mutations were confirmed with bidirectional sequencing. In 189 melanomas, the frequency of KIT mutations for acral melanomas was 23%, mucosal melanomas 16%, conjunctival melanomas 8%, cutaneous melanoma 2%, and choroidal tumors 0%.

There have been a few case series and reports claiming dramatic regression of melanoma after treatment with imatinib.[102] In 2007, Antonescu and colleagues[103] published their series of patients with anal melanoma, specifically looking at KIT mutations and the response to targeted therapy. In this cohort of 20 patients, a KIT exon 11 L576P substitution was identified in 3 patients. In 2010, Handolias and colleagues[104] published a series of 32 patients with mucosal or acral melanomas who were screened for KIT mutations. Of the 32 specimens, 23 were metastatic and 9 were primary tumors and all were tested for KIT mutations in exons 11, 13, and 17. Of the acral melanomas, 6% had a KIT mutation, whereas 38% of the mucosal melanomas had mutations. Four patients in this series were treated: 3 with imatinib and 1 with sorafenib. Two of the patients treated with imatinib had a partial response and 1 had progressive disease. The patient treated with sorafenib had stability of disease. The investigators noted that 3 of the patients developed central nervous system progression, which may be caused by the limited penetration of small molecule kinase inhibitors into the brain.

Guo and colleagues[105] presented work on their phase 2 trial of imatinib in patients with stage IV melanoma with KIT mutation or amplification. In this trial, 43 patients were eligible and underwent testing for KIT mutations, including exons 9, 11, 13, 17, and 18. Patients received 400 mg/d and were allowed to escalate to 600 mg/d or 800 mg/d with disease progression, with a primary end point of median PFS and 6-month PFS rate. Of the 43 patients, 21 had acral melanomas and 11 had mucosal melanomas. At a median of 12 months, the median PFS was 3.5 months and the 6-month PFS rate was 37%. Ten patients achieved partial response, and 13 had stable disease. Tumor regression was observed in 42% of patients.

Recently, results of a phase 2 trial in 295 patients with melanomas screened for KIT mutations and treated with imatinib (400 mg twice daily) have been published.[106] In this study, KIT amplification was identified in 295 patients, who included: 85 patients with acral melanomas, 93 with mucosal melanomas, and 87 with melanomas arising in chronically sun-damaged skin. Of these patients, 28 were treated, 13 with mucosal melanoma, 10 with acral melanoma, and 5 with melanoma arising from chronically sun-damaged skin. Two patients achieved durable CRs, 2 achieved durable partial responses, 2 achieved transient partial responses, and 5 achieved stability of disease lasting more than 12 weeks. Overall durable response rate was 16%, with a median time to progression of 12 weeks and a median overall survival of 46.3 weeks.

Minor and colleagues[107] evaluated the use of the multikinase inhibitor sunitinib in 12 patients identified to harbor a mutation in KIT, BRAF, or NRAS. Sunitinib is a potent multikinase inhibitor of both KIT and VEGF receptors. In this study, they initially screened tissue in 90 eligible patients with stage IV melanoma for mutations or amplification in KIT, BRAF, NRAS, and GNAQ. Melanoma subtypes consisted of acral (n = 22), mucosal (n = 30), and CSD (n = 38). Similar to other reports, there were fewer BRAF mutations in mucosal melanomas. No tissues had a GNAQ mutation. Of the acral melanomas, mutations were identified in KIT (14%), BRAF (32%), and NRAS (27%). Of mucosal melanomas, mutations were identified in KIT (17%), BRAF (3%), and NRAS (7%). In CSD melanomas, mutations were identified in KIT (5%), BRAF (34%), and NRAS (13%). Staining assay for CD117 was positive in 31% of samples tested. Of the 10 KIT mutated samples, 8 expressed CD117, the other 2 were negative for CD117; however, 70% of cases with KIT overexpression did not show mutations in KIT. In 12 patients found to have KIT mutations, therapy was initiated with sunitinib. Of the 12 patients, 10 were evaluable for response and showed 1 CR, 3 partial responses, 1 with stability of disease, and 5 with progressive disease.

Overall, KIT mutations occur infrequently in unselected patients with melanoma, and KIT-directed therapy has been disappointing compared with the experience with selective BRAF inhibitors. Although KIT may be mutated in some melanomas, the association with inhibition seems to be more complex, because response to therapy may not occur even when a mutation is identified.[106] Possible alternatives include attempts at targeting NRAS, including both P13K and MEK.[24,93,108]

SUMMARY

Recent advances in the systemic therapy for melanoma have profoundly altered the outlook for patients afflicted with advanced stages of this increasingly prevalent disease. Effective immunotherapy is associated with infrequent and slowly developing responses, which may result in durable remission of disease at the expense of significant autoimmune toxicities. Targeted therapies are associated with high response rates and rapid tumor regression; however, the responses tend to be short-lived. The armamentarium will broaden with the development of newer agents. The issue of intrinsic and acquired resistance to targeted therapies must be addressed. Future investigations will seek to find rational combinations of existing therapies. Previously ineffective therapies, such as many of the vaccines, may be useful when used in combination with immunomodulating agents. There is already tantalizing preclinical work suggesting that immunotherapies and targeted therapies may synergize.[109–111] Robust biomarkers need to be identified in order to increase the probability that the individual patient is likely to benefit from a specific therapeutic strategy.[112] The culmination of decades of basic and translational research into tangible clinical end points in the therapy for melanoma is cause for celebration and will be fertile grounds for further investigation.

REFERENCES

1. Simard EP, Ward EM, Siegel R, et al. Cancers with increasing incidence trends in the United States: 1999 through 2008. CA Cancer J Clin 2012;62:118–28.
2. Siegel R, Naishadham D, Jemal A. Cancer statistics, 2013. CA Cancer J Clin 2013;63:11–30.

3. Lens MB, Dawes M. Global perspectives of contemporary epidemiological trends of cutaneous malignant melanoma. Br J Dermatol 2004;150:179–85.
4. Balch CM, Gershenwald JE, Soong SJ, et al. Final version of 2009 AJCC melanoma staging and classification. J Clin Oncol 2009;27:6199–206.
5. Middleton MR, Grob JJ, Aaronson N, et al. Randomized phase III study of temozolomide versus dacarbazine in the treatment of patients with advanced metastatic malignant melanoma. J Clin Oncol 2000;18:158–66.
6. Eggermont AM, Kirkwood JM. Re-evaluating the role of dacarbazine in metastatic melanoma: what have we learned in 30 years? Eur J Cancer 2004;40:1825–36.
7. Garbe C, Eigentler TK, Keilholz U, et al. Systematic review of medical treatment in melanoma: current status and future prospects. Oncologist 2011;16:5–24.
8. Rosenberg SA. Progress in human tumour immunology and immunotherapy. Nature 2001;411:380–4.
9. Rosenberg SA, Yang JC, White DE, et al. Durability of complete responses in patients with metastatic cancer treated with high-dose interleukin-2: identification of the antigens mediating response. Ann Surg 1998;228:307–19.
10. Steinman RM, Banchereau J. Taking dendritic cells into medicine. Nature 2007;449:419–26.
11. Mueller DL, Jenkins MK, Schwartz RH. Clonal expansion versus functional clonal inactivation: a costimulatory signalling pathway determines the outcome of T cell antigen receptor occupancy. Annu Rev Immunol 1989;7:445–80.
12. Rosenberg SA, Yang JC, Restifo NP. Cancer immunotherapy: moving beyond current vaccines. Nat Med 2004;10:909–15.
13. Klebanoff CA, Acquavella N, Yu Z, et al. Therapeutic cancer vaccines: are we there yet? Immunol Rev 2011;239:27–44.
14. Schwartzentruber DJ, Lawson DH, Richards JM, et al. gp100 Peptide vaccine and interleukin-2 in patients with advanced melanoma. N Engl J Med 2011;364:2119–27.
15. Stopeck AT, Jones A, Hersh EM, et al. Phase II study of direct intralesional gene transfer of allovectin-7, an HLA-B7/beta2-microglobulin DNA-liposome complex, in patients with metastatic melanoma. Clin Cancer Res 2001;7:2285–91.
16. Bedikian AY, Richards J, Kharkevitch D, et al. A phase 2 study of high-dose Allovectin-7 in patients with advanced metastatic melanoma. Melanoma Res 2010;20:218–26.
17. Gonzalez R, Hutchins L, Nemunaitis J, et al. Phase 2 trial of Allovectin-7 in advanced metastatic melanoma. Melanoma Res 2006;16:521–6.
18. Schreiber RD, Old LJ, Smyth MJ. Cancer immunoediting: integrating immunity's roles in cancer suppression and promotion. Science 2011;331:1565–70.
19. Khong HT, Restifo NP. Natural selection of tumor variants in the generation of "tumor escape" phenotypes. Nat Immunol 2002;3:999–1005.
20. Roman M, Martin-Orozco E, Goodman JS, et al. Immunostimulatory DNA sequences function as T helper-1-promoting adjuvants. Nat Med 1997;3:849–54.
21. Liu BL, Robinson M, Han ZQ, et al. ICP34.5 deleted herpes simplex virus with enhanced oncolytic, immune stimulating, and anti-tumour properties. Gene Ther 2003;10:292–303.
22. Senzer NN, Kaufman HL, Amatruda T, et al. Phase II clinical trial of a granulocyte-macrophage colony-stimulating factor-encoding, second-generation oncolytic herpesvirus in patients with unresectable metastatic melanoma. J Clin Oncol 2009;27:5763–71.
23. Rosenberg SA, Restifo NP, Yang JC, et al. Adoptive cell transfer: a clinical path to effective cancer immunotherapy. Nat Rev Cancer 2008;8:299–308.

24. Gattinoni L, Powell DJ Jr, Rosenberg SA, et al. Adoptive immunotherapy for cancer: building on success. Nat Rev Immunol 2006;6:383–93.

25. Rosenberg SA, Yang JC, Sherry RM, et al. Durable complete responses in heavily pretreated patients with metastatic melanoma using T-cell transfer immunotherapy. Clin Cancer Res 2011;17:4550–7.

26. Park TS, Rosenberg SA, Morgan RA. Treating cancer with genetically engineered T cells. Trends Biotechnol 2011;29:550–7.

27. Morgan RA, Dudley ME, Wunderlich JR, et al. Cancer regression in patients after transfer of genetically engineered lymphocytes. Science 2006;314:126–9.

28. Robbins PF, Morgan RA, Feldman SA, et al. Tumor regression in patients with metastatic synovial cell sarcoma and melanoma using genetically engineered lymphocytes reactive with NY-ESO-1. J Clin Oncol 2011;29:917–24.

29. Morgan RA, Chinnasamy N, Abate-Daga D, et al. Cancer regression and neurological toxicity following anti-MAGE-A3 TCR gene therapy. J Immunother 2013; 36:133–51.

30. Burns WR, Zhao Y, Frankel TL, et al. A high molecular weight melanoma-associated antigen-specific chimeric antigen receptor redirects lymphocytes to target human melanomas. Cancer Res 2010;70:3027–33.

31. Lo AS, Ma Q, Liu DL, et al. Anti-GD3 chimeric sFv-CD28/T-cell receptor zeta designer T cells for treatment of metastatic melanoma and other neuroectodermal tumors. Clin Cancer Res 2010;16:2769–80.

32. Rosenberg SA, Lotze MT, Muul LM, et al. Observations on the systemic administration of autologous lymphokine-activated killer cells and recombinant interleukin-2 to patients with metastatic cancer. N Engl J Med 1985;313:1485–92.

33. Lotze MT, Chang AE, Seipp CA, et al. High-dose recombinant interleukin 2 in the treatment of patients with disseminated cancer. Responses, treatment-related morbidity, and histologic findings. JAMA 1986;256:3117–24.

34. Cipponi A, Wieers G, van Baren N, et al. Tumor-infiltrating lymphocytes: apparently good for melanoma patients. But why? Cancer Immunol Immunother 2011; 60:1153–60.

35. Lenschow DJ, Walunas TL, Bluestone JA. CD28/B7 system of T cell costimulation. Annu Rev Immunol 1996;14:233–58.

36. Mellman I, Coukos G, Dranoff G. Cancer immunotherapy comes of age. Nature 2011;480:480–9.

37. Brunet JF, Denizot F, Luciani MF, et al. A new member of the immunoglobulin superfamily–CTLA-4. Nature 1987;328:267–70.

38. Lindsten T, Lee KP, Harris ES, et al. Characterization of CTLA-4 structure and expression on human T cells. J Immunol 1993;151:3489–99.

39. Krummel MF, Allison JP. CTLA-4 engagement inhibits IL-2 accumulation and cell cycle progression upon activation of resting T cells. J Exp Med 1996;183: 2533–40.

40. Walunas TL, Bakker CY, Bluestone JA. CTLA-4 ligation blocks CD28-dependent T cell activation. J Exp Med 1996;183:2541–50.

41. Chambers CA, Kuhns MS, Egen JG, et al. CTLA-4-mediated inhibition in regulation of T cell responses: mechanisms and manipulation in tumor immunotherapy. Annu Rev Immunol 2001;19:565–94.

42. Ahmadzadeh M, Johnson LA, Heemskerk B, et al. Tumor antigen-specific CD8 T cells infiltrating the tumor express high levels of PD-1 and are functionally impaired. Blood 2009;114:1537–44.

43. Wherry EJ, Ha SJ, Kaech SM, et al. Molecular signature of CD8+ T cell exhaustion during chronic viral infection. Immunity 2007;27:670–84.

44. Wing K, Onishi Y, Prieto-Martin P, et al. CTLA-4 control over Foxp3+ regulatory T cell function. Science 2008;322:271–5.
45. Maker AV, Phan GQ, Attia P, et al. Tumor regression and autoimmunity in patients treated with cytotoxic T lymphocyte-associated antigen 4 blockade and inter-leukin 2: a phase I/II study. Ann Surg Oncol 2005;12:1005–16.
46. Weber J, Thompson JA, Hamid O, et al. A randomized, double-blind, placebo-controlled, phase II study comparing the tolerability and efficacy of ipilimumab administered with or without prophylactic budesonide in patients with unresect-able stage III or IV melanoma. Clin Cancer Res 2009;15:5591–8.
47. Wolchok JD, Neyns B, Linette G, et al. Ipilimumab monotherapy in patients with pretreated advanced melanoma: a randomised, double-blind, multicentre, phase 2, dose-ranging study. Lancet Oncol 2010;11:155–64.
48. O'Day SJ, Maio M, Chiarion-Sileni V, et al. Efficacy and safety of ipilimumab monotherapy in patients with pretreated advanced melanoma: a multicenter single-arm phase II study. Ann Oncol 2010;21:1712–7.
49. Hodi FS, O'Day SJ, McDermott DF, et al. Improved survival with ipilimumab in patients with metastatic melanoma. N Engl J Med 2010;363:711–23.
50. Robert C, Thomas L, Bondarenko I, et al. Ipilimumab plus dacarbazine for pre-viously untreated metastatic melanoma. N Engl J Med 2011;364:2517–26.
51. Prieto PA, Yang JC, Sherry RM, et al. CTLA-4 blockade with ipilimumab: long-term follow-up of 177 patients with metastatic melanoma. Clin Cancer Res 2012;18:2039–47.
52. Keir ME, Butte MJ, Freeman GJ, et al. PD-1 and its ligands in tolerance and im-munity. Annu Rev Immunol 2008;26:677–704.
53. Barber DL, Wherry EJ, Masopust D, et al. Restoring function in exhausted CD8 T cells during chronic viral infection. Nature 2006;439:682–7.
54. Hino R, Kabashima K, Kato Y, et al. Tumor cell expression of programmed cell death-1 ligand 1 is a prognostic factor for malignant melanoma. Cancer 2010; 116:1757–66.
55. Dong H, Strome SE, Salomao DR, et al. Tumor-associated B7-H1 promotes T-cell apoptosis: a potential mechanism of immune evasion. Nat Med 2002;8:793–800.
56. Brahmer JR, Tykodi SS, Chow LQ, et al. Safety and activity of anti-PD-L1 anti-body in patients with advanced cancer. N Engl J Med 2012;366:2455–65.
57. Topalian SL, Hodi FS, Brahmer JR, et al. Safety, activity, and immune correlates of anti-PD-1 antibody in cancer. N Engl J Med 2012;366:2443–54.
58. Miller AJ, Mihm MC Jr. Melanoma. N Engl J Med 2006;355:51–65.
59. Gray-Schopfer V, Wellbrock C, Marais R. Melanoma biology and new targeted therapy. Nature 2007;445:851–7.
60. Peyssonnaux C, Eychène A. The Raf/MEK/ERK pathway: new concepts of acti-vation. Biol Cell 2001;93:53–62.
61. Davies H, Bignell GR, Cox C, et al. Mutations of the BRAF gene in human can-cer. Nature 2002;417:949–54.
62. Pollock PM, Meltzer PS. A genome-based strategy uncovers frequent BRAF mu-tations in melanoma. Cancer Cell 2002;2:5–7.
63. Terai K, Matsuda M. The amino-terminal B-Raf-specific region mediates calcium-dependent homo- and hetero-dimerization of Raf. EMBO J 2006;25: 3556–64.
64. Sullivan RJ, Flaherty K. MAP kinase signaling and inhibition in melanoma. Onco-gene 2013;32(19):2373–9.
65. Hauschild A, Agarwala SS, Trefzer U, et al. Results of a phase III, randomized, placebo-controlled study of sorafenib in combination with carboplatin and

paclitaxel as second-line treatment in patients with unresectable stage III or stage IV melanoma. J Clin Oncol 2009;27:2823–30.

66. Sosman JA, Kim KB, Schuchter L, et al. Survival in BRAF V600-mutant advanced melanoma treated with vemurafenib. N Engl J Med 2012;366:707–14.

67. Chapman PB, Hauschild A, Robert C, et al. Improved survival with vemurafenib in melanoma with BRAF V600E mutation. N Engl J Med 2011;364:2507–16.

68. Zambon A, Niculescu-Duvaz D, Niculescu-Duvaz I, et al. BRAF as a therapeutic target: a patent review (2006-2012). Expert Opin Ther Pat 2013;23:155–64.

69. Ascierto PA, Kirkwood JM, Grob JJ, et al. The role of BRAF V600 mutation in melanoma. J Transl Med 2012;10:85.

70. Rinderknecht JD, Goldinger SM, Rozati S, et al. RASopathic skin eruptions during vemurafenib therapy. PLoS One 2013;8(3):e58721.

71. Boussemart L, Routier E, Mateus C, et al. Prospective study of cutaneous side-effects associated with the BRAF inhibitor vemurafenib: a study of 42 patients. Ann Oncol 2013;24(6):1691–7.

72. Cichowski K, Jänne PA. Drug discovery: inhibitors that activate. Nature 2010; 464:358–9.

73. Hatzivassiliou G, Song K, Yen I, et al. RAF inhibitors prime wild-type RAF to activate the MAPK pathway and enhance growth. Nature 2010;464:431–5.

74. Heidorn SJ, Milagre C, Whittaker S, et al. Kinase-dead BRAF and oncogenic RAS cooperate to drive tumor progression through CRAF. Cell 2010;140: 209–21.

75. Lacouture ME, Duvic M, Hauschild A, et al. Analysis of dermatologic events in vemurafenib-treated patients with melanoma. Oncologist 2013;18:314–22.

76. Fedorenko IV, Paraiso KH, Smalley KS. Acquired and intrinsic BRAF inhibitor resistance in BRAF V600E mutant melanoma. Biochem Pharmacol 2011;82:201–9.

77. Hauschild A, Grob JJ, Demidov LV, et al. Dabrafenib in BRAF-mutated metastatic melanoma: a multicentre, open-label, phase 3 randomised controlled trial. Lancet 2012;380:358–65.

78. Mittapalli RK, Vaidhyanathan S, Dudek AZ, et al. Mechanisms limiting distribution of the BRAFV600E inhibitor dabrafenib to the brain: implications for the treatment of melanoma brain metastases. J Pharmacol Exp Ther 2012;344(3):655–64.

79. Rochet NM, Dronca RS, Kottschade LA, et al. Melanoma brain metastases and vemurafenib: need for further investigation. Mayo Clin Proc 2012;87:976–81.

80. Falchook GS, Long GV, Kurzrock R, et al. Dabrafenib in patients with melanoma, untreated brain metastases, and other solid tumours: a phase 1 dose-escalation trial. Lancet 2012;379:1893–901.

81. Preusser M, Berghoff AS, Schadendorf D, et al. Brain metastasis: opportunity for drug development? Curr Opin Neurol 2012;25:786–94.

82. Giroux S. Overcoming acquired resistance to kinase inhibition: the cases of EGFR, ALK and BRAF. Bioorg Med Chem Lett 2013;23:394–401.

83. Sullivan RJ, Flaherty KT. Resistance to BRAF-targeted therapy in melanoma. Eur J Cancer 2013;49(6):1297–304.

84. Nazarian R, Shi H, Wang Q, et al. Melanomas acquire resistance to B-RAF(V600E) inhibition by RTK or N-RAS upregulation. Nature 2010;468:973–7.

85. Poulikakos PI, Persaud Y, Janakiraman M, et al. RAF inhibitor resistance is mediated by dimerization of aberrantly spliced BRAF(V600E). Nature 2011;480: 387–90.

86. Das Thakur M, Salangsang F, Landman AS, et al. Modelling vemurafenib resistance in melanoma reveals a strategy to forestall drug resistance. Nature 2013; 494:251–5.

87. Le K, Blomain E, Rodeck U, et al. Selective RAF inhibitor impairs ERK1/2 phosphorylation and growth in mutant NRAS, vemurafenib-resistant melanoma cells. Pigment Cell Melanoma Res 2013;26(4):509–17.
88. Johannessen CM, Boehm JS, Kim SY, et al. COT drives resistance to RAF inhibition through MAP kinase pathway reactivation. Nature 2010;468:968–72.
89. Flaherty KT, Robert C, Hersey P, et al. Improved survival with MEK inhibition in BRAF-mutated melanoma. N Engl J Med 2012;367:107–14.
90. Falchook GS, Lewis KD, Infante JR, et al. Activity of the oral MEK inhibitor trametinib in patients with advanced melanoma: a phase 1 dose-escalation trial. Lancet Oncol 2012;13:782–9.
91. Kim KB, Kefford R, Pavlick AC, et al. Phase II study of the MEK1/MEK2 inhibitor Trametinib in patients with metastatic BRAF-mutant cutaneous melanoma previously treated with or without a BRAF inhibitor. J Clin Oncol 2013;31: 482–9.
92. Flaherty KT, Infante JR, Daud A, et al. Combined BRAF and MEK inhibition in melanoma with BRAF V600 mutations. N Engl J Med 2012;367:1694–703.
93. McArthur GA, Ribas A. Targeting oncogenic drivers and the immune system in melanoma. J Clin Oncol 2013;31:499–506.
94. Shull AY, Latham-Schwark A, Ramasamy P, et al. Novel somatic mutations to PI3K pathway genes in metastatic melanoma. PLoS One 2012;7:e43369.
95. Chen B, Tardell C, Higgins B, et al. BRAFV600E negatively regulates the AKT pathway in melanoma cell lines. PLoS One 2012;7:e42598.
96. Villanueva J, Vultur A, Lee JT, et al. Acquired resistance to BRAF inhibitors mediated by a RAF kinase switch in melanoma can be overcome by cotargeting MEK and IGF-1R/PI3K. Cancer Cell 2010;18:683–95.
97. Liu F, Cao J, Wu J, et al. Stat3 targeted therapies overcome the acquired resistance to vemurafenib in melanomas. J Invest Dermatol 2013;133:2041–9.
98. Atefi M, von Euw E, Attar N, et al. Reversing melanoma cross-resistance to BRAF and MEK inhibitors by co-targeting the AKT/mTOR pathway. PLoS One 2011;6:e28973.
99. Britten CD. PI3K and MEK inhibitor combinations: examining the evidence in selected tumor types. Cancer Chemother Pharmacol 2013;71(6):1395–409.
100. Curtin JA, Busam K, Pinkel D, et al. Somatic activation of KIT in distinct subtypes of melanoma. J Clin Oncol 2006;24:4340–6.
101. Beadling C, Jacobson-Dunlop E, Hodi FS, et al. KIT gene mutations and copy number in melanoma subtypes. Clin Cancer Res 2008;14:6821–8.
102. Hodi FS, Friedlander P, Corless CL, et al. Major response to imatinib mesylate in KIT-mutated melanoma. J Clin Oncol 2008;26:2046–51.
103. Antonescu CR, Busam KJ, Francone TD, et al. L576P KIT mutation in anal melanomas correlates with KIT protein expression and is sensitive to specific kinase inhibition. Int J Cancer 2007;121:257–64.
104. Handolias D, Hamilton AL, Salemi R, et al. Clinical responses observed with imatinib or sorafenib in melanoma patients expressing mutations in KIT. Br J Cancer 2010;102:1219–23.
105. Guo J, Si L, Kong Y, et al. Phase II, open-label, single-arm trial of imatinib mesylate in patients with metastatic melanoma harboring c-Kit mutation or amplification. J Clin Oncol 2011;29:2904–9.
106. Carvajal RD, Antonescu CR, Wolchok JD, et al. KIT as a therapeutic target in metastatic melanoma. JAMA 2011;305:2327–34.
107. Minor DR, Kashani-Sabet M, Garrido M, et al. Sunitinib therapy for melanoma patients with KIT mutations. Clin Cancer Res 2012;18:1457–63.

108. Kelleher FC, McArthur GA. Targeting NRAS in melanoma. Cancer J 2012;18: 132–6.
109. Koya RC, Mok S, Otte N, et al. BRAF inhibitor vemurafenib improves the anti-tumor activity of adoptive cell immunotherapy. Cancer Res 2012;72:3928–37.
110. Frederick DT, Piris A, Cogdill AP, et al. BRAF inhibition is associated with enhanced melanoma antigen expression and a more favorable tumor microen-vironment in patients with metastatic melanoma. Clin Cancer Res 2013;19: 1225–31.
111. Liu C, Peng W, Xu C, et al. BRAF inhibition increases tumor infiltration by T cells and enhances the antitumor activity of adoptive immunotherapy in mice. Clin Cancer Res 2013;19:393–403.
112. Ascierto PA, Kalos M, Schaer DA, et al. Biomarkers for immunostimulatory monoclonal antibodies in combination strategies for melanoma and other tumor types. Clin Cancer Res 2013;19:1009–20.

Targeted Therapy for Cancer
The Gastrointestinal Stromal Tumor Model

Vinod P. Balachandran, MD, Ronald P. DeMatteo, MD*

KEYWORDS

- Gastrointestinal stromal tumor • Sarcoma • KIT • Imatinib • Tyrosine kinase

KEY POINTS

- Gastrointestinal stromal tumors (GISTs) are unique solid tumors because they are driven predominantly by oncogenic mutations in KIT or PDGFRA tyrosine kinases.
- Surgery is the most effective treatment for localized, primary GIST. Adjuvant tyrosine kinase inhibition (TKI) with imatinib substantially decreases recurrence rates but does not seem to affect overall survival.
- Imatinib is initial therapy for metastatic GIST; however, acquired mutations frequently lead to resistance after initial responses. The role of surgery and TKI in metastatic GIST remains unclear.
- Imatinib dose escalation, sunitinib, and regorafenib are the initial therapeutic options for imatinib-resistant GIST, with many novel TKIs under investigation.
- Preclinical data suggest that antitumor effects of imatinib in GIST are partially dependent on host immune responses. Combination imatinib and immunotherapy may be effective in GIST and other solid tumors.

INTRODUCTION

Gastrointestinal stromal tumor (GIST) is the most common sarcoma, accounting for approximately 18% of all sarcomas and 1% of all intestinal neoplasms.[1] The annual incidence of GIST as determined by population-based studies is approximately 10 cases per million.[2–4] GISTs have historically portended a poor prognosis. Up to 50% of patients have recurrent disease 5 years after complete resection. Median survival in metastatic GIST used to be approximately 9 months because it is inherently resistant to chemotherapy and radiation.[5–7] The discovery of oncogenic tyrosine kinase mutations in GIST, and the successful application of kinase inhibitor therapies, have made GIST a model of targeting aberrant signal transduction to treat cancer. Lessons learned from this approach have allowed new insight into the molecular

Disclosures: the authors have nothing to disclose.
Department of Surgery, Memorial Sloan-Kettering Cancer Center, 1275 York Avenue, New York, NY 10065, USA
* Corresponding author.
E-mail address: dematter@mskcc.org

Surg Oncol Clin N Am 22 (2013) 805–821
http://dx.doi.org/10.1016/j.soc.2013.06.001
1055-3207/13/$ – see front matter © 2013 Elsevier Inc. All rights reserved.

biology and mechanisms of resistance of kinase-driven cancers. It has spurred development of novel targeted inhibitors and uncovered exciting possibilities for combination therapy with other systemic agents.

ONCOGENIC KINASE MUTATIONS AND GIST PATHOGENESIS
KIT

In 1998, 2 important discoveries were made that furthered our understanding of GIST biology. Hirota and colleagues[8] described their landmark discovery of gain-of-function mutations in KIT in 5 patients with GIST. They hypothesized that these were oncogenic driver mutations, because Ba/F3 lymphoid cells transfected with mutant KIT cDNA underwent malignant transformation. Shortly thereafter, 2 groups[9,10] reported that 95% of GISTs are immunohistochemically positive for the receptor tyrosine kinase KIT, also known as CD117. Since then, a causal relationship between KIT mutations and GIST pathogenesis has been further supported by many lines of evidence. Mutant KIT induces constitutive kinase activation without ligand binding.[8,11,12] KIT mutations have been discovered in very small GISTs, suggesting that it occurs as a very early event.[13,14] GIST tumor extracts almost universally show phosphorylated KIT.[15] Transgenic Kit knock-in mouse models develop spindle cell tumors that are morphologically similar to human GIST.[16,17] KIT blockade in vitro and in vivo inhibits tumor growth.[12,18–21]

KIT, a receptor tyrosine kinase, binds KIT ligand (stem cell factor), which results in receptor dimerization, phosphorylation, and activation of downstream signaling pathways that promote cell proliferation and survival. It is now known that 70% to 80% of GISTs harbor a KIT mutation that induces constitutive kinase activation. Mutations most commonly occur in the juxtamembrane domain in exon 11 (**Fig. 1**, **Table 1**), which normally inhibits the kinase activation loop in the absence of ligand binding. Exon 11 mutations include in-frame deletions, insertions, and substitutions, but deletions are the most common. Mutations also occur in the extracellular domains (exons 8 [rarely] and 9), and infrequently in the kinase domains (exons 13 and 17) (see **Fig. 1**, see **Table 1**).[22] The downstream signaling pathways activated include the MAPK, PI3K-AKT, and STAT3 pathways, which lead to inhibition of apoptosis and cell proliferation.[22] Recently, ETV1, a lineage survival factor in interstitial cells of Cajal, the hypothesized cell of origin for GIST, was shown to cooperate with activated KIT to induce GIST tumorigenesis.[23]

Platelet-Derived Growth Factor Receptor α

Approximately one-third of GISTs that do not have a mutation in KIT (8% of all GISTs) harbor a mutation in a closely related tyrosine kinase, platelet-derived growth factor receptor α (PDGFRA).[24,25] PDGFRA and KIT mutations are mutually exclusive in GIST. Like mutations in KIT, PDGFRA mutations are found in its juxtamembrane domain (see **Fig. 1**, see **Table 1**), adenosine triphosphate–binding domain, or activation loop, and cause ligand-independent receptor activation. An oncogenic role for these mutations in GIST has followed evidence similar to that for KIT: mutant PDGFRA induces ligand-independent receptor activation, and PDGFRA inhibition induces cellular arrest.[24–26] However, PDGFRA mutant GISTs do have unique clinical profiles, including gastric location, epithelioid morphology, variable KIT expression, and a more indolent clinical course.[27]

Wild-Type GIST

10% to 15% of tumors do not have mutations in KIT and PDGFRA (wild-type [WT] GIST). Other mutations that may contribute to tumorigenesis have been recently

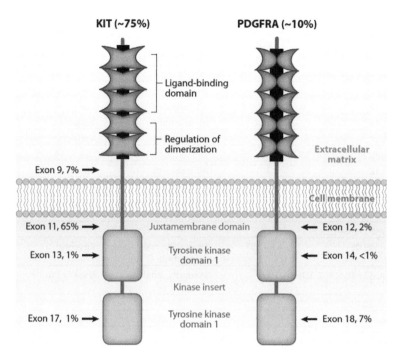

KIT (~75%)   **PDGFRA (~10%)**

- Ligand-binding domain

- Regulation of dimerization

Extracellular matrix

Exon 9, 7% →

Cell membrane

Exon 11, 65% →   Juxtamembrane domain   ← Exon 12, 2%

Exon 13, 1% →   Tyrosine kinase domain 1   ← Exon 14, <1%

Kinase insert

Exon 17, 1% →   Tyrosine kinase domain 1   ← Exon 18, 7%

Fig. 1. Schematic structures of KIT and PDGFR. The percentages indicate the frequency of mutations detected in each exon of the gene that encodes for the protein. (*From* Joensuu H, DeMatteo RP. The management of gastrointestinal stromal tumors: a model for targeted and multidisciplinary therapy of malignancy. Annu Rev Med 2012;63:249; with permission.)

uncovered (see **Table 1**). Similar to *BRAF* mutations in melanoma, papillary thyroid cancer, and colorectal cancer, GIST *BRAF* mutations have also been identified in 7% to 15% of WT GISTS within the exon 15 V600E hot-spot.[28,29] BRAF proteins and constituents of the MAPK signaling pathway can stimulate cell growth independent of KIT and are a possible cause of resistance to KIT and PDGFRA kinase inhibitors. Mutations in the succinate dehydrogenase (SDH) respiratory chain complex have also been discovered in WT GIST. *SDH* mutations were initially identified in the germline in subunits *SDHB, SDHC,* and *SDHD,* predisposing affected individuals to GIST and paraganglionomas (Carney-Stratakis syndrome). *SDH* mutations have since been identified in 12% of WT GIST (see **Table 1**).[30] Mutations in *SDHA* have also since been reported.[31] The precise oncogenic role of *SDH* mutations in GIST remains to be elucidated. Expression of insulin-like growth factor 1 receptor, which signals through MAPK and PI3K-AKT pathways, has also been detected and may contribute to GIST pathogenesis.[32] WT GISTs are also found in 7% of patients with neurofibromatosis type I, who harbor germline mutations in the neurofibromin 1 gene (see **Table 1**).[33]

TARGETING KINASE PATHWAYS IN GIST

Until 2000, outcomes in patients with metastatic GIST were poor. Median survival was approximately 9 months, and responses to conventional chemotherapy was

Table 1
Molecular classification of GIST

Gene	Incidence (%)	Anatomic Location	Imatinib Sensitivity
Mutations in *KIT* (80%)			
Exon 9	7	Small intestine, colon	Yes, consider 800 mg/d
Exon 11	65	All locations	Yes
Exon 13	1	All locations	Variable
Exon 17	1	All locations	Variable
Mutations in *PDGFRA* (5%–8%)			
Exon 12	2	All locations	Yes
Exon 14	<1	Stomach	Yes
Exon 18	7	Stomach, mesentery, omentum	D842V insensitive, most other sensitive
Wild Type (12%–15%)			
BRAF V600E	7–15[a]	Stomach, small intestine	Possibly
SDHA, SDHB, SDHC, SDHD	12[a]	Stomach, small intestine	Usually not
Familiar GIST			
KIT, rarely *PDGFRA*	Very rare	Small intestine	Usually not
Syndromic GIST			
Unknown gene (Carney triad)	Very rare	Stomach	Usually not
SDHB, SDHC, SDHD (Carney-Stratakis)	Rare	Stomach	Usually not
NF1 (neurofibromatosis 1)	Rare	Small intestine	Usually not

[a] % of wild-type GISTs.

Data from Joensuu H, DeMatteo RP. The management of gastrointestinal stromal tumors: a model for targeted and multidisciplinary therapy of malignancy. Annu Rev Med 2012;63:247–58.

less than 5%.[5–7] The discovery of oncogenic *KIT* mutations in GIST coincided with the successful clinical development and application of the tyrosine kinase inhibitor (TKI) imatinib (Gleevec) for the treatment of chronic myelogenous leukemia. It was noted that the kinases KIT and ABL shared structural similarity, prompting the first clinical application of imatinib in a 50-year-old woman with advanced GIST, which was met with a dramatic clinical response.[34] This experience led to phase I, II, and 2 international phase III trials to investigate the benefit of imatinib in the metastatic setting. Overall, imatinib achieved disease control in 70% to 85% of patients with KIT-positive GIST, with a median progression-free-survival of 20 to 24 months, and an estimated overall survival (OS) greater than 36 months (**Fig. 2**).[6,7,35,36] The advent of imatinib therapy for metastatic GIST has dramatically altered prognosis: median survival is 5 years with 34% of patients surviving more than 9 years.[33] Imatinib is first-line treatment in patients with metastatic GIST, and treatment is recommended to continue indefinitely if there is clinical benefit, because interruption is associated with high rate of relapse.[37]

Paralleling the success in GIST, a molecular approach to systemic therapy has been adopted in many other solid tumors. Genomic analyses have uncovered biologically

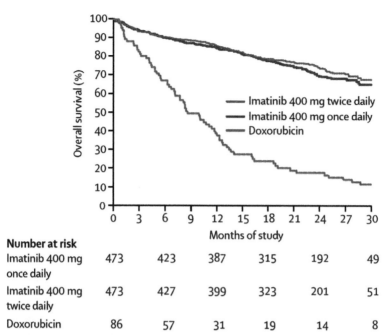

Fig. 2. OS for study population of EORTC 62005 compared with historical controls from EORTC database. (*From* Verweij J, Casali PG, Zalcberg J, et al. Progression-free survival in gastrointestinal stromal tumors with high-dose imatinib: randomized trial. Lancet 2004;364(9440):1131; with permission.)

relevant and druggable kinase mutations in other solid malignancies. Although the success achieved in these cancers has not replicated the GIST success, it has validated a molecular approach to systemic treatment and has heralded kinase-based therapies as an integral component of cancer care (**Table 2**).

Table 2
Tyrosine kinase mutations and targeted agents in solid tumors

Gene	Tumor	Agent
KIT	Melanoma, seminoma, small cell lung cancer, synovial sarcoma, thymic carcinoma	Imatinib[80–88]
PDGFRA	Dermatofibrosarcoma protuberans	Imatinib[89,90]
EGFR	Non–small cell lung cancer Squamous cell, ovarian, renal cell, and colorectal cancer, glioblastoma multiforme	Gefitinib, erlotinib[91–95] Erlotinib,[96] gefitinib,[97] lapatanib,[98] cetuximab[99] Panitumumab[100]
BRAF	Melanoma, papillary thyroid cancer, colon cancer	Vemurafenib[101,102]
HER-2	Breast cancer, lung cancer	Trastuzumab[103,104]
VEGFR	Non–small cell lung, breast, prostate, renal, colorectal	Bevacizumab, vascular endothelial growth factor inhibitors[105]
RET	Multiple endocrine neoplasia 2A, 2B, familial medullary thyroid cancer, radiation-associated papillary thyroid cancer	Cabozantinib,[106] vandetanib,[107] sorafenib[108]

ASSESSING RESPONSE TO KINASE THERAPY

Responses to systemic therapy in solid tumors have traditionally been assessed using the response evaluation criteria in solid tumors (RECIST), which incorporates unidirectional tumor size. However, assessing responses using RECIST has been shown to be insensitive in GIST.[38] Positron emission tomography (PET) scans had traditionally been used to assess continuing responses to TKI treatment, because significant decreases in fluorodeoxyglucose signal are seen within 24 hours in patients responding to imatinib.[39] However, Choi and colleagues[40,41] proposed using computed tomography to determine tumor size and density in assessing treatment response; responding tumors show homogeneous and hypodense features, losing solid elements and neovascularity. The Choi criteria correlate with PET, are superior to RECIST, and are a significant improvement in our understanding of assessing clinical responses to systemic agents in solid tumors.

COMBINING TARGETED THERAPY WITH SURGERY
Adjuvant Imatinib

Although TKI therapy induces tumor regression in most patients, it rarely induces complete responses. Even long-term TKI therapy fails to eradicate GIST cells, with viable tumor cells detected even in tumors with good histologic responses.[42] In contrast, surgery for patients with primary GIST without metastases cures more than 50% of patients.[43] In a double-blind, placebo-controlled, multicenter, randomized trial, the American College of Surgeons Oncology Group (ACOSOG) reported that 1 year of adjuvant imatinib after resection of GISTs at least 3 cm in size significantly improved 1-year recurrence-free survival (RFS) (83% in placebo arm vs 98% in imatinib arm, **Fig. 3**).[44] Based on these results, the US Food and Drug Administration (FDA) approved imatinib for use in the adjuvant setting. Recently, it was shown that patients at high risk of recurrence treated with 3 years of adjuvant imatinib after surgical

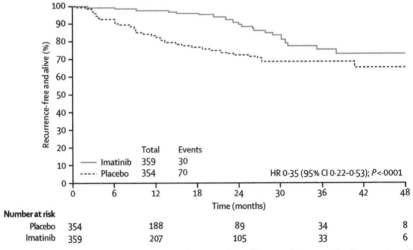

Fig. 3. RFS in the ACOSOG trial Z9001 evaluating the efficacy of 1 year of adjuvant imatinib compared with placebo. (*From* DeMatteo RP, Ballman KV, Antonescu CR, et al. Adjuvant imatinib mesylate after resection of localized, primary gastrointestinal stromal tumor; a randomized, double-blind, placebo-controlled trial. Lancet 2009;373(9669):1100; with permission.)

resection have 5-year RFS and OS rates of 65.6% and 92%, respectively, compared with 47.9% and 81.7% in patients treated with 1 year of adjuvant imatinib.[45] However, there was no difference in disease-specific survival between 1 and 3 years of therapy. An additional phase III trial is examining the outcomes after 2 years of adjuvant imatinib after surgery. A phase II, nonrandomized, multicenter trial is also evaluating the efficacy of 5 years of adjuvant imatinib after complete resection of primary GIST. The success of adjuvant imatinib in GIST ranks with trastuzumab as one of the most successful applications of kinase inhibitor therapy for the adjuvant treatment of solid tumors.[46]

Neoadjuvant Imatinib

When primary GIST seems borderline resectable or unresectable, neoadjuvant imatinib treatment may allow for tumor shrinkage and a subsequent R0 resection. Preliminary phase II trials have shown the safety and efficacy of preoperative imatinib.[47–49] However, there are no published phase III data on neoadjuvant imatinib for unresectable GIST. This is an area of ongoing investigation.

MOLECULAR BIOLOGY AND RISK STRATIFICATION

Similar to other sarcomas, tumor size, mitotic index, and location have been shown to determine biological aggressiveness in GIST.[50] However, the discovery of oncogenic kinase mutations has allowed new insight into links between molecular biology and clinical behavior. It is now clear that recurrence patterns after primary resection are also governed by mutation type: deletion and insertion mutations in *KIT* exon 11 and exon 9 confer higher recurrence rates compared with other mutations.[50,51] Within exon 11 mutations, deletions (specifically in amino acids 557 or 558) have worse outcome.[50,52,53] Our understanding of risk stratification to predict the natural history of resected disease is achieved through prognostic nomograms. We developed a nomogram predicting 2-year and 5-year RFS factoring tumor size, mitotic index, and location (**Fig. 4**).[54] Dei Tos and colleagues[55] have reported a nomogram

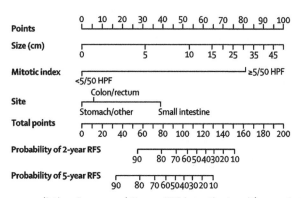

Fig. 4. Nomogram predicting 2-year and 5-year RFS in patients with resected primary GIST. Points are assigned based on tumor size, mitotic index, and site by drawing an upward vertical line to the points bar. Based on the sum of the points generated, a downward vertical line is drawn from the total points line to calculate 2-year and 5-year RFS. (*From* Gold JS, Gonen M, Gutierrez A, et al. Development and validation of a prognostic nomogram for recurrence-free survival after complete surgical resection of localized primary gastrointestinal stromal tumor: a retrospective analysis. Lancet Oncol 2009;10:1045–52; with permission.)

predicting 10-year OS. The relationship between mutation type, adjuvant imatinib, and other factors in the nomogram remain unclear.

TKI RESISTANCE

Although most patients initially respond to TKI therapy, most develop resistance. More than 50% of patients develop disease progression by 2 years.[56] Primary resistance, defined as progression within the first 6 months of treatment, occurs in 10% of patients. Resistance is linked to kinase genotype and TKI sensitivity: patients with *KIT* exon 11 or 9 mutation or WT GISTs have a 5%, 16%, and 23% probability of showing primary imatinib resistance.[57] PDGFRA D842V mutations are strongly resistant to imatinib in vitro and in vivo. The mechanism of primary resistance remains unclear.

Patients with secondary resistance develop disease progression after an initial benefit from imatinib, predominantly because of secondary mutations in the identical gene and allele as the primary oncogenic driver mutation.[20,33,56,58–63] More than 80% of drug-resistant GIST tumors harbor secondary mutations.[33,64–66] Secondary mutations may disrupt imatinib binding, or stabilize the active conformation of the KIT kinase.[56,60] The mechanism of development of second site mutations remains unclear. Long-term imatinib therapy can also lead to polyclonal acquired resistance, whereby different tumor nodules acquire different secondary mutations, and progress independently.[20,56,67,68] In addition, up to one-third of secondary resistant GISTs lack secondary mutations, in which possible mechanisms of resistance include *KIT* genomic amplification and alternate tyrosine kinase activation.[42] These findings have provided invaluable insight into a common end point of kinase inhibitor therapy in solid tumors and have guided the development of second-line TKIs. However, the genetic complexity of acquired resistance argues against second-line TKI monotherapy providing durable clinical benefit.

STRATEGIES TO COMBAT TKI RESISTANCE
Second-Line TKIs

Imatinib dose escalation is the initial recommendation for patients progressing on imatinib, because 20% to 30% of patients may have 1 year or more of disease control.[36] Multiple salvage TKIs are in development to combat imatinib resistance (**Table 3**). Sunitinib, a TKI that inhibits KIT, PDGFRA, PDGFRB, FMS-like tyrosine kinase 3 receptor, RET, and vascular endothelial growth factor receptors (VEGFR) 1, 2, and 3, is the second-line TKI of choice in patients with generalized disease progression who have

Table 3
New targeted agents under investigation for GIST

TKIs	Molecular Target	Development Phase
Nilotinib	KIT, PDGFR, BCR-ABL[109–111]	III
Dasatinib	KIT, ABL, SRC[112]	III
Sorafenib	KIT, PDGFR, VEGFR, BRAF[113–115]	II
Regorafenib	KIT, PDGFRA, VEGFR, BRAF, FLT-3, Raf-1[73,116]	III
Masitinib	KIT, PDGFR, LYN[70,117]	III
Pazopanib	KIT, PDGFRA, VEGFR	II
Vatalanib	KIT, PDGFRA, VEGFR[72,118]	II
Crenolanib	PDGFRA D842 V[119]	II

failed imatinib dose escalation or who are imatinib intolerant. Demetri and colleagues[69] reported that patients with imatinib-resistant GIST treated with sunitinib had a median time to progression of 27.3 weeks compared with 6.4 weeks for placebo. Despite the remarkable success with imatinib, results with second-line TKIs in GIST have been poor, underscoring the need for new treatment strategies.[70–73] Regorafenib was recently approved by the FDA as a third-line agent.[73]

Surgery and TKI Therapy for Metastatic Disease

TKI therapy has been combined with surgery in the metastatic setting. We found that metastatic GIST patients with focal resistance (1 tumor growing) on imatinib who were treated with surgery had a 2-year OS of 36% compared with 100% in patients with imatinib-responsive or stable tumors. Patients with multifocal resistance (>1 tumor growing) had a 1-year OS of 36%.[74] Other groups have also reported a lack of clinical benefit for patients progressing on imatinib treated with surgery.[75,76] Identifying the patient cohort and quantifying the precise benefit from surgery after imatinib in the metastatic setting remains an area needing further examination.

Combination Targeted Therapy and Immunotherapy

In addition to inhibition of oncogenic signaling pathways, targeted agents are potent immunomodulators. They promote dendritic cell maturation and T-cell priming, increase death receptor expression on tumor cells, sensitizing them to immune-mediated tumor clearance, and diminish tumor-induced immunosuppression.[77] The immune system has also been shown to be important in GIST. In GIST patients treated with imatinib, progression-free survival correlated with GIST, progression-free survival correlated with IFN-γ secretion by natural killer cells in the blood.[78] We reported that the antitumor effects of imatinib, previously believed to act exclusively via oncogenic kinase inhibition in tumor cells, rely partially on indirect effects of the immune system. Using a mouse model of spontaneous GIST, we found that imatinib therapy activated $CD8^+$ T cells and induced inhibitory regulatory T-cell (Treg) apoptosis, thereby increasing the intratumoral $CD8^+$ T-cell/Treg ratio, a hallmark of immunologic outcome.[79] The mechanism relied on imatinib inhibiting tumor-cell expression of the immunosuppressive enzyme indoleamine 2,3-dioxygenase (IDO), by reducing expression of the transcription factor ETV4, and disrupting its ability to bind the IDO promoter. Extending these findings in vivo, we correlated the intratumoral $CD8^+$ T-cell/ Treg ratio to imatinib response and intratumoral IDO expression in freshly analyzed human GISTs. Our results link acquired resistance to imatinib to restoration of intratumoral immunosuppression. Hence, molecular and immune resistance in GIST seem to be intertwined. To investigate whether imatinib synergizes with immune modulating agents, we combined imatinib therapy with blockade of cytotoxic T-lymphocyte-associated antigen 4 (CTLA-4), a known T-cell and IDO modulator. Tumor size was significantly decreased in mouse GIST compared with either treatment alone. These data show the rationale and potential of combining targeted therapy with immunotherapy to improve outcomes in not only GIST but also other solid tumors treated with TKIs. We are conducting a phase I trial sponsored by the National Cancer Institute examining the effects of CTLA-4 inhibition with dasatinib in GIST and other sarcomas. Multiple other groups are investigating combining targeted agents and immune agents, including a phase II trial examining vemurafenib and CTLA-4 blockade in patients with melanoma who have V600E *BRAF* mutations.[77]

SUMMARY

GISTs are unique tumors, arising largely due to oncogenic mutations in *KIT* or *PDGFRA* tyrosine kinases. Although surgery remains the most effective treatment, the remarkable clinical success achieved with kinase inhibition has made GIST one of the most successful examples of targeted therapy for the treatment of cancer. The insight gained from this approach has allowed a deeper understanding of the molecular biology driving kinase dependent cancers, and the adaptations to kinase inhibition, linking genotype to phenotype. Mutation tailored kinase inhibition with second generation TKI's, and combination immunotherapy to harness the effects of TKIs remain exciting areas of investigation.

REFERENCES

1. Ducimetiere F, Lurkin A, Ranchere-Vince D, et al. Incidence of sarcoma histotypes and molecular subtypes in a prospective epidemiological study with central pathology review and molecular testing. PLoS One 2011;6(8): e20294.
2. Nilsson B, Bumming P, Meis-Kindblom JM, et al. Gastrointestinal stromal tumors: the incidence, prevalence, clinical course, and prognostication in the preimatinib mesylate era–a population-based study in western Sweden. Cancer 2005; 103(4):821–9.
3. Steigen SE, Eide TJ. Trends in incidence and survival of mesenchymal neoplasm of the digestive tract within a defined population of northern Norway. APMIS 2006;114(3):192–200.
4. Mucciarini C, Rossi G, Bertolini F, et al. Incidence and clinicopathologic features of gastrointestinal stromal tumors. A population-based study. BMC Cancer 2007;7:230.
5. DeMatteo RP, Lewis JJ, Leung D, et al. Two hundred gastrointestinal stromal tumors: recurrence patterns and prognostic factors for survival. Ann Surg 2000;231(1):51–8.
6. Demetri GD, von Mehren M, Blanke CD, et al. Efficacy and safety of imatinib mesylate in advanced gastrointestinal stromal tumors. N Engl J Med 2002; 347(7):472–80.
7. Verweij J, Casali PG, Zalcberg J, et al. Progression-free survival in gastrointestinal stromal tumours with high-dose imatinib: randomised trial. Lancet 2004; 364(9440):1127–34.
8. Hirota S, Isozaki K, Moriyama Y, et al. Gain-of-function mutations of c-kit in human gastrointestinal stromal tumors. Science 1998;279(5350):577–80.
9. Kindblom LG, Remotti HE, Aldenborg F, et al. Gastrointestinal pacemaker cell tumor (GIPACT): gastrointestinal stromal tumors show phenotypic characteristics of the interstitial cells of Cajal. Am J Pathol 1998;152(5): 1259–69.
10. Sarlomo-Rikala M, Kovatich AJ, Barusevicius A, et al. CD117: a sensitive marker for gastrointestinal stromal tumors that is more specific than CD34. Mod Pathol 1998;11(8):728–34.
11. Heinrich MC, Griffith DJ, Druker BJ, et al. Inhibition of c-kit receptor tyrosine kinase activity by STI 571, a selective tyrosine kinase inhibitor. Blood 2000; 96(3):925–32.
12. Tuveson DA, Willis NA, Jacks T, et al. STI571 inactivation of the gastrointestinal stromal tumor c-KIT oncoprotein: biological and clinical implications. Oncogene 2001;20(36):5054–8.

13. Corless CL, McGreevey L, Haley A, et al. KIT mutations are common in incidental gastrointestinal stromal tumors one centimeter or less in size. Am J Pathol 2002;160(5):1567–72.
14. Agaimy A, Wunsch PH, Hofstaedter F, et al. Minute gastric sclerosing stromal tumors (GIST tumorlets) are common in adults and frequently show c-KIT mutations. Am J Surg Pathol 2007;31(1):113–20.
15. Rubin BP, Singer S, Tsao C, et al. KIT activation is a ubiquitous feature of gastrointestinal stromal tumors. Cancer Res 2001;61(22):8118–21.
16. Sommer G, Agosti V, Ehlers I, et al. Gastrointestinal stromal tumors in a mouse model by targeted mutation of the kit receptor tyrosine kinase. Proc Natl Acad Sci U S A 2003;100(11):6706–11.
17. Rubin BP, Antonescu CR, Scott-Browne JP, et al. A knock-in mouse model of gastrointestinal stromal tumor harboring kit K641E. Cancer Res 2005;65(15):6631–9.
18. Nakatani H, Kobayashi M, Jin T, et al. STI571 (Glivec) inhibits the interaction between c-KIT and heat shock protein 90 of the gastrointestinal stromal tumor cell line, GIST-T1. Cancer Sci 2005;96(2):116–9.
19. Tarn C, Skorobogatko YV, Taguchi T, et al. Therapeutic effect of imatinib in gastrointestinal stromal tumors: AKT signaling dependent and independent mechanisms. Cancer Res 2006;66(10):5477–86.
20. Heinrich MC, Corless CL, Blanke CD, et al. Molecular correlates of imatinib resistance in gastrointestinal stromal tumors. J Clin Oncol 2006;24(29):4764–74.
21. Rossi F, Ehlers I, Agosti V, et al. Oncogenic Kit signaling and therapeutic intervention in a mouse model of gastrointestinal stromal tumor. Proc Natl Acad Sci U S A 2006;103(34):12843–8.
22. Rubin BP, Heinrich MC, Corless CL. Gastrointestinal stromal tumour. Lancet 2007;369(9574):1731–41.
23. Chi P, Chen Y, Zhang L, et al. ETV1 is a lineage survival factor that cooperates with KIT in gastrointestinal stromal tumours. Nature 2010;467(7317):849–53.
24. Heinrich MC, Corless CL, Duensing A, et al. PDGFRA activating mutations in gastrointestinal stromal tumors. Science 2003;299(5607):708–10.
25. Hirota S, Ohashi A, Nishida T, et al. Gain-of-function mutations of platelet-derived growth factor receptor alpha gene in gastrointestinal stromal tumors. Gastroenterology 2003;125(3):660–7.
26. Kang HJ, Nam SW, Kim H, et al. Correlation of KIT and platelet-derived growth factor receptor alpha mutations with gene activation and expression profiles in gastrointestinal stromal tumors. Oncogene 2005;24(6):1066–74.
27. Lasota J, Dansonka-Mieszkowska A, Sobin LH, et al. A great majority of GISTs with PDGFRA mutations represent gastric tumors of low or no malignant potential. Lab Invest 2004;84(7):874–83.
28. Agaram NP, Wong GC, Guo T, et al. Novel V600E BRAF mutations in imatinib-naive and imatinib-resistant gastrointestinal stromal tumors. Genes Chromosomes Cancer 2008;47(10):853–9.
29. Hostein I, Faur N, Primois C, et al. BRAF mutation status in gastrointestinal stromal tumors. Am J Clin Pathol 2010;133(1):141–8.
30. Janeway KA, Kim SY, Lodish M, et al. Defects in succinate dehydrogenase in gastrointestinal stromal tumors lacking KIT and PDGFRA mutations. Proc Natl Acad Sci U S A 2011;108(1):314–8.
31. Pantaleo MA, Astolfi A, Indio V, et al. SDHA loss-of-function mutations in KIT-PDGFRA wild-type gastrointestinal stromal tumors identified by massively parallel sequencing. J Natl Cancer Inst 2011;103(12):983–7.

32. Lasota J, Wang Z, Kim SY, et al. Expression of the receptor for type I insulin-like growth factor (IGF1R) in gastrointestinal stromal tumors: an immunohistochemical study of 1078 cases with diagnostic and therapeutic implications. Am J Surg Pathol 2013;37(1):114–9.

33. Corless CL, Barnett CM, Heinrich MC. Gastrointestinal stromal tumours: origin and molecular oncology. Nat Rev Cancer 2011;11(12):865–78.

34. Joensuu H, Roberts PJ, Sarlomo-Rikala M, et al. Effect of the tyrosine kinase inhibitor STI571 in a patient with a metastatic gastrointestinal stromal tumor. N Engl J Med 2001;344(14):1052–6.

35. van Oosterom AT, Judson I, Verweij J, et al. Safety and efficacy of imatinib (STI571) in metastatic gastrointestinal stromal tumours: a phase I study. Lancet 2001;358(9291):1421–3.

36. Blanke CD, Rankin C, Demetri GD, et al. Phase III randomized, intergroup trial assessing imatinib mesylate at two dose levels in patients with unresectable or metastatic gastrointestinal stromal tumors expressing the kit receptor tyrosine kinase: S0033. J Clin Oncol 2008;26(4):626.

37. Le Cesne A, Ray-Coquard I, Bui BN, et al. Discontinuation of imatinib in patients with advanced gastrointestinal stromal tumours after 3 years of treatment: an open-label multicentre randomised phase 3 trial. Lancet Oncol 2010;11(10): 942–9.

38. Benjamin RS, Choi H, Macapinlac HA, et al. We should desist using RECIST, at least in GIST. J Clin Oncol 2007;25(13):1760–4.

39. Van den Abbeele AD, Badawi RD. Use of positron emission tomography in oncology and its potential role to assess response to imatinib mesylate therapy in gastrointestinal stromal tumors (GISTs). Eur J Cancer 2002;38(Suppl 5):S60–5.

40. Choi H. Critical issues in response evaluation on computed tomography: lessons from the gastrointestinal stromal tumor model. Curr Oncol Rep 2005; 7(4):307–11.

41. Choi H, Charnsangavej C, Faria SC, et al. Correlation of computed tomography and positron emission tomography in patients with metastatic gastrointestinal stromal tumor treated at a single institution with imatinib mesylate: proposal of new computed tomography response criteria. J Clin Oncol 2007;25(13): 1753–9.

42. Antonescu CR. The GIST paradigm: lessons for other kinase-driven cancers. J Pathol 2011;223(2):251–61.

43. Joensuu H, DeMatteo RP. The management of gastrointestinal stromal tumors: a model for targeted and multidisciplinary therapy of malignancy. Annu Rev Med 2012;63:247–58.

44. DeMatteo RP, Ballman KV, Antonescu CR, et al. Adjuvant imatinib mesylate after resection of localised, primary gastrointestinal stromal tumour: a randomised, double-blind, placebo-controlled trial. Lancet 2009;373(9669):1097–104.

45. Joensuu H, Eriksson M, Sundby Hall K, et al. One vs three years of adjuvant imatinib for operable gastrointestinal stromal tumor: a randomized trial. J Am Med Assoc 2012;307(12):1265–72.

46. Romond EH, Perez EA, Bryant J, et al. Trastuzumab plus adjuvant chemotherapy for operable HER2-positive breast cancer. N Engl J Med 2005; 353(16):1673–84.

47. McAuliffe JC, Hunt KK, Lazar AJ, et al. A randomized, phase II study of preoperative plus postoperative imatinib in GIST: evidence of rapid radiographic response and temporal induction of tumor cell apoptosis. Ann Surg Oncol 2009;16(4):910–9.

48. Doyon C, Sideris L, Leblanc G, et al. Prolonged therapy with imatinib mesylate before surgery for advanced gastrointestinal stromal tumor results of a phase II trial. Int J Surg Oncol 2012;2012:761576.
49. Wang D, Zhang Q, Blanke CD, et al. Phase II trial of neoadjuvant/adjuvant imatinib mesylate for advanced primary and metastatic/recurrent operable gastrointestinal stromal tumors: long-term follow-up results of Radiation Therapy Oncology Group 0132. Ann Surg Oncol 2012;19(4):1074–80.
50. DeMatteo RP, Gold JS, Saran L, et al. Tumor mitotic rate, size, and location independently predict recurrence after resection of primary gastrointestinal stromal tumor (GIST). Cancer 2008;112(3):608–15.
51. Singer S, Rubin BP, Lux ML, et al. Prognostic value of KIT mutation type, mitotic activity, and histologic subtype in gastrointestinal stromal tumors. J Clin Oncol 2002;20(18):3898–905.
52. Wardelmann E, Losen I, Hans V, et al. Deletion of Trp-557 and Lys-558 in the juxtamembrane domain of the c-kit protooncogene is associated with metastatic behavior of gastrointestinal stromal tumors. Int J Cancer 2003;106(6):887–95.
53. Martin J, Poveda A, Llombart-Bosch A, et al. Deletions affecting codons 557-558 of the c-KIT gene indicate a poor prognosis in patients with completely resected gastrointestinal stromal tumors: a study by the Spanish Group for Sarcoma Research (GEIS). J Clin Oncol 2005;23(25):6190–8.
54. Gold J, Gönen M, Gutiérrez A, et al. Development and validation of a prognostic nomogram for recurrence-free survival after complete surgical resection of localised primary gastrointestinal stromal tumour: a retrospective analysis. Lancet Oncol 2009;10:1045–52.
55. Rossi S, Miceli R, Messerini L, et al. Natural history of imatinib-naive GISTs: a retrospective analysis of 929 cases with long-term follow-up and development of a survival nomogram based on mitotic index and size as continuous variables. Am J Surg Pathol 2011;35(11):1646–56.
56. Antonescu CR, Besmer P, Guo T, et al. Acquired resistance to imatinib in gastrointestinal stromal tumor occurs through secondary gene mutation. Clin Cancer Res 2005;11(11):4182–90.
57. Heinrich MC, Corless CL, Demetri GD, et al. Kinase mutations and imatinib response in patients with metastatic gastrointestinal stromal tumor. J Clin Oncol 2003;21(23):4342–9.
58. Chen LL, Trent JC, Wu EF, et al. A missense mutation in KIT kinase domain 1 correlates with imatinib resistance in gastrointestinal stromal tumors. Cancer Res 2004;64(17):5913–9.
59. Wakai T, Kanda T, Hirota S, et al. Late resistance to imatinib therapy in a metastatic gastrointestinal stromal tumour is associated with a second KIT mutation. Br J Cancer 2004;90(11):2059–61.
60. Debiec-Rychter M, Cools J, Dumez H, et al. Mechanisms of resistance to imatinib mesylate in gastrointestinal stromal tumors and activity of the PKC412 inhibitor against imatinib-resistant mutants. Gastroenterology 2005;128(2):270–9.
61. Grimpen F, Yip D, McArthur G, et al. Resistance to imatinib, low-grade FDG-avidity on PET, and acquired KIT exon 17 mutation in gastrointestinal stromal tumour. Lancet Oncol 2005;6(9):724–7.
62. Wardelmann E, Thomas N, Merkelbach-Bruse S, et al. Acquired resistance to imatinib in gastrointestinal stromal tumours caused by multiple KIT mutations. Lancet Oncol 2005;6(4):249–51.

63. Koyama T, Nimura H, Kobayashi K, et al. Recurrent gastrointestinal stromal tumor (GIST) of the stomach associated with a novel c-kit mutation after imatinib treatment. Gastric Cancer 2006;9(3):235–9.

64. Liegl B, Kepten I, Le C, et al. Heterogeneity of kinase inhibitor resistance mechanisms in GIST. J Pathol 2008;216(1):64–74.

65. Lim KH, Huang MJ, Chen LT, et al. Molecular analysis of secondary kinase mutations in imatinib-resistant gastrointestinal stromal tumors. Med Oncol 2008;25(2):207–13.

66. Nishida T, Kanda T, Nishitani A, et al. Secondary mutations in the kinase domain of the KIT gene are predominant in imatinib-resistant gastrointestinal stromal tumor. Cancer Sci 2008;99(4):799–804.

67. Wardelmann E, Merkelbach-Bruse S, Pauls K, et al. Polyclonal evolution of multiple secondary KIT mutations in gastrointestinal stromal tumors under treatment with imatinib mesylate. Clin Cancer Res 2006;12(6):1743–9.

68. Loughrey MB, Waring PM, Dobrovic A, et al. Polyclonal resistance in gastrointestinal stromal tumor treated with sequential kinase inhibitors. Clin Cancer Res 2006;12(20 Pt 1):6205–6 [author reply: 6206–7].

69. Demetri GD, van Oosterom AT, Garrett CR, et al. Efficacy and safety of sunitinib in patients with advanced gastrointestinal stromal tumour after failure of imatinib: a randomised controlled trial. Lancet 2006;368(9544):1329–38.

70. Le Cesne A, Blay JY, Bui BN, et al. Phase II study of oral masitinib mesilate in imatinib-naive patients with locally advanced or metastatic gastro-intestinal stromal tumour (GIST). Eur J Cancer 2010;46(8):1344–51.

71. Benjamin RS, Schoffski P, Hartmann JT, et al. Efficacy and safety of motesanib, an oral inhibitor of VEGF, PDGF, and Kit receptors, in patients with imatinib-resistant gastrointestinal stromal tumors. Cancer Chemother Pharmacol 2011; 68(1):69–77.

72. Joensuu H, De Braud F, Grignagni G, et al. Vatalanib for metastatic gastrointestinal stromal tumour (GIST) resistant to imatinib: final results of a phase II study. Br J Cancer 2011;104(11):1686–90.

73. Demetri GD, Reichardt P, Kang YK, et al. Efficacy and safety of regorafenib for advanced gastrointestinal stromal tumours after failure of imatinib and sunitinib (GRID): an international, multicentre, randomised, placebo-controlled, phase 3 trial. Lancet 2013;381(9863):295–302.

74. DeMatteo RP, Maki RG, Singer S, et al. Results of tyrosine kinase inhibitor therapy followed by surgical resection for metastatic gastrointestinal stromal tumor. Ann Surg 2007;245(3):347–52.

75. Raut CP, Posner M, Desai J, et al. Surgical management of advanced gastrointestinal stromal tumors after treatment with targeted systemic therapy using kinase inhibitors. J Clin Oncol 2006;24(15):2325–31.

76. Gronchi A, Fiore M, Miselli F, et al. Surgery of residual disease following molecular-targeted therapy with imatinib mesylate in advanced/metastatic GIST. Ann Surg 2007;245(3):341–6.

77. Vanneman M, Dranoff G. Combining immunotherapy and targeted therapies in cancer treatment. Nat Rev Cancer 2012;12(4):237–51.

78. Ménard C, Blay JY, Borg C, et al. Natural killer cell IFN-gamma levels predict long-term survival with imatinib mesylate therapy in gastrointestinal stromal tumor-bearing patients. Cancer Res 2009;69(8):3563–9.

79. Balachandran VP, Cavnar MJ, Zeng S, et al. Imatinib potentiates antitumor T cell responses in gastrointestinal stromal tumor through the inhibition of Ido. Nat Med 2011;17(9):1094–100.

80. Curtin JA, Busam K, Pinkel D, et al. Somatic activation of KIT in distinct subtypes of melanoma. J Clin Oncol 2006;24(26):4340–6.
81. Beadling C, Jacobson-Dunlop E, Hodi FS, et al. KIT gene mutations and copy number in melanoma subtypes. Clin Cancer Res 2008;14(21):6821–8.
82. Carvajal RD, Antonescu CR, Wolchok JD, et al. KIT as a therapeutic target in metastatic melanoma. J Am Med Assoc 2011;305(22):2327–34.
83. Kemmer K, Corless CL, Fletcher JA, et al. KIT mutations are common in testicular seminomas. Am J Pathol 2004;164(1):305–13.
84. Pedersini R, Vattemi E, Mazzoleni G, et al. Complete response after treatment with imatinib in pretreated disseminated testicular seminoma with overexpression of c-KIT. Lancet Oncol 2007;8(11):1039–40.
85. Johnson BE, Fischer T, Fischer B, et al. Phase II study of imatinib in patients with small cell lung cancer. Clin Cancer Res 2003;9(16 Pt 1):5880–7.
86. Boldrini L, Ursino S, Gisfredi S, et al. Expression and mutational status of c-kit in small-cell lung cancer: prognostic relevance. Clin Cancer Res 2004;10(12 Pt 1): 4101–8.
87. Tamborini E, Bonadiman L, Greco A, et al. Expression of ligand-activated KIT and platelet-derived growth factor receptor beta tyrosine kinase receptors in synovial sarcoma. Clin Cancer Res 2004;10(3):938–43.
88. Strobel P, Hartmann M, Jakob A, et al. Thymic carcinoma with overexpression of mutated KIT and the response to imatinib. N Engl J Med 2004;350(25): 2625–6.
89. Simon MP, Pedeutour F, Sirvent N, et al. Deregulation of the platelet-derived growth factor B-chain gene via fusion with collagen gene COL1A1 in dermatofibrosarcoma protuberans and giant-cell fibroblastoma. Nat Genet 1997;15(1): 95–8.
90. Rutkowski P, Van Glabbeke M, Rankin CJ, et al. Imatinib mesylate in advanced dermatofibrosarcoma protuberans: pooled analysis of two phase II clinical trials. J Clin Oncol 2010;28(10):1772–9.
91. Kris MG, Natale RB, Herbst RS, et al. Efficacy of gefitinib, an inhibitor of the epidermal growth factor receptor tyrosine kinase, in symptomatic patients with non-small cell lung cancer: a randomized trial. J Am Med Assoc 2003; 290(16):2149–58.
92. Lynch TJ, Bell DW, Sordella R, et al. Activating mutations in the epidermal growth factor receptor underlying responsiveness of non-small-cell lung cancer to gefitinib. N Engl J Med 2004;350(21):2129–39.
93. Pao W, Miller V, Zakowski M, et al. EGF receptor gene mutations are common in lung cancers from "never smokers" and are associated with sensitivity of tumors to gefitinib and erlotinib. Proc Natl Acad Sci U S A 2004;101(36):13306–11.
94. Paez JG, Janne PA, Lee JC, et al. EGFR mutations in lung cancer: correlation with clinical response to gefitinib therapy. Science 2004;304(5676):1497–500.
95. Shepherd FA, Rodrigues Pereira J, Ciuleanu T, et al. Erlotinib in previously treated non-small-cell lung cancer. N Engl J Med 2005;353(2):123–32.
96. Cohen EE, Davis DW, Karrison TG, et al. Erlotinib and bevacizumab in patients with recurrent or metastatic squamous-cell carcinoma of the head and neck: a phase I/II study. Lancet Oncol 2009;10(3):247–57.
97. Pautier P, Joly F, Kerbrat P, et al. Phase II study of gefitinib in combination with paclitaxel (P) and carboplatin (C) as second-line therapy for ovarian, tubal or peritoneal adenocarcinoma (1839IL/0074). Gynecol Oncol 2010;116(2):157–62.
98. Rini BI. Lapatinib therapy for patients with advanced renal cell carcinoma. Nat Clin Pract Oncol 2008;5(11):626–7.

99. Cunningham D, Humblet Y, Siena S, et al. Cetuximab monotherapy and cetuximab plus irinotecan in irinotecan-refractory metastatic colorectal cancer. N Engl J Med 2004;351(4):337–45.

100. Peeters M, Price TJ, Cervantes A, et al. Randomized phase III study of panitumumab with fluorouracil, leucovorin, and irinotecan (FOLFIRI) compared with FOLFIRI alone as second-line treatment in patients with metastatic colorectal cancer. J Clin Oncol 2010;28(31):4706–13.

101. Bollag G, Hirth P, Tsai J, et al. Clinical efficacy of a RAF inhibitor needs broad target blockade in BRAF-mutant melanoma. Nature 2010;467(7315):596–9.

102. Chapman PB, Hauschild A, Robert C, et al. Improved survival with vemurafenib in melanoma with BRAF V600E mutation. N Engl J Med 2011;364(26): 2507–16.

103. Slamon DJ, Leyland-Jones B, Shak S, et al. Use of chemotherapy plus a monoclonal antibody against HER2 for metastatic breast cancer that overexpresses HER2. N Engl J Med 2001;344(11):783–92.

104. Oxnard GR, Binder A, Janne PA. New targetable oncogenes in non-small-cell lung cancer. J Clin Oncol 2013;31:1097–104.

105. Krause DS, Van Etten RA. Tyrosine kinases as targets for cancer therapy. N Engl J Med 2005;353(2):172–87.

106. Kurzrock R, Sherman SI, Ball DW, et al. Activity of XL184 (Cabozantinib), an oral tyrosine kinase inhibitor, in patients with medullary thyroid cancer. J Clin Oncol 2011;29(19):2660–6.

107. Wells SA Jr, Robinson BG, Gagel RF, et al. Vandetanib in patients with locally advanced or metastatic medullary thyroid cancer: a randomized, double-blind phase III trial. J Clin Oncol 2012;30(2):134–41.

108. Lam ET, Ringel MD, Kloos RT, et al. Phase II clinical trial of sorafenib in metastatic medullary thyroid cancer. J Clin Oncol 2010;28(14):2323–30.

109. Sawaki A, Nishida T, Doi T, et al. Phase 2 study of nilotinib as third-line therapy for patients with gastrointestinal stromal tumor. Cancer 2011;117:4633–41.

110. Cauchi C, Somaiah N, Engstrom PF, et al. Evaluation of nilotinib in advanced GIST previously treated with imatinib and sunitinib. Cancer Chemother Pharmacol 2012;69(4):977–82.

111. Reichardt P, Blay JY, Gelderblom H, et al. Phase III study of nilotinib versus best supportive care with or without a TKI in patients with gastrointestinal stromal tumors resistant to or intolerant of imatinib and sunitinib. Ann Oncol 2012; 23(7):1680–7.

112. Demetri GD, Lo Russo P, MacPherson IR, et al. Phase I dose-escalation and pharmacokinetic study of dasatinib in patients with advanced solid tumors. Clin Cancer Res 2009;15(19):6232–40.

113. Wilhelm SM, Carter C, Tang L, et al. BAY 43-9006 exhibits broad spectrum oral antitumor activity and targets the RAF/MEK/ERK pathway and receptor tyrosine kinases involved in tumor progression and angiogenesis. Cancer Res 2004; 64(19):7099–109.

114. Italiano A, Cioffi A, Coco P, et al. Patterns of care, prognosis, and survival in patients with metastatic gastrointestinal stromal tumors (GIST) refractory to first-line imatinib and second-line sunitinib. Ann Surg Oncol 2012;19(5):1551–9.

115. Park SH, Ryu MH, Ryoo BY, et al. Sorafenib in patients with metastatic gastrointestinal stromal tumors who failed two or more prior tyrosine kinase inhibitors: a phase II study of Korean gastrointestinal stromal tumors study group. Invest New Drugs 2012;30(6):2377–83.

116. George S, Wang Q, Heinrich MC, et al. Efficacy and safety of regorafenib in patients with metastatic and/or unresectable GI stromal tumor after failure of imatinib and sunitinib: a multicenter phase II trial. J Clin Oncol 2012;30(19): 2401–7.

117. Soria JC, Massard C, Magne N, et al. Phase 1 dose-escalation study of oral tyrosine kinase inhibitor masitinib in advanced and/or metastatic solid cancers. Eur J Cancer 2009;45(13):2333–41.

118. Joensuu H, De Braud F, Coco P, et al. Phase II, open-label study of PTK787/ ZK222584 for the treatment of metastatic gastrointestinal stromal tumors resistant to imatinib mesylate. Ann Oncol 2008;19(1):173–7.

119. Heinrich MC, Griffith D, McKinley A, et al. Crenolanib inhibits the drug-resistant PDGFRA D842V mutation associated with imatinib-resistant gastrointestinal stromal tumors. Clin Cancer Res 2012;18(16):4375–84.

Advances in Molecular and Clinical Subtyping of Breast Cancer and Their Implications for Therapy

Karen A. Cadoo, MB, BCh, BAO[a], Tiffany A. Traina, MD[b],
Tari A. King, MD[c],*

KEYWORDS

- Breast cancer • Intrinsic subtypes • Endocrine therapy • HER2 positive
- Triple negative • Resistance

KEY POINTS

- The intrinsic subtypes of breast cancer have enhanced understanding of the molecular drivers underlying subgroups of tumors.
- Endocrine receptor–positive breast cancer may develop resistance to antiestrogen therapy, and therapies to overcome this resistance are being developed.
- The management of HER2 (human epidermal growth factor receptor 2)-positive breast cancer has been revolutionized by the development of HER2 targeting drugs.
- In triple-negative breast cancer, there are no currently validated targeted therapies; however, several novel approaches are being investigated.

INTRODUCTION

Breast cancer represents a complex and heterogenous group of diseases with distinct morphologic and molecular features.[1,2] Most patients present with early-stage disease, and a proportion of these are cured with local therapy alone. Accurate identification of patients who are at risk for recurrent or metastatic disease, and the selection of appropriate systemic interventions for these patients, has helped to improve survival.

Disclosures: The authors have nothing to disclose.
[a] Breast Cancer Medicine Service, Memorial Sloan-Kettering Cancer Center, Weill Medical College of Cornell University, New York, NY 10065, USA; [b] Breast Cancer Medicine Service, Memorial Sloan-Kettering Cancer Center, Department of Medicine, Weill Medical College of Cornell University, New York, NY 10065, USA; [c] Breast Service, Department of Surgery, Memorial Sloan-Kettering Cancer Center, Weill Medical College of Cornell University, New York, NY 10065, USA
* Corresponding author.
E-mail address: kingt@mskcc.org

Surg Oncol Clin N Am 22 (2013) 823–840
http://dx.doi.org/10.1016/j.soc.2013.06.006
1055-3207/13/$ – see front matter © 2013 Elsevier Inc. All rights reserved.

The risk of recurrence has traditionally been estimated by amalgamating clinico-pathologic features, including tumor size, histologic grade, lymph node involvement, estrogen receptor (ER), progesterone receptor (PR), and human epidermal growth factor receptor 2 (HER2) receptor status. Patients stratified into a high-risk category are often advised to undergo systemic therapy; however, this approach overtreats some patients, exposing them to the potential for significant toxicity without corresponding benefit. In contrast, some tumors that have low-risk features may subsequently recur. It is clear that these clinicopathologic criteria incompletely represent underlying tumor biology.[3] Significant effort has been made over the last decade to investigate the molecular drivers of breast tumors. Through better understanding of breast cancer biology, the ability to prognosticate and predict treatment benefit in early-stage disease, and to overcome resistance to therapy and improve survival in metastatic breast cancer (MBC), is becoming a reality.

INTRINSIC SUBTYPES OF BREAST CANCER

Perou and Sorlie and colleagues[4,5] used gene expression profiling to group breast cancers into 5 distinct molecular classes or intrinsic subtypes, termed luminal A, luminal B, basal-like, HER2-enriched, and normal-like subtypes. A further subtype, claudin-low, was recently identified.[6] This classification reflects clinical subdivisions based on ER and HER2 status[2] but, independent of these variables, it identifies groups with differing survival[4,5,7,8] and treatment responses (**Fig. 1**).[9–12]

Luminal A and Luminal B

Luminal A is the most common subgroup and accounts for 40% to 60% of breast cancers.[1,12] These tumors are predominantly ER+/PR+ and HER2−, with low histologic grade and low expression of proliferative genes, including Ki67.[2,12] They are associated with lower relapse rate and longer survival from the time of that relapse, compared with the other subtypes.[13,14] Luminal B cancers, in common with luminal A, express high levels of luminal cytokeratins and are predominantly ER+, although they have lower expression of ER-related genes.[5] They make up 15% of breast cancers[1] and, in contrast with luminal A tumors, are more aggressive, with significantly poorer prognosis.[1,5,8,14] In addition, the TP53 pathway is conserved in luminal A but frequently inactivated in the luminal B subtype.[14] Luminal B tumors are histologically high grade and have increased expression of proliferation genes (eg, Ki67 and cyclin B1) with variable PR and HER2 status.[12] The management of luminal A tumors is centered on antiendocrine strategies,[12] and this subtype is less responsive to chemotherapy.[15] Although luminal B tumors are also ER+, a significant number do not respond to antiestrogen therapy[16] and instead show greater response to chemotherapy.[12]

HER2 Enriched

The HER2-enriched subtype makes up 10% of breast cancers[1] and is characterized by high expression of HER2 and related genes.[14] This subtype is associated with increased coexpression of proliferative genes and has high genomic instability.[14] Although chemosensitive,[11] the HER2-enriched subtype was a poor prognosis category[8] until the introduction of HER2-targeted drugs.[14,17] There is incomplete concordance between histologic and intrinsic subtyping, with only 70% of HER2-enriched tumors by microarray showing protein overexpression.[18,19] For tumors that are HER2 enriched but clinically HER2−, the role of anti-HER2 therapy is unclear.[19] In addition, a significant number of clinically HER2+ tumors belong to the luminal B

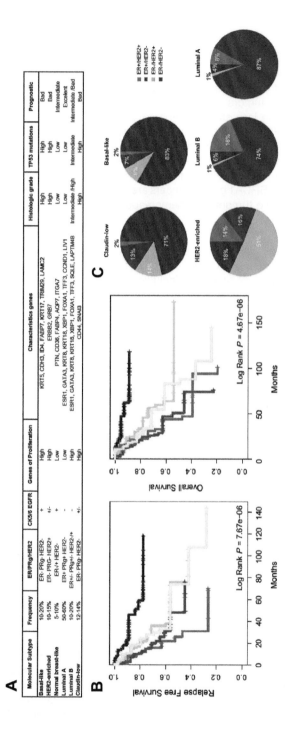

Fig. 1. (A) Features of molecular subtypes of breast cancer; (B) Kaplan-Meier curves of disease-free survival and overall survival based on the UNC337 database. Dark blue, luminal A; light blue, luminal B; red, basal-like; pink, HER2-enriched; yellow, claudin-low; (C) distribution of ER and HER2 in the different subtypes of breast cancer based on mRNA expression. (*From* Eroles P, Bosch A, Perez-Fidalgo JA, et al. Molecular biology in breast cancer: intrinsic subtypes and signaling pathways. Cancer Treat Rev 2012;38(6):699; with permission.)

cluster, and these are associated with better prognosis than those that are HER2 enriched.[18]

Basal-like

Basal-like breast cancers (BLBCs) express genes characteristic of normal breast myoepithelial cells, such as cytokeratins 5, 6, and 17.[20] These tumors represent 10% to 25% of breast cancers, are highly proliferative, and have a high rate of p53 mutations.[19] Basal-like tumors are associated with increased genetic complexity and are purported to be less stable compared with other breast subtypes.[21] They do not express ER/PR or HER2, and overlap with the clinically defined triple-negative breast cancers (TNBCs).[21] However, these terms are not synonymous. Not all tumors with a basal-like gene expression profile are triple negative; 15% to 45% express ER and HER2 or both.[21] In contrast, only 85% of TNBCs have a basal-like molecular phenotype.[21] BRCA1 breast cancers are associated with the basal-like sub-group.[1,19] Although these tumors are chemoresponsive,[11] they have shown a poor prognosis across several studies.[1,5,20,22,23]

Claudin-low

Claudin-low tumors make up 7% to 14%[24] of breast cancers and have low expression of genes involved in cell-cell adhesion, including claudin 3, 4, 7, and E-cadherin.[9] These tumors have metaplastic and medullary differentiation, and they predominantly present as TNBC.[9,19] However, there is incomplete concordance, with 15% of claudin-low breast cancers expressing ER and 15% overexpressing HER2.[24] These tumors may also be associated with BRCA1 mutations.[19] Claudin-low tumors do not show high expression of proliferation genes, but they also have a poor prognosis.[9] These tumors are unique in being enriched for epithelial-to-mesenchymal transition markers, and have a significant immune cell infiltrate and cancer stem cell–like features.[9,19] Claudin-low tumor response to chemotherapy is intermediate between that of basal-like and luminal subtypes.[9,19]

Normal-like

The normal-like subset expresses genes characteristic of adipose tissue[12] and represents 3% to 10% of breast cancers.[24] These tumors are frequently ER+ and have low levels of proliferative genes and low tumor cellularity.[24] The prognosis of this group is reported to be intermediate, with better survival than all but luminal A breast cancers.[12] There is controversy as to the significance of this group, and it has been suggested that it represents technical artifact.[25]

The identification of these molecular signatures has reshaped understanding of breast cancer and helps to inform the search for novel therapies.[2,12] However, this classification is a work in progress, requiring refinement and standardization before it can be incorporated into clinical practice and decision making.[12,15,25,26] Further intrinsic subtypes, such as interferon-rich and molecular apocrine, have been proposed, but the significance of these groups remains unknown.[26]

Several tools have been developed in an attempt to use molecular profiling to prognosticate and predict benefit from therapy. The PAM50 assay classifies tumor samples into intrinsic subtypes and predicts risk of relapse. However, it lacks validation and is not ready for clinical decision making.[25,26] Several multigene signatures have also been developed that can risk stratify and predict therapeutic response to varying degrees. These multigene signatures include MammaPrint, OncotypeDx, Theros/MGI, MapQuant Dx, Rotterdam/Veridex 76-gene, and the wound-response gene signatures.[27] MammaPrint is a prognostic test[28–30] that has been granted US Food and Drug Administration approval for assessment of breast cancer recurrence risk in tumors that are lymph node negative, less than 5 cm, and either ER positive or ER negative. OncotypeDx applies to ER-positive, primarily node-negative breast cancer, and can predict risk of recurrence and likelihood of benefit from chemotherapy.[31,32] It has also shown similar predictive power in retrospective analysis of lymph node–positive patients.[33] Both tests are currently in clinical use; however, the Evaluation of Genomic Applications in Practice and Prevention (EGAPP) working group assessment found that further evaluation of these technologies is required.[25] Prospective validation is ongoing with the MINDACT (MammaPrint), TAILORx (OncotypeDx), and RxPONDER (OncotypeDx, in patients with 1–3 positive lymph nodes) studies.

Therefore, despite the progress and better understanding of the drivers of this disease, from a clinical management perspective, breast cancer remains divided into 3 therapeutic categories:

1. ER+ disease, which is targeted with antiendocrine strategies
2. HER2+ disease, which is treated with HER2-targeted agents
3. Triple-negative breast cancer, which lacks validated targeted therapy options and is treated with traditional cytotoxic therapy.

This article discusses how translational research has led to the development of targeted therapies based on the drivers of specific subgroups of breast cancer.

ER-POSITIVE BREAST CANCER
Endocrine Therapy

Targeting the ER is well established in the treatment of early and advanced ER+ breast cancer. This approach was pioneered in the 19th Century when Beatson[34] noted tumor responses in women with advanced breast cancer treated with oophorectomy. With the identification of the ER, it was subsequently possible to select patients likely to benefit from antiendocrine therapy. Tamoxifen, a selective ER modulator, was approved in the late 1970s for the treatment of postmenopausal women with MBC.[35] Later, its role in preventing disease recurrence was established, and tamoxifen was incorporated into adjuvant therapy, for all women with ER+ breast cancer.[35] In the mid-1990s, anastrozole was the first aromatase inhibitor (AI) developed for postmenopausal women with ER+ MBC. Shortly afterward, it too was approved for adjuvant use. Other AIs, letrozole and exemestane, followed and are applied in both the metastatic and adjuvant settings. The AIs have shown increased efficacy compared with tamoxifen, but their benefit is limited to postmenopausal women based on their mechanism of action, which causes a paradoxic estrogen surge in women with functioning ovaries.[36] Fulvestrant, a selective ER downregulator, was subsequently developed for postmenopausal women with progression of ER+ breast cancer following antiestrogen therapy.[35] In premenopausal women, tamoxifen remains the first-line antiendocrine strategy in both the adjuvant and metastatic setting. The role of ovarian suppression has been explored, and, in premenopausal women with MBC, the combination of tamoxifen with ovarian suppression improves survival.[37] The role of ovarian suppression in the adjuvant setting is less clear, and the results of the Suppression of Ovarian Function Plus Either Tamoxifen or Exemestane Compared With Tamoxifen Alone in Treating Premenopausal Women With Hormone-Responsive Breast Cancer (SOFT) study are awaited.

Despite these effective antiendocrine strategies, several patients develop treatment resistance—in adjuvant patients with the development of metastatic disease or, in the context of MBC, progression of disease in the face of ongoing therapy.[38,39] This may be caused by de novo resistance (ie, having never responded to antiestrogen therapy) or acquired resistance shown by refractory disease following an initial period of response. Extensive efforts have been made to better elucidate mechanisms of resistance to identify potential therapeutic targets that may overcome this resistance.

Signaling downstream of ER involves multiple crosstalking and potentially compensatory pathways, including mitogen-activated protein kinase (MAPK), phosphatidylinositide 3-kinase (PI3K)/AKT/mammalian target of rapamycin (mTOR), epidermal growth factor receptor (EGFR), insulinlike growth factor receptor (IGF-IR), fibroblast growth factor (FGF) receptor, and Src (**Fig. 2**).[39,40] Inhibition of the ER may cause upregulation of these alternative pathways, driving resistance to therapy.[39]

mTOR

Increased activity of PI3K/AKT is associated with endocrine resistance in breast cancer cells.[41] There has been significant interest in targeting mTOR, a downstream mediator of this pathway, using inhibitors developed for transplant immunotherapy and kidney cancer. Inhibition of mTOR restored sensitivity to endocrine therapy in breast cancer cells.[42,43] The randomized phase III study BOLERO-2 examined the combination of everolimus (an mTOR inhibitor) and exemestane versus exemestane alone in women with progressive metastatic disease following an AI.[38] Everolimus significantly improved progression-free survival (PFS) from 4.1 to 10.6 months (hazard ratio, 0.36;

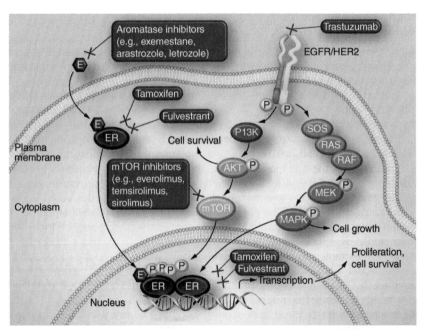

Fig. 2. Binding of estrogen to the intracellular ER leads to proliferation and cell survival. Antiendocrine therapy with tamoxifen, AIs, or fulvestrant blocks this signaling. However, there is crosstalk between the ER pathway and other growth factor pathways including the EGFR and HER2 pathway, and activation of these pathways is implicated in resistance to antiendocrine therapy. (*From* Gnant M. Overcoming endocrine resistance in breast cancer: importance of mTOR inhibition. Expert Rev Anticancer Ther 2012;12(12):1580. © Future Science Group (2012); with permission.)

95% confidence interval [CI], 0.27 to 0.47; $P<.001$). This improvement came with additional toxicity, notably an increase in greater than or equal to grade 3 stomatitis, anemia, dyspnea, hyperglycemia, and pneumonitis.[38] TAMRAD, a phase II study of tamoxifen with or without everolimus, also included women who had resistance to an AI. This trial met its primary end point of improved clinical benefit rate (6-month clinical benefit rate, 61% vs 42%). In addition, there was improved time to progression and overall survival (OS) with the combination supporting the benefit of mTOR inhibition seen in BOLERO-2.[44] A phase I/II study of the combination of an alternative mTOR inhibitor, sirolimus, and tamoxifen similarly improved PFS in women who were previously treated with antiestrogen therapy and in the first-line setting.[45]

In contrast, the HORIZON study, which combined the mTOR inhibitor, temsirolimus, with letrozole as first-line therapy for MBC, was terminated for futility in PFS.[46] Patient population differences may account for these contrasting results,[47] because women in BOLERO-2 and TAMRAD had endocrine-resistant disease, whereas the HORIZON study was conducted in the first-line setting. It is also possible that inadequate temsirolimus dosing may have contributed to the disappointing outcome because lower-than-anticipated adverse events were observed.[48] Significant heterogeneity across ER+ breast cancers[14] likely influences drivers of resistance and response to any given therapy. A more specific biomarker than ER status may be required to select patients who will respond to mTOR inhibition.

PIK3CA

There is also interest in targeting PI3K, the upstream driver of the PIK3-AKT-mTOR pathway. PI3K is commonly mutated in breast cancer, and activation of this pathway has been implicated in acquired and de novo resistance to endocrine therapy. There is crosstalk between the ER and PI3K/AKT pathways; however, they also signal independently, suggesting that dual pathway targeting may be required to optimize outcomes.[49] The phase III trial, BELLE-2, is exploring the role of the PI3K inhibitor BKM120 with fulvestrant in women who have progressive ER+ MBC following an AI (NCT01610284).[50] An ongoing phase II trial (NCT01437566) is studying fulvestrant with or without GDC0941, an alternative PI3K inhibitor in a similar population. This study is also examining the role of PI3K mutational status as a potential biomarker. The outcome of these studies will further inform the role of targeting this pathway.

HER2

In addition to mTOR inhibition, overexpression of the HER2 proto-oncogene has been clinically validated as a mediator of resistance to endocrine therapy.[51] However, this applies to a small subgroup because only 10% of ER+ breast cancers are also HER2 positive. HER2-driven resistance to antiendocrine therapy is mediated via decreased ER level and increased ER phosphorylation, altered ER transcription, and activated downstream PI3K/AKT and MAPK pathways.[40] Dual targeting of both ER and HER2 overcomes this resistance in preclinical models.[52] Increased HER2 signaling is seen in 20% of HER2− patients relapsing on tamoxifen, although conversion to clinically HER2+ disease is rare.[53] Crosstalk between the HER2 and ER pathways is thought to drive endocrine therapy resistance. In ER+ HER2− cell lines with acquired resistance, lapatinib, an oral tyrosine kinase inhibitor of HER2, was able to restore sensitivity.[53] The phase III TAnDEM study randomized women with ER+ HER2+ MBC to anastrozole with or without trastuzumab, a monoclonal antibody to HER2.[54] The combination improved response rate (RR) and PFS. A 4.6-month improvement in OS did not achieve statistical significance; however, 70% of patients on anastrozole crossed over to receive trastuzumab on disease progression. In another phase III study, lapatinib with letrozole improved response and PFS in women with ER+ HER2+ disease.[55] There was no benefit with the addition of lapatinib to letrozole in women who had ER+ HER2− disease.

EGFR

EGFR contributes to endocrine resistance in preclinical models; however, clinical trials targeting this pathway have had only moderate success.[40] A phase II study showed improved PFS with the addition of gefitinib to anastrozole as first-line therapy for ER+ MBC.[56] Another phase II trial of gefitinib monotherapy showed a clinical benefit rate of 54% in tamoxifen-resistant MBC.[57] Another phase II study of tamoxifen with gefitinib had a numerically improved PFS with the EGFR inhibitor, but there was no benefit in patients who had received prior endocrine therapy.[58] In addition, a phase II study of anastrozole and the EGFR/HER2/HER3 inhibitor AZD8931 has been closed for futility.[59] The role of EGFR inhibitors in this setting is therefore not well defined. Biomarkers to better predict response to EGFR inhibition may lead to appropriate patient selection for this targeted therapy.

HER2-POSITIVE BREAST CANCER

The HER2 gene, also known as HER2/neu or c-erbB2, is located on chromosome 17q. HER2 belongs to the ErbB family of receptor tyrosine kinases, which normally regulate a series of cellular processes, including proliferation and growth.[60] The HER2 gene is a proto-oncogene, a normal gene with the potential to become an oncogene as a result of molecular alterations, such as mutation, amplification, or overexpression of its protein product. The HER2 protein is overexpressed and/or its gene is amplified in approximately 20% of invasive breast cancers, and it is associated with a more aggressive biology, increased risk for progression of disease, and decreased OS.[61,62] Advances in translational science have led to the development of several therapies that target HER2, including the monoclonal antibody trastuzumab and the small-molecule tyrosine kinase inhibitor (TKI) lapatinib; however, many tumors either exhibit de novo resistance to anti-HER2 therapy or acquire resistance over time, leading to disease progression and shortened survival for patients. More recently, novel agents with varying mechanisms of action have been described, and emerging data indicate that combinations of anti-HER2 agents may overcome resistance.

Trastuzumab

Trastuzumab is a humanized recombinant monoclonal antibody that binds to the external domain of HER2. On binding, trastuzumab downregulates the ligand-independent HER2 dimerization and growth factor signaling cascades downstream of HER2, including the PI3K/AKT/mTOR pathway.[63–65] Trastuzumab mediates several antitumor mechanisms, including induction of an immune response to tumor through antibody-dependent cellular cytotoxicity, blockade of cleavage of the HER2 receptor, as well as downregulating ligand-independent HER2 dimers.

The clinical benefit of trastuzumab for patients with tumors that are HER2 positive (amplified or overexpressed) was first shown in 2001 in a pivotal phase III randomized trial in which the addition of trastuzumab to chemotherapy was associated with higher overall RRs, and improved PFS and OS, in patients with MBC.[66] In 2005 trastuzumab was introduced in the adjuvant setting following publication of the results from several large phase III trials showing that the addition of 1 year of trastuzumab to postoperative chemotherapy decreased risk of recurrence by approximately one-half, and decreased risk of death from breast cancer by one-third.[67,68] Longer follow-up from these studies has shown sustained benefits, and 1 year of therapy remains the standard of care. In the preoperative setting, the addition of trastuzumab to chemotherapy has been associated with an increase in the rates of pathologic complete response (pCR), from 22% to 44% in the NeOAdjuvant Heceptin Study[69] and, similarly, from 16% to 32% in the phase III GeparQuattro Study,[70] leading to the acceptance of chemotherapy plus trastuzumab as standard of care in the neoadjuvant setting for women with HER2-positive breast cancer.

The molecular basis for resistance to trastuzumab, either de novo or acquired, has been difficult to elucidate, in part because of the difficulty in obtaining tumor samples after tumor progression, and in part because trastuzumab has multiple modes of pharmacologic action. Several laboratory models of resistance to trastuzumab have been reported, including hyperactivation of the PI3K/AKT/mTOR pathway through loss of the phosphatidylinositol phosphate 3'-phosphatase (PTEN) tumor suppressor or mutational activation of PIK3CA, and alteration of HER2 expression either through overt loss of overexpression or through induction of a cleaved form of HER2 that lacks the extracellular domain.[71–75] In a study of biopsy specimens from patients with tumors progressing on trastuzumab therapy, we found evidence for changes that activate PI3K/AKT signaling, but little evidence for loss of HER2 expression, suggesting that continued targeting of HER2 along with cotargeting of the PI3K/AKT pathway may represent a rational therapeutic approach.[76]

Lapatinib

Lapatinib is an oral reversible, small-molecule dual inhibitor of both the EGFR (HER1) and HER2 kinases. In 2007 it was approved for use in trastuzumab-refractory HER2-positive MBC. Preclinical evidence suggests that lapatinib exerts its antitumor effects by inducing growth arrest and/or apoptosis, as well as by blocking downstream MAPK and AKT signaling pathways. Synergism for the combination of lapatinib and trastuzumab in HER2-positive disease has been shown in the metastatic setting[77] and in the neoadjuvant setting by increased rates of pCR.[78] The Adjuvant Lapatinib and/or Trastuzumab Treatment Optimization (ALTTO) study is expected to refine the treatment algorithm for HER2-positive breast cancer in the adjuvant setting.[79]

Other Anti-HER2 Agents

Pertuzumab is a humanized monoclonal antibody that binds to an alternate extracellular domain of the HER2 receptor. Antibody binding prevents receptor dimerization and ligand-activated signaling with other growth factor receptors. Similar to lapatinib, recent studies have shown an improvement in PFS in the metastatic setting with the combination of pertuzumab and trastuzumab,[80,81] and increased rates of pCR in the neoadjuvant setting.[82]

The novel antibody drug conjugate, ado-trastuzumab emtansine (also called T-DM1), which couples trastuzumab with a chemotherapeutic agent with a microtubule binding effect similar to vinca alkaloids, was recently approved for HER2-positive metastatic disease,[83] and a range of compounds to overcome resistance by targeting heat shock protein 90, a molecular chaperone required for the stabilization of cellular proteins, are under development.

In addition, as described earlier, possible mechanisms of resistance to trastuzumab include loss of PTEN and/or activation of the PI3K/AKT signaling pathway, and these observations have led to investigation of the role of mTOR, which is a downstream component of the PTEN/PI3K pathway. As such, mTOR inhibitors, such as everolimus, are under investigation for HER2-positive MBC.

TNBC

TNBCs are defined as tumors that do not express ER, PR, or HER2. There is significant overlap between TNBC and BLBCs; however, these terms refer to different methods of classifying tumors. BLBC is defined by a gene expression signature and has immunohistochemical surrogates, which include epithelial cytokeratins 5/6, 14, 17, EGFR, and lack of ER, PR, and HER2.[23] Both TNBC and BLBC are more likely to recur early with visceral metastases and shorter OS.[84] There is an unmet need to better understand the drivers of this breast cancer subtype because the usual antiendocrine and anti-HER2 targeted therapies are ineffective, and traditional cytotoxic chemotherapy seems to be insufficient.

Recent gene expression profiling of TNBCs has shown molecular heterogeneity, dividing TNBC into 6 subtypes: 2 basal-like (basal-like 1, basal-like 2); immunomodulatory; mesenchymal; mesenchymal stem–like; and luminal androgen receptor (AR).[85] Each of these subtypes seems to have unique molecular drivers that may allow rational selection of actionable targets in select subpopulations of TNBC (**Fig. 3**). Select examples of targeted therapies for some of these subgroups are discussed later.

Platinum Chemotherapy

Basal-like 1 and 2 subtypes are enriched with cell cycle and cell division pathways as well as DNA damage response pathways.[85] Preclinical evidence suggests platinum-based therapy for TNBC and, in particular, BRCA1-associated malignancy is of benefit because it causes DNA cross-link strand breaks. In cells that lack homologous repair (ie, BRCA1-associated breast cancers), carboplatin or cisplatin have been hypothesized to have particular anticancer activity by leveraging the vulnerability of the cancer cell to DNA damage.

In a recent retrospective neoadjuvant study, 12 women with BRCA1-associated breast cancer, most of whom had TNBC, received single-agent cisplatin for 4 cycles.[86] Eighty-three percent of women treated with cisplatin achieved a pCR, in contrast with retrospective data showing that ~10% to 22% of patients with BRCA1-associated breast cancer achieved pCR with conventional anthracycline-based or taxane-based therapy. It is difficult to draw definitive conclusions from this small retrospective study; however, these data show robust activity of platinum agents in BRCA-associated TNBC. However, in a prospective neoadjuvant cisplatin study conducted in women with TNBC not enriched for BRCA mutation carriers, 18 of 28 patients experienced clinical response to therapy and only 6 achieved pCR (21%).[87] Two of those 6 had germline BRCA1 mutations. This more modest pCR rate is more typical of what is generally observed with neoadjuvant chemotherapy, and may reflect TNBC sensitivity to chemotherapy in general rather than platinums in particular.

The Translational Breast Cancer Research Consortium (TBCRC) conducted a multicenter, single-arm, phase II study of single-agent platinum in metastatic TNBC.[88] This nonrandomized trial observed an overall RR of ~30% and a clinical benefit rate of 34% with either carboplatin or cisplatin in the first-line or second-line treatment of metastatic TNBC. Investigators concluded that platinums are active and well tolerated for treatment of metastatic TNBC, but ongoing correlative studies involving BRCA mutation and p63/p73 analyses may help to better predict who will benefit most from this approach.

EGFR Inhibitors

The mesenchymal stem–like subtype is enriched for genes responsible for cell motility, cellular differentiation, and growth pathways. There are also genes representing

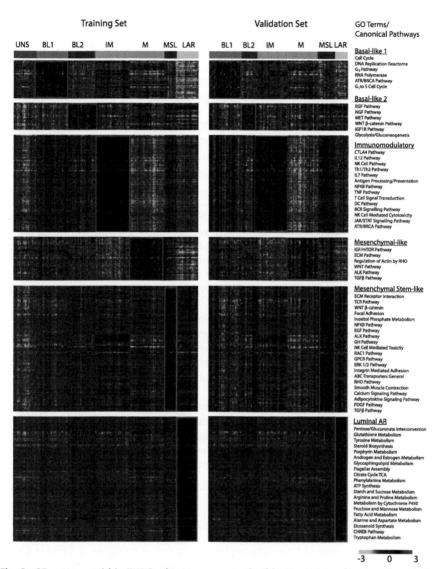

Training Set	Validation Set	GO Terms/ Canonical Pathways
UNS BL1 BL2 IM M MSL LAR	BL1 BL2 IM M MSL LAR	

Basal-like 1
Cell Cycle
DNA Replication Reactome
G_2 Pathway
RNA Polymerase
ATR/BRCA Pathway
G_1 to S Cell Cycle

Basal-like 2
EGF Pathway
NGF Pathway
MET Pathway
WNT β-catenin Pathway
IGF1R Pathway
Glycolysis/Gluconeogenesis

Immunomodulatory
CTLA4 Pathway
IL12 Pathway
NK Cell Pathway
Th1/Th2 Pathway
IL7 Pathway
Antigen Processing/Presentation
NFKB Pathway
TNF Pathway
T Cell Signal Transduction
DC Pathway
BCR Signalling Pathway
NK Cell Mediated Cytotoxicity
JAK/STAT Signalling Pathway
ATR/BRCA Pathway

Mesenchymal-like
IGF/mTOR Pathway
ECM Pathway
Regulation of Actin by RHO
WNT Pathway
ALK Pathway
TGFβ Pathway

Mesenchymal Stem-like
ECM Receptor Interaction
TCR Pathway
WNT β-catenin
Focal Adhesion
Inositol Phosphate Metabolism
NFKB Pathway
EGF Pathway
ALK Pathway
GH Pathway
NK Cell Mediated Toxicity
RAC1 Pathway
GPCR Pathway
ERK 1/2 Pathway
Integrin Mediated Adhesion
ABC Transporters General
RHO Pathway
Smooth Muscle Contraction
Calcium Signaling Pathway
Adipocytokine Signaling Pathway
PDGF Pathway
TGFβ Pathway

Luminal AR
Pentose/Glucuronate Interconversion
Glutathione Metabolism
Tyrosine Metabolism
Steroid Biosynthesis
Porphyrin Metabolism
Androgen and Estrogen Metabolism
Glycosphingolipid Metabolism
Flagellar Assembly
Citrate Cycle TCA
Phenylalanine Metabolism
ATP Synthesis
Starch and Sucrose Metabolism
Arginine and Proline Metabolism
Metabolism by Cytochrome P450
Fructose and Mannose Metabolism
Fatty Acid Metabolism
Alanine and Aspartate Metabolism
Eicosanoid Synthesis
CHREB Pathway
Tryptophan Metabolism

-3   0   3

Fig. 3. GE patterns within TNBC subtypes are reproducible. Heat maps showing the relative gene expression (log$_2$, −3 to 3) of the top differentially expressed genes ($P<.05$) in each subtype in the training set (*left*) and the same differentially expressed genes used to predict the best-fit TNBC subtype of the validation set (*right*). Overlapping gene ontology (GO) terms for top canonical pathways in both the training and validation sets as determined by gene set enrichment analysis are shown to the right of the heat maps. (*From* Lehmann BD, Bauer JA, Chen X, et al. Identification of human triple-negative breast cancer subtypes and preclinical models for selection of targeted therapies. J Clin Invest 2011;121(7):2755; with permission.)

growth factor signaling pathways such as EGFR.[85] Numerous studies have explored EGFR inhibitors for the treatment of unselected TNBC, with mixed results. Cetuximab monotherapy was compared with the combination of cetuximab and carboplatin in a phase II study by the TBCRC for the treatment of metastatic TNBC.[89] Cetuximab monotherapy offered a small clinical benefit of 10% but, in combination with carboplatin, the clinical benefit rate increased to 27%. In contrast, another phase II study compared irinotecan and carboplatin with or without cetuximab.[90] In this trial, the addition of cetuximab increased overall RR from 30% to 49%. The BALI-1 trial recently randomized 173 patients with metastatic TNBC to cisplatin monotherapy or in combination with cetuximab.[91] The addition of cetuximab offered a statistically significant improvement in PFS from 1.5 to 3.7 months (hazard ratio, 0.675; P = .032) as well as a doubling of the overall RR (10.3% vs 20.0%). Modest gains from EGFR inhibition may be a function of study designs that included unselected populations of patients with TNBC rather than those that express a molecular profile that predicts response. This approach remains under investigation.

Targeting the AR in TNBC

Several groups have described a subset of TNBCs that seem to have an endocrine-driven gene expression signature.[85,92,93] However, rather than growth being driven by ER or PR, these cancers show androgen-dependent growth, which can be diminished with the use of an antiandrogen therapy such as flutamide.[85,92] This preclinical observation was translated recently into the first prospective multicenter clinical trial testing androgen inhibition with oral bicalutamide in patients with MBC selected by AR status: AR+ ER/PR− (TBCRC011). The trial successfully met its prespecified efficacy end point, achieving a clinical benefit rate of 20%.[94] Treatment was well tolerated and now offers select patients with TNBC with AR dependency a treatment option other than cytotoxic chemotherapy. Several ongoing studies are now testing the next-generation antiandrogens developed for the treatment of prostate cancer, such as abiraterone acetate and enzalutamide, in this setting.[95]

TNBC is a heterogeneous subtype of breast cancer that differs from ER-driven or HER2-driven cancers. At present, conventional cytotoxic chemotherapy remains the standard of care for patients with TNBC because there is not a proven effective targeted therapy. However, several potential therapies are under investigation based on molecular drivers of TNBC that may offer improved clinical outcomes through precision medicine.

SUMMARY

The identification of intrinsic molecular subtypes of breast cancer has greatly enhanced understanding of the differing biology of tumor subtypes, informing therapeutic targeting and clinical trial design. Management of ER+ breast cancer is primarily centered on antiendocrine therapy. However, tumors frequently develop resistance to this strategy. Significant progress has been made in elucidating the mechanisms of this resistance, and the addition of an mTOR inhibitor, everolimus, to exemestane is now approved for women with ER+ MBC. HER2+ breast cancer has traditionally been associated with a poor prognosis; however, outcomes in this subgroup have been revolutionized by the development of HER2 targeting agents. The recent addition of pertuzumab and T-DM1 to the armamentarium will further improve survival for women with HER2+ disease. Cytotoxic chemotherapy remains the standard of care for patients with TNBC. However, based on an understanding of molecular drivers, several novel therapies are currently being investigated in this subtype. In particular, the identification of a subgroup of tumors that show androgen-dependent growth, which can be targeted with antiandrogen therapy, has shown promise in early-phase studies.

As further progress is made in translating molecular profiling into clinical practice, the challenge is to establish drivers of sensitivity and resistance within subgroups of breast cancer, which will enable the identification of the optimum pathways to target for individual patients, allowing their care to be better tailored.

REFERENCES

1. Sorlie T, Tibshirani R, Parker J, et al. Repeated observation of breast tumor subtypes in independent gene expression data sets. Proc Natl Acad Sci U S A 2003;100(14):8418–23.
2. Sotiriou C, Pusztai L. Gene-expression signatures in breast cancer. N Engl J Med 2009;360(8):790–800.
3. Sotiriou C, Piccart MJ. Taking gene-expression profiling to the clinic: when will molecular signatures become relevant to patient care? Nat Rev Cancer 2007; 7(7):545–53.
4. Perou CM, Sorlie T, Eisen MB, et al. Molecular portraits of human breast tumours. Nature 2000;406(6797):747–52.
5. Sorlie T, Perou CM, Tibshirani R, et al. Gene expression patterns of breast carcinomas distinguish tumor subclasses with clinical implications. Proc Natl Acad Sci U S A 2001;98(19):10869–74.
6. Herschkowitz JI, Simin K, Weigman VJ, et al. Identification of conserved gene expression features between murine mammary carcinoma models and human breast tumors. Genome Biol 2007;8(5):R76.
7. Hu Z, Fan C, Oh DS, et al. The molecular portraits of breast tumors are conserved across microarray platforms. BMC Genomics 2006;7:96.
8. O'Brien KM, Cole SR, Tse CK, et al. Intrinsic breast tumor subtypes, race, and long-term survival in the Carolina Breast Cancer Study. Clin Cancer Res 2010; 16(24):6100–10.
9. Prat A, Parker JS, Karginova O, et al. Phenotypic and molecular characterization of the claudin-low intrinsic subtype of breast cancer. Breast Cancer Res 2010; 12(5):R68.
10. Carey LA, Dees EC, Sawyer L, et al. The triple negative paradox: primary tumor chemosensitivity of breast cancer subtypes. Clin Cancer Res 2007;13(8): 2329–34.
11. Rouzier R, Perou CM, Symmans WF, et al. Breast cancer molecular subtypes respond differently to preoperative chemotherapy. Clin Cancer Res 2005; 11(16):5678–85.
12. Eroles P, Bosch A, Perez-Fidalgo JA, et al. Molecular biology in breast cancer: intrinsic subtypes and signaling pathways. Cancer Treat Rev 2012;38(6): 698–707.
13. Kennecke H, Yerushalmi R, Woods R, et al. Metastatic behavior of breast cancer subtypes. J Clin Oncol 2010;28(20):3271–7.
14. Cancer Genome Atlas Network. Comprehensive molecular portraits of human breast tumours. Nature 2012;490(7418):61–70.
15. Gnant M, Harbeck N, Thomssen C. St. Gallen 2011: Summary of the consensus discussion. Breast Care (Basel) 2011;6(2):136–41.
16. Creighton CJ. The molecular profile of luminal B breast cancer. Biologics 2012; 6:289–97.
17. Colozza M, de Azambuja E, Cardoso F, et al. Breast cancer: achievements in adjuvant systemic therapies in the pre-genomic era. Oncologist 2006;11(2): 111–25.

18. Parker JS, Mullins M, Cheang MC, et al. Supervised risk predictor of breast cancer based on intrinsic subtypes. J Clin Oncol 2009;27(8):1160–7.
19. Perou CM. Molecular stratification of triple-negative breast cancers. Oncologist 2011;16(Suppl 1):61–70.
20. Carey LA, Perou CM, Livasy CA, et al. Race, breast cancer subtypes, and survival in the Carolina Breast Cancer Study. JAMA 2006;295(21):2492–502.
21. Rakha EA, Reis-Filho JS, Ellis IO. Basal-like breast cancer: a critical review. J Clin Oncol 2008;26(15):2568–81.
22. Rakha EA, El-Rehim DA, Paish C, et al. Basal phenotype identifies a poor prognostic subgroup of breast cancer of clinical importance. Eur J Cancer 2006; 42(18):3149–56.
23. Nielsen TO, Hsu FD, Jensen K, et al. Immunohistochemical and clinical characterization of the basal-like subtype of invasive breast carcinoma. Clin Cancer Res 2004;10(16):5367–74.
24. Prat A, Perou CM. Deconstructing the molecular portraits of breast cancer. Mol Oncol 2011;5(1):5–23.
25. Gokmen-Polar Y, Badve S. Molecular profiling assays in breast cancer: are we ready for prime time? Oncology (Williston Park) 2012;26(4):350–7, 61.
26. Guiu S, Michiels S, Andre F, et al. Molecular subclasses of breast cancer: how do we define them? The IMPAKT 2012 Working Group Statement. Ann Oncol 2012;23(12):2997–3006.
27. Colombo PE, Milanezi F, Weigelt B, et al. Microarrays in the 2010s: the contribution of microarray-based gene expression profiling to breast cancer classification, prognostication and prediction. Breast Cancer Res 2011;13(3):212.
28. van de Vijver MJ, He YD, van't Veer LJ, et al. A gene-expression signature as a predictor of survival in breast cancer. N Engl J Med 2002;347(25): 1999–2009.
29. Buyse M, Loi S, van't Veer L, et al. Validation and clinical utility of a 70-gene prognostic signature for women with node-negative breast cancer. J Natl Cancer Inst 2006;98(17):1183–92.
30. Mook S, Schmidt MK, Weigelt B, et al. The 70-gene prognosis signature predicts early metastasis in breast cancer patients between 55 and 70 years of age. Ann Oncol 2010;21(4):717–22.
31. Paik S, Tang G, Shak S, et al. Gene expression and benefit of chemotherapy in women with node-negative, estrogen receptor-positive breast cancer. J Clin Oncol 2006;24(23):3726–34.
32. Paik S, Shak S, Tang G, et al. A multigene assay to predict recurrence of tamoxifen-treated, node-negative breast cancer. N Engl J Med 2004;351(27): 2817–26.
33. Albain KS, Barlow WE, Shak S, et al. Prognostic and predictive value of the 21-gene recurrence score assay in postmenopausal women with node-positive, oestrogen-receptor-positive breast cancer on chemotherapy: a retrospective analysis of a randomised trial. Lancet Oncol 2010;11(1):55–65.
34. Beatson GT. On the treatment of inoperable cases of carcinoma of the mamma: suggestions for a new method of treatment with illustrative cases. Lancet 1896; 2:104–7.
35. Sainsbury R. The development of endocrine therapy for women with breast cancer. Cancer Treat Rev 2013;39(5):507–17.
36. Chang J, Fan W. Endocrine therapy resistance: current status, possible mechanisms and overcoming strategies. Anticancer Agents Med Chem 2013;13(3): 464–75.

37. Klijn JG, Beex LV, Mauriac L, et al. Combined treatment with buserelin and tamoxifen in premenopausal metastatic breast cancer: a randomized study. J Natl Cancer Inst 2000;92(11):903–11.

38. Baselga J, Campone M, Piccart M, et al. Everolimus in postmenopausal hormone-receptor-positive advanced breast cancer. N Engl J Med 2012; 366(6):520–9.

39. Gnant M. Overcoming endocrine resistance in breast cancer: importance of mTOR inhibition. Expert Rev Anticancer Ther 2012;12(12):1579–89.

40. Roop RP, Ma CX. Endocrine resistance in breast cancer: molecular pathways and rational development of targeted therapies. Future Oncol 2012;8(3):273–92.

41. Clark AS, West K, Streicher S, et al. Constitutive and inducible Akt activity promotes resistance to chemotherapy, trastuzumab, or tamoxifen in breast cancer cells. Mol Cancer Ther 2002;1(9):707–17.

42. deGraffenried LA, Friedrichs WE, Russell DH, et al. Inhibition of mTOR activity restores tamoxifen response in breast cancer cells with aberrant Akt Activity. Clin Cancer Res 2004;10(23):8059–67.

43. Ghayad SE, Bieche I, Vendrell JA, et al. mTOR inhibition reverses acquired endocrine therapy resistance of breast cancer cells at the cell proliferation and gene-expression levels. Cancer Sci 2008;99(10):1992–2003.

44. Bachelot T, Bourgier C, Cropet C, et al. Randomized phase II trial of everolimus in combination with tamoxifen in patients with hormone receptor-positive, human epidermal growth factor receptor 2-negative metastatic breast cancer with prior exposure to aromatase inhibitors: a GINECO study. J Clin Oncol 2012;30(22): 2718–24.

45. Bhattacharyya GS, Biswas J, Singh JK, et al. Reversal of tamoxifen resistance (hormone resistance) by addition of sirolimus (mTOR inhibitor) in metastatic breast cancer. European Multidisciplinary Cancer Conference, Stockholm. September 23–27, 2011. [abstract LBA16].

46. Wolff AC, Lazar AA, Bondarenko I, et al. Randomized phase III placebo-controlled trial of letrozole plus oral temsirolimus as first-line endocrine therapy in postmenopausal women with locally advanced or metastatic breast cancer. J Clin Oncol 2013;31(2):195–202.

47. Dees EC, Carey LA. Improving endocrine therapy for breast cancer: it's not that simple. J Clin Oncol 2013;31(2):171–3.

48. Rugo HS, Keck S. Reversing hormone resistance: have we found the golden key? J Clin Oncol 2012;30(22):2707–9.

49. Miller TW, Balko JM, Arteaga CL. Phosphatidylinositol 3-kinase and antiestrogen resistance in breast cancer. J Clin Oncol 2011;29(33):4452–61.

50. Baselga J, Campone M, Cortes J, et al. Phase III randomized study of the oral pan-PI3K inhibitor BKM120 with fulvestrant in postmenopausal women with HR+/HER2– locally advanced or metastatic breast cancer resistant to aromatase inhibitor – BELLE-2. Cancer Res 2012;72(Suppl 24) [abstract OT2-3-09].

51. Fox EM, Arteaga CL, Miller TW. Abrogating endocrine resistance by targeting ERalpha and PI3K in breast cancer. Front Oncol 2012;2:145.

52. Cortes J, Baselga J. How to treat hormone receptor-positive, human epidermal growth factor receptor 2-amplified breast cancer. J Clin Oncol 2009;27(33): 5492–4.

53. Leary AF, Drury S, Detre S, et al. Lapatinib restores hormone sensitivity with differential effects on estrogen receptor signaling in cell models of human epidermal growth factor receptor 2-negative breast cancer with acquired endocrine resistance. Clin Cancer Res 2010;16(5):1486–97.

54. Kaufman B, Mackey JR, Clemens MR, et al. Trastuzumab plus anastrozole versus anastrozole alone for the treatment of postmenopausal women with human epidermal growth factor receptor 2-positive, hormone receptor-positive metastatic breast cancer: results from the randomized phase III TAnDEM study. J Clin Oncol 2009;27(33):5529–37.

55. Johnston S, Pippen J Jr, Pivot X, et al. Lapatinib combined with letrozole versus letrozole and placebo as first-line therapy for postmenopausal hormone receptor-positive metastatic breast cancer. J Clin Oncol 2009;27(33):5538–46.

56. Cristofanilli M, Valero V, Mangalik A, et al. Phase II, randomized trial to compare anastrozole combined with gefitinib or placebo in postmenopausal women with hormone receptor-positive metastatic breast cancer. Clin Cancer Res 2010; 16(6):1904–14.

57. Gutteridge E, Agrawal A, Nicholson R, et al. The effects of gefitinib in tamoxifen-resistant and hormone-insensitive breast cancer: a phase II study. Int J Cancer 2010;126(8):1806–16.

58. Osborne CK, Neven P, Dirix LY, et al. Gefitinib or placebo in combination with tamoxifen in patients with hormone receptor-positive metastatic breast cancer: a randomized phase II study. Clin Cancer Res 2011;17(5):1147–59.

59. Study of Anastrozole +/- AZD8931 in Postmenopausal Women With Endocrine Therapy Naive Breast Cancer (MINT). ClinicalTrials.gov Identifier: NCT01151215. Available at: http://clinicaltrials.gov/ct2/show/NCT01151215. Accessed March 10, 2013.

60. Hudis CA. Trastuzumab–mechanism of action and use in clinical practice. N Engl J Med 2007;357(1):39–51.

61. Slamon DJ, Clark GM, Wong SG, et al. Human breast cancer: correlation of relapse and survival with amplification of the HER-2/neu oncogene. Science 1987;235(4785):177–82.

62. Slamon DJ, Godolphin W, Jones LA, et al. Studies of the HER-2/neu proto-oncogene in human breast and ovarian cancer. Science 1989;244(4905): 707–12.

63. Junttila TT, Akita RW, Parsons K, et al. Ligand-independent HER2/HER3/PI3K complex is disrupted by trastuzumab and is effectively inhibited by the PI3K inhibitor GDC-0941. Cancer Cell 2009;15(5):429–40.

64. Cuello M, Ettenberg SA, Clark AS, et al. Down-regulation of the erbB-2 receptor by trastuzumab (herceptin) enhances tumor necrosis factor-related apoptosis-inducing ligand-mediated apoptosis in breast and ovarian cancer cell lines that overexpress erbB-2. Cancer Res 2001;61(12):4892–900.

65. Yakes FM, Chinratanalab W, Ritter CA, et al. Herceptin-induced inhibition of phosphatidylinositol-3 kinase and Akt Is required for antibody-mediated effects on p27, cyclin D1, and antitumor action. Cancer Res 2002;62(14):4132–41.

66. Slamon DJ, Leyland-Jones B, Shak S, et al. Use of chemotherapy plus a mono-clonal antibody against HER2 for metastatic breast cancer that overexpresses HER2. N Engl J Med 2001;344(11):783–92.

67. Piccart-Gebhart MJ, Procter M, Leyland-Jones B, et al. Trastuzumab after adju-vant chemotherapy in HER2-positive breast cancer. N Engl J Med 2005;353(16): 1659–72.

68. Romond EH, Perez EA, Bryant J, et al. Trastuzumab plus adjuvant chemo-therapy for operable HER2-positive breast cancer. N Engl J Med 2005; 353(16):1673–84.

69. Gianni L, Eiermann W, Semiglazov V, et al. Neoadjuvant chemotherapy with tras-tuzumab followed by adjuvant trastuzumab versus neoadjuvant chemotherapy

alone, in patients with HER2-positive locally advanced breast cancer (the NOAH trial): a randomised controlled superiority trial with a parallel HER2-negative cohort. Lancet 2010;375(9712):377–84.

70. Untch M, Rezai M, Loibl S, et al. Neoadjuvant treatment with trastuzumab in HER2-positive breast cancer: results from the GeparQuattro study. J Clin Oncol 2010;28(12):2024–31.

71. Esteva FJ, Guo H, Zhang S, et al. PTEN, PIK3CA, p-AKT, and p-p70S6K status: association with trastuzumab response and survival in patients with HER2-positive metastatic breast cancer. Am J Pathol 2010;177(4):1647–56.

72. Berns K, Horlings HM, Hennessy BT, et al. A functional genetic approach identifies the PI3K pathway as a major determinant of trastuzumab resistance in breast cancer. Cancer Cell 2007;12(4):395–402.

73. Nagata Y, Lan KH, Zhou X, et al. PTEN activation contributes to tumor inhibition by trastuzumab, and loss of PTEN predicts trastuzumab resistance in patients. Cancer Cell 2004;6(2):117–27.

74. Mittendorf EA, Wu Y, Scaltriti M, et al. Loss of HER2 amplification following trastuzumab-based neoadjuvant systemic therapy and survival outcomes. Clin Cancer Res 2009;15(23):7381–8.

75. Scaltriti M, Rojo F, Ocana A, et al. Expression of p95HER2, a truncated form of the HER2 receptor, and response to anti-HER2 therapies in breast cancer. J Natl Cancer Inst 2007;99(8):628–38.

76. Chandarlapaty S, Sakr RA, Giri D, et al. Frequent mutational activation of the PI3K-AKT pathway in trastuzumab-resistant breast cancer. Clin Cancer Res 2012;18(24):6784–91.

77. Blackwell KL, Burstein HJ, Storniolo AM, et al. Randomized study of lapatinib alone or in combination with trastuzumab in women with ErbB2-positive, trastuzumab-refractory metastatic breast cancer. J Clin Oncol 2010;28(7):1124–30.

78. Baselga J, Bradbury I, Eidtmann H, et al. Lapatinib with trastuzumab for HER2-positive early breast cancer (NeoALTTO): a randomised, open-label, multicentre, phase 3 trial. Lancet 2012;379(9816):633–40.

79. ALTTO (Adjuvant Lapatinib And/Or Trastuzumab Treatment Optimisation) Study; BIG 2–06/N063D. ClinicalTrials.gov Identifier: NCT00490139. Available at: http://clinicaltrials.gov/ct2/show/NCT00490139. Accessed March 27, 2013.

80. Baselga J, Gelmon KA, Verma S, et al. Phase II trial of pertuzumab and trastuzumab in patients with human epidermal growth factor receptor 2-positive metastatic breast cancer that progressed during prior trastuzumab therapy. J Clin Oncol 2010;28(7):1138–44.

81. Baselga J, Cortes J, Kim SB, et al. Pertuzumab plus trastuzumab plus docetaxel for metastatic breast cancer. N Engl J Med 2012;366(2):109–19.

82. Gianni L, Pienkowski T, Im YH, et al. Efficacy and safety of neoadjuvant pertuzumab and trastuzumab in women with locally advanced, inflammatory, or early HER2-positive breast cancer (NeoSphere): a randomised multicentre, open-label, phase 2 trial. Lancet Oncol 2012;13(1):25–32.

83. Thompson CA. CMS tackles patients' use of home medications at hospitals, MTM program fulfillment. Am J Health Syst Pharm 2013;70(7):562–5.

84. Dent R, Trudeau M, Pritchard KI, et al. Triple-negative breast cancer: Clinical features and patterns of recurrence. Clin Cancer Res 2007;13(15):4429–34.

85. Lehmann BD, Bauer JA, Chen X, et al. Identification of human triple-negative breast cancer subtypes and preclinical models for selection of targeted therapies. J Clin Invest 2011;121(7):2750–67.

86. Byrski T, Gronwald J, Huzarski T, et al. Pathologic complete response rates in young women with BRCA1-positive breast cancers after neoadjuvant chemotherapy. J Clin Oncol 2010;28(3):375–9.

87. Silver DP, Richardson AL, Eklund AC, et al. Efficacy of neoadjuvant cisplatin in triple-negative breast cancer. J Clin Oncol 2010;28(7):1145–53.

88. Isakoff SJ, Goss PE, Mayer EL, et al. TBCRC009: A multicenter phase II study of cisplatin or carboplatin for metastatic triple-negative breast cancer and evaluation of p63/p73 as a biomarker of response. J Clin Oncol 2011;29(15, Suppl) [abstract 1025].

89. Carey LA, Rugo HS, Marcom PK, et al. TBCRC 001: randomized phase II study of cetuximab in combination with carboplatin in stage IV triple-negative breast cancer. J Clin Oncol 2012;30(21):2615–23.

90. O'Shaughnessy J, Weckstein D, Vukelja S. Preliminary results of a randomized phase II study of weekly irinotecan/carboplatin with or without cetuximab in patients with metastatic breast cancer. Breast Cancer Res Treat 2007;106:S32 [abstract 308, presented data at SABCS 2007].

91. Baselga J, Stemmer S, Pego A. Cetuximab + cisplatin in estrogen receptor-negative, progesterone receptor-negative, HER2-negative (triple-negative) metastatic breast cancer: results of the randomized phase II BALI-1 trial. Cancer Res 2010;70(24, Suppl 2):PD01–01. Presented data at SABCS 2010.

92. Doane AS, Danso M, Lal P, et al. An estrogen receptor-negative breast cancer subset characterized by a hormonally regulated transcriptional program and response to androgen. Oncogene 2006;25(28):3994–4008.

93. Farmer P, Bonnefoi H, Becette V, et al. Identification of molecular apocrine breast tumours by microarray analysis. Oncogene 2005;24(29):4660–71.

94. Gucalp A, Tolaney S, Isakoff S. Targeting the androgen receptor (AR) in women with AR+ ER-/PR- metastatic breast cancer (MBC). J Clin Oncol 2012;30(Suppl) [abstract 1006].

95. Ng CH, Macpherson I, Rea D, et al. Phase I/II trial of abiraterone acetate (AA) in estrogen receptor (ERα) or androgen receptor (AR) positive metastatic breast cancer (MBC). Presented at the ESMO 2012 Conference, Vienna, September 28-October 2, 2012.

Biomarkers and Targeted Therapeutics in Colorectal Cancer

Ari N. Meguerditchian, MD, MSc, FRCS[a], Kelli Bullard Dunn, MD[b],*

KEYWORDS

- Colorectal cancer • Molecular biology • APC • p53 • Loss of heterozygosity
- Microsatellite instability • CPG-island methylation

KEY POINTS

- Genetic mutations in colorectal cancer (CRC) result in oncogene activation with uncontrolled cellular proliferation (ras, myc, src, and erbB2), or tumor-suppressor gene deletion with uncontrolled cell growth (APC, DCC, and p53).
- Loss of heterozygosity is characterized by chromosomal deletions and tumor aneuploidy. A key example of this occurs in the chromosome 18q region, deleted in up to 70% of CRCs.
- CRCs can also arise from mutations in the microsatellite instability pathway, characterized by errors in mismatch repair during DNA replication; these are seen in both hereditary and sporadic tumors.
- In the CpG-island methylation pathway, genes do not accumulate mutations; instead they are activated or inactivated by methylation (epigenetic alteration).
- MicroRNAs are posttranscriptional regulators. Abnormal microRNA expression profiles accompany every aspect of CRC transformation.

INTRODUCTION

Significant advances in molecular biology have resulted in a better understanding of the genetic defects and molecular abnormalities associated with the development and progression of colorectal cancer (CRC). Efforts to translate this knowledge into clinical applications have led to exciting developments in biomarker development. The National Institutes of Health defines a biomarker as "a characteristic that is objectively measured and evaluated as an indicator of normal biological processes, pathogenic processes, or pharmacologic responses to a therapeutic intervention."[1]

Disclosures: The authors have nothing to disclose.
[a] Department of Surgery, McGill University, 687 Pine Avenue West, Room S7.30, Montreal, Quebec H3A 1A1, Canada; [b] James Graham Brown Cancer Center, University of Louisville, 529 South Jackson Street, Suite 429, Louisville, KY 40292, USA
* Corresponding author.
E-mail address: kbdunn01@louisville.edu

Patient-specific and tumor-specific molecular signatures may represent the ideal CRC biomarkers, by allowing[2]:

- Risk stratification
- Accurate prognostic assessment
- Personalized treatment planning
- Development of targeted agents
- Accurate evaluation of treatment response

As multimodal treatment of colorectal cancer progressively shifts toward targeted therapy based on these molecular biomarkers, it is important for the cancer surgeon to have a thorough understanding of recent advances in colorectal molecular oncology. The purpose of the article is 3-fold:

1. To provide a survey of the key molecular abnormalities relevant to CRCs
2. To review details of the clinical relevance of these abnormalities
3. To demonstrate through a specific example of a molecular abnormality the process of translational research

ADENOMA-CARCINOMA SEQUENCE

Colorectal carcinoma is thought to develop from adenomatous polyps following the accumulation of mutations in what has come to be known as the adenoma-carcinoma sequence (**Fig. 1**). Adenomatous polyps arise when mechanisms normally regulating epithelial renewal are disrupted. Cellular proliferation usually occurs exclusively at the crypt base, and cells undergo terminal differentiation with eventual apoptosis as they move toward the surface of the lumen. As the polyp increases in size it becomes more dysplastic, and cells ultimately acquire invasive potential. In addition to animal models and numerous epidemiologic and clinical observational studies, the validity of this model is confirmed by large, well-designed clinical trials

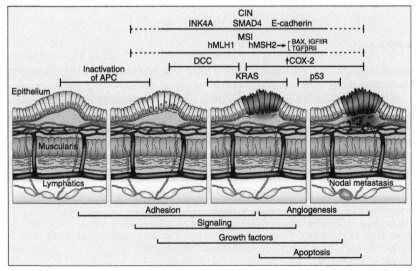

Fig. 1. Adenoma-carcinoma sequence and associated molecular alterations in colorectal cancer. (*From* Compton C, Hawk E, Grochow L, et al. Colon cancer. In: Abeloff MD, Armitage JO, Niederhuber JE, et al, editors. Abeloff's clinical oncology. 4th edition. Philadelphia: Churchill Livingstone; 2008; with permission.)

that demonstrate a reduction of CRC in patients having undergone endoscopic polypectomy.[3]

Vogelstein and colleagues[4–6] characterized the molecular basis for this multistep process whereby each additional genetic event confers a survival advantage to the epithelial cell. According to this model, the accumulation of genetic mutations rather than their specific sequence ultimately determines tumor behavior (see **Fig. 1**). Inherited colon cancer syndromes such as hereditary nonpolyposis colon cancer (HNPCC) and familial adenomatous polyposis (FAP) result from germline mutations, whereas sporadic cancers arise from the accumulation of multiple somatic mutations.

TYPES OF MUTATIONS

Genetic mutations can result in either activation of oncogenes or inactivation of tumor-suppressor genes.

Oncogenes

Oncogenes are normal cellular genes involved in cell-cycle regulation and growth. After acquiring a mutation, these genes become constitutively activated and result in uncontrolled cellular proliferation.[7] These mutations are referred to as "gain of function" mutations, because they activate what was initially a normal gene function. Oncogenes associated with sporadic CRC include ras, myc, src, and erbB2.[8–15]

The ras oncogene

The ras oncogene exists in 3 variants, of which K-ras is the most commonly involved in CRC.[16] Ras mutations are seen in 50% of adenomas larger than 1 cm and up to 50% of sporadic CRCs.[4] A signaling molecule in the epidermal growth factor receptor (EGFR) pathway, K-ras regulates cellular signal transduction, by acting as a one-way switch for the transmission of extracellular growth signals to the nucleus. The K-ras gene product is a G protein involved in intracellular signal transduction. When active, K-ras binds guanosine triphosphate (GTP); hydrolysis of GTP to guanosine diphosphate (GDP) then inactivates the G protein.[17] Mutation of K-ras results in an inability to hydrolyze GTP, thus leaving the G protein permanently active, which leads to uncontrolled cell division.[16]

Tumor-Suppressor Genes

In their normal state, tumor-suppressor genes inhibit the cell cycle. Their deletion or loss of function results in uncontrolled cell growth. Unlike proto-oncogenes, tumor-suppressor gene function is lost only when both alleles of the gene are mutated. Common examples encountered in CRC include APC, DCC, and p53.

The APC gene

Defects in the APC gene (located on chromosome 5q) were first described in patients with FAP, and are now known to be present in 80% of sporadic CRCs as well. Loss of APC gene function appears to be a very early and critical event in the development of CRC. Mutations in both alleles are necessary to initiate polyp formation, leading to sporadic CRC.[18,19] The majority of these mutations are premature stop codons, resulting in a truncated APC protein. In FAP, a single germline mutation is required. The site of mutation correlates with the clinical severity of the disease. For example, mutations in either the 3' or 5' end of the gene result in attenuated forms of FAP, whereas mutations in the center of the gene result in more virulent disease. Therefore, knowledge of the specific mutation in a family may help guide clinical decision making.

It is thought that the abnormal APC gene promotes tumor formation through the Wnt (Wingless-type) signal transduction pathway involved in supporting intestinal epithelial renewal (**Fig. 2**). The mutation results in an abnormal accumulation of β-catenin in the cell's nucleus, which binds and activates the transcriptional factor Tcf-4. Because the β-catenin/Tcf-4 construct is a switch controlling proliferation versus differentiation of intestinal crypt cells, overactivation of the switch prevents cells from either entering G1 arrest or undergoing terminal differentiation, and induces resistance to apoptosis.[20–25]

APC inactivation alone does not result in a carcinoma. Instead, this mutation sets the stage for the accumulation of genetic damage that results in malignancy. Additional mutations may include activation or inactivation of a variety of genes.

The p53 gene

The tumor-suppressor gene p53 has been well characterized in several malignancies. It acts as a transcriptional activator of at least 20 inhibitory genes and seems to be crucial in initiating a variety of growth-limiting responses including cell-cycle arrest to facilitate DNA repair, apoptosis, and differentiation.[26–28] Because of this critical function in preventing propagation of cells with damaged genetic material, p53 has been referred to as the "guardian of the genome."[29] Mutations in p53 are present in 75% of CRCs.[30] Inactivation occurs by a mutation of one allele followed by loss of the remaining wild-type gene,[31–33] and appears to be a late event in the majority of CRCs.[4,34] In addition, according to an international study of 3583 CRCs, the frequency of p53 mutations increases with advancing disease stage.[35]

The DCC gene

Point mutations in the DCC ("deleted in colon cancer") gene have been identified on chromosome 18q21 in CRCs.[5,36] DCC is thought to have a role in cell-cell or cell-matrix interactions.[37,38] Loss of DCC expression may be of prognostic value in patients with node-negative CRC. Five-year survival rates for patients with stage II

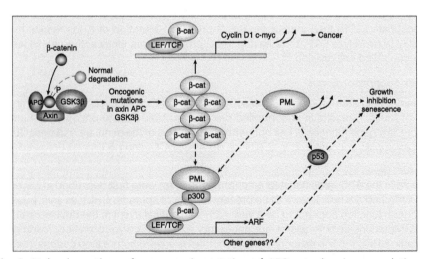

Fig. 2. Molecular pathway for oncogenic mutation of APC: cytoplasmic accumulation of β-catenin, activation of TCF complex, and consequent activation target genes promoting cell proliferation. (*From* Compton C, Hawk E, Grochow L, et al. Colon cancer. In: Abeloff MD, Armitage JO, Niederhuber JE, et al, editors. Abeloff's clinical oncology. 4th edition. Philadelphia: Churchill Livingstone; 2008; with permission.)

CRCs that lack DCC expression are worse than for those that express it, more closely approximating those of patients with stage III (node-positive) disease.[39,40]

MOLECULAR PATHWAYS TO COLORECTAL TUMORIGENESIS

The mutations involved in CRC pathogenesis and progression are now recognized to accumulate via 1 of 3 major genetic pathways:

- The loss of heterozygosity (LOH)/chromosomal instability pathway
- The microsatellite instability (MSI)/defective mismatch repair (MMR) pathway
- The CpG-island methylation/serrated methylated pathway (CIMP)

These pathways are useful for understanding the mechanisms underlying carcinogenesis; however, they are not mutually exclusive.

Loss of Heterozygosity/Chromosomal Instability Pathway

First described in patients with FAP, the LOH pathway is characterized by chromosomal deletions and tumor aneuploidy. Most CRCs appear to arise from mutations through this pathway. A key example of LOH occurs in the region of chromosome 18q, which has been found to be deleted in up to 70% of CRCs. DCC and SMAD4 are located in this region.[41–43] As described earlier, DCC is a tumor-suppressor gene thought to be involved in differentiation and cellular adhesion in CRC. SMAD4 functions in the signaling cascade of transforming growth factor β and β-catenin (also a downstream effector of the APC gene). Tumors arising from the LOH pathway tend to occur in the more distal colon, often have chromosomal aneuploidy, and are associated with a poorer prognosis.

Microsatellite Instability/Defective Mismatch Repair Pathway

Fifteen percent to 20% of CRCs arise from mutations in the MSI pathway, which is characterized by errors in mismatch repair during DNA replication. These errors were first described in HNPCC (Lynch syndrome), but are now known to be present in sporadic tumors as well. Several genes seem crucial in recognizing and repairing DNA replication errors. These MMR genes include MSH2, MLH1, PMS1, PMS2, and MSH6.[44] A mutation in 1 of these genes predisposes a cell to additional mutations, which may occur in proto-oncogenes or tumor-suppressor genes. Most HNPCCs are associated with MLH1 or MSH2 gene abnormalities, whereas sporadic cancers are associated with mutations of the MLH1 gene.[45] Accumulation of these errors leads to genomic instability and ultimately to carcinogenesis. Microsatellites are regions of the genome particularly susceptible to replication error, because short base-pair segments are repeated multiple times. A mutation in an MMR gene produces variable lengths of these repetitive sequences, a finding called MSI.

Tumors associated with a high degree of microsatellite instability (MSI-H) appear to have biological characteristics different to those of tumors that result from the LOH pathway. The majority of HNPCC as well as about 15% of sporadic CRCs have MSI-H tumors. MSI-H tumors are more likely to be right sided and are associated with a better prognosis than tumors that arise from the LOH pathway and are microsatellite stable, even if they more often are poorly differentiated.[46]

CpG-Island Methylation Pathway

In the recently described CIMP pathway, genes do not accumulate mutations (deletions or insertions of bases); instead they are activated or inactivated by methylation. This process has been called epigenetic alteration to differentiate it from the more traditional genetic alterations or true mutations. In normal cells, methylation is a critical process for gene-expression regulation. In cancer, aberrant methylation (either hyper-methylation or hypomethylation), usually of a promoter region, results in abnormal activation or inactivation of genes (including MMR enzymes).[47–50] This abnormal gene silencing or activation results in a phenotype similar to that seen in the case of a true gene mutation. Consequently, CRCs with a high frequency of methylation of promoter islands are referred to as CIMP+ tumors. This pathway has also been called the serrated methylated pathway because of the observation that serrated polyps often harbor aberrant methylation, in contrast to adenomatous polyps that are more often associated with mutations in the APC gene (LOH pathway).[51,52] In addition to abnormal methylation, this pathway is characterized by mutations in the BRAF kinase gene, which is an uncommon finding in traditional adenomas but a typical one in serrated adenomas.[53–55]

CLINICAL IMPLICATIONS

In addition to advancing our understanding of the pathogenesis of CRC, the characterization of these molecular pathways also has important clinical implications with regard to:

- Risk stratification
- Accurate prognostication
- Tumor-specific treatment planning
- Accurate evaluation of treatment response
- Targeted therapy

Risk Stratification and Prognostic Prediction

MSI-H CRCs have a distinct biological behavior: they are more often localized to the right colon, have a higher grade and mucinous component, have more necrosis, and bear a larger load of tumor-infiltrating lymphocytes.[56,57] Thibodeau and colleagues[58] and Lothe and colleagues[59] initially observed that these tumors had a more favorable prognostic profile in 1993; however, these findings were based on small, retrospective series comprising patients with tumors of stage I to IV, without regard to adjuvant or palliative systemic therapy. Since then, well-designed, large studies of nonmetastatic CRC patients have shown that while MSI-H tumors were more often locally advanced (T4), they were less frequently associated with positive lymph nodes and metastatic spread.[60–62] In a cohort of 2141 patients with stage II to stage III CRC, Sinicrope and colleagues[63] showed that disease-free survival and overall survival were significantly better in MSI-H cases, with a hazard ratio of 0.73 (95% confidence interval [CI] 0.59–0.91) and 0.73 (95% CI 0.59–0.90), respectively. In addition, a large meta-analysis of 7642 patients with CRC from 32 studies confirmed the survival advantage of MSI-H tumors, regardless of stage (relative risk of death 0.65; 95% CI 0.59–0.71).[64] As such, MSI-H status represents the best prognostic marker to date for CRC.

By contrast, other well-characterized molecular abnormalities in CRC have not been shown to have any prognostic value. For example, although K-ras mutations have consistently been shown to predict lack of response to anti-EGFR targeted therapy, they do not have any meaningful prognostic role in terms of clinical outcomes.[65]

Tumor-Specific Treatment Planning

Emerging data about prognostic biomarkers suggest that that molecular abnormalities should have a predictive value in determining the efficacy of adjuvant systemic therapy in CRC.[57] However, to date few of the known biomarkers have proved to be useful for predicting treatment response. MSI status has been most widely studied, and does appear to predict response to 5-fluorouracil (5-FU)-based chemotherapy. Kim and colleagues[66] and Ribic and colleagues[67] have demonstrated in retrospective studies that patients with MSI-H CRC experience no benefit with 5-FU–based regimens. The data from these studies showed that only patients with low-degree MSI CRC (microsatellite stable) had improved outcomes with the use of adjuvant 5-FU–based chemotherapy.[66,67] Therefore, MSI testing is increasingly being performed on CRC tissue samples to help guide decision making about adjuvant therapy in stage II and stage III disease. A prospective randomized trial (ECOG 5202) is currently under way to determine the value of MSI and 18q LOH status in predicting response to therapy with FOLFOX6.[68]

Although MSI-H is currently the only biomarker that predicts response to adjuvant therapy for stage III CRC, several other biomarkers are proving to be useful in predicting response to treatment in stage IV disease. Tyrosine kinase inhibitors (TKIs) are increasingly being used to treat metastatic CRC. Although some patients respond well to these agents, others do not. It is now known that K-ras status largely predicts response to anti-EGFR/TKI therapy (eg, cetuximab, panitumumab). Several trials have shown that the objective response in K-ras wild-type tumors can be as high as 44%, whereas the response in K-ras mutant tumors is essentially zero (CRYSTAL trial, OPUS trial).[69–76] A recent meta-analysis of 12 trials confirmed the value of first-line, second-line, and even third-line therapy with anti-EGFR monoclonal antibodies combined with 5-FU exclusively in wild-type K-ras cases.[77] As such, it is now considered standard of care to K-ras type all stage IV patients who are being considered for anti-EGFR therapy. Despite good response to anti-EGFR therapy in wild-type K-ras tumors, many of these patients fail to respond or develop resistance. Recent evidence shows that in addition to determining KRAS status, testing for BRAF, NRAS, and PI3KCA exon-20 mutations could improve response rates to cetuximab by identifying patients who would most likely benefit from the addition of this drug to systemic chemotherapy.[78–80]

Other biomarkers also have been studied for the ability to predict response to therapy, but none have proved to be as robust as K-ras. For example, using archival material, Barratt and colleagues[81] demonstrated that LOH at 1 or more chromosome 17p and 18q sites was predictive of FU-based treatment response. However, in the context of a prospective study assessing the relevance of irinotecan in 1264 patients with stage III colon cancer, Bertagnolli and colleagues[82] showed only a statistically nonsignificant trend toward improved outcomes in MSI-H patients treated with irinotecan. Similarly, Kim and colleagues[83] determined that MMR status and p53 positivity were not significantly predictive of outcomes in patients treated with 5-FU and oxaliplatin. These findings highlight the fact that molecular profiling for determination of systemic treatment requires a more refined understanding before mainstream clinical application is achieved. In particular, homogeneous groups of patients based on compatible risk profiles and equivalent cancer regimens need to be enrolled.

Molecular Profiling and Evaluation of Treatment Response

It is increasingly being recognized that no single biomarker will prove to be the "holy grail" for prognostic assessment, treatment planning, and response assessment. Rather, there is currently an intense research focus in identifying patterns of gene expression that are meaningful in terms of clinical outcomes. This type of molecular profiling has been most widely studied in breast cancer, but is rapidly growing to include a variety of other malignancies (including CRC), and the pharmaceutical industry has shown great interest developing products that predict prognosis and response to treatment. For example, OncotypeDx Colon (Genomic Health, Redwood City, CA) is a 12-gene profile that provides a composite prognostic recurrence score.[84,85] Until recently, evidence was limited to validation studies presented mostly as meeting abstracts. These validation studies represent retrospective analyses on a subset of the patients from the prospectively designed QUASAR trial. Within the constraints of these limitations, recent publications have shown that the OncotypeDx Colon assay is a valid predictor of relapse-free survival but is not a valid predictor of treatment response.[86,87] A similar product, ColoPrint (Agendia, Irvine, CA), is an 18-gene profile that stratifies CRC patients into high-risk and low-risk categories.[88–90] Finally, other approaches such as improved detection of micrometastases have been proposed. Reverse transcriptase–polymerase chain reaction for guanylyl cyclase C (GUCY2C), for example, has been shown to "upstage" patients by detecting nodal metastases that were otherwise undetected by traditional pathologic methods.[91] Although these new molecular profiling methods clearly hold promise in predicting prognosis, none have yet been shown to predict response to therapy. As such, their clinical utility in directing treatment decisions will require further study.[68]

Targeted Therapy

In addition to identifying molecules that may predict prognosis and response to therapy, research efforts are increasingly focused on identifying molecular targets for tumor-specific therapy. Several molecular targets hold promise in CRC. TKIs (anti-EGFR and anti-BRAF), discussed earlier, have been the most widely studied. Angiogenesis inhibitors (anti–vascular endothelial growth factor [VEGF]) also have shown promise in treating a variety of cancers, but results in CRC have been mixed. Bevacizumab (Avastin), an anti–VEGF-A antibody, first showed efficacy in metastatic disease and has been used as both first-line and second-line therapy in stage IV CRC.[92,93] The BRiTE (Bevacizumab Regimens' Investigation of Treatment Effects) study recently examined the efficacy of bevacizumab combined with chemotherapy as first-line treatment for metastatic CRC. At 20 months, progression-free survival was observed in 22% of patients who had received bevacizumab, whereas disease progression was seen in 79% of the patients. In addition, 66% of patients died during the study period, and 12% either withdrew from the study or were lost to follow-up.[94] In addition to these sobering outcomes, toxicity is not insignificant, and the long-term benefit of bevacizumab therapy in CRC remains to be seen.

Another recent molecule of interest is focal adhesion kinase (FAK). FAK is a nonreceptor tyrosine kinase that was first identified at the sites of adhesion between cells and the extracellular matrix.[95] FAK is known to be overexpressed in metastatic colon cancer, and phosphorylated (activated) FAK is also increased in colorectal tumor cells. Given its apparent role in tumorigenesis and overexpression in many types of cancers, FAK inhibition seems an appropriate approach to targeted cancer treatment. Recent work has shown that FAK inhibition with small-molecule inhibitors decreases colon cancer cell growth both in vitro and in vivo. Moreover, dual inhibition with other molecules such as hyaluronan synthase (HAS) appears to have synergistic effects on growth. These preclinical data suggest that FAK inhibition may offer another therapeutic target for treating patients with CRC.[96,97]

MICRORNAS, A NEW AVENUE FOR TREATMENT

MicroRNAs represent a specific class of noncoding RNA molecules, and are, in fact, 18- to 24-nucleotide posttranscriptional regulators and stabilizers of mRNA

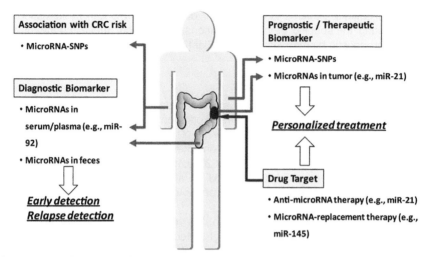

Fig. 3. Potential microRNA-based screening, and diagnostic and therapeutic strategies for colorectal cancer. (*From* Schetter AJ, Okayama H, Harris CC. The role of micro RNAs in colorectal cancer. Cancer J 2012;18(3):245; with permission.)

expression.[98] MicroRNAs play a role in multiple physiologic cellular processes, such as migration, proliferation, differentiation, and apoptosis. Abnormal microRNA expression profiles accompany cancer transformation and are involved in almost every aspect of tumor biology (**Fig. 3**).[99,100] There seems to be a strong connection between an inflammatory microenvironment, altered microRNA expression, and eventual cancerization. Some microRNAs act as inflammatory mediators while others can act as either oncogenes or tumor suppressors, depending on the cellular environment in which they are expressed. MicroRNAs have potential as biomarkers and therapeutic targets in CRC, as they are systematically altered in CRC[101] and fit consistently with the stepwise multihit model of colorectal carcinogenesis.[102] Single-nucleotide polymorphisms disrupt microRNA and therefore increase an individual's susceptibility to CRC.[103] MicroRNAs may offer the possibility of early diagnosis, as they have been shown to be present in circulating blood as well as stools.[104] Moreover, they are currently being evaluated as prognostic and predictive classifiers. MicroRNA mR21 overexpression has been shown to be associated with worse prognosis,[105–107] in addition to chemoresistance to a 5-FU–based regimen.[108] Although there is still much to be done in terms of prospective validation of these observations, microRNA-related diagnostic and therapeutic strategies offer great potential in the management of CRC.

SUMMARY

A multistep, complex process of genetic changes drives transformation from normal colonic epithelium to invasive cancer. Specific and unique germline mutations are associated with common inherited colon cancer syndromes such as FAP and HNPCC. Sporadic CRCs result from the stepwise accumulation of multiple somatic mutations. APC gene mutations (whether germline or somatic) are seen in most CRCs and appear to be an early occurrence. Subsequent genetic events diverge, depending on the molecular pathway leading to genetic instability: LOH, MSI, and CpG-island methylation. The identification of specific genetic mutations responsible for CRC has direct clinical implications. Patients at high risk for developing CRC can be identified via genetic testing for specific germline mutations. In addition, these mutations also represent prognostic biomarkers and potential therapeutic targets.

REFERENCES

1. Verma M, Dunn BK, Ross S, et al. Early detection and risk assessment: proceedings and recommendations from the Workshop on Epigenetics in Cancer Prevention. Ann N Y Acad Sci 2003;983:298–319.
2. Verma M, Srivastava S. New cancer biomarkers deriving from NCI early detection research. Recent Results Cancer Res 2003;163:72–84 [discussion: 264–66].
3. Zauber AG, Winawer SJ, O'Brien MJ, et al. Colonoscopic polypectomy and long-term prevention of colorectal-cancer deaths. N Engl J Med 2012;366: 687–96.
4. Vogelstein B, Fearon ER, Hamilton SR, et al. Genetic alterations during colorectal-tumor development. N Engl J Med 1988;319:525–32.
5. Fearon ER, Cho KR, Nigro JM, et al. Identification of a chromosome 18q gene that is altered in colorectal cancers. Science 1990;247:49–56.
6. Leslie A, Carey FA, Pratt NR, et al. The colorectal adenoma-carcinoma sequence. Br J Surg 2002;89:845–60.
7. Sherr CJ. Cancer cell cycles. Science 1996;274:1672–7.
8. Irby RB, Mao W, Coppola D, et al. Activating SRC mutation in a subset of advanced human colon cancers. Nat Genet 1999;21:187–90.
9. Kapitanovic S, Radosevic S, Kapitanovic M, et al. The expression of p185(HER-2/neu) correlates with the stage of disease and survival in colorectal cancer. Gastroenterology 1997;112:1103–13.
10. Cartwright C. Intestinal cell growth control: role of Src tyrosine kinases. Gastroenterology 1998;114:1335–8.
11. Forgacs I. Oncogenes and gastrointestinal cancer. Gut 1988;29:417–21.
12. Hamilton SR. The molecular genetics of colorectal neoplasia. Gastroenterology 1993;105:3–7.
13. Sikora K. Cancer genes in gastrointestinal malignancy. Baillieres Clin Gastroenterol 1990;4:135–50.
14. Tahara E. Genetic alterations in human gastrointestinal cancers. The application to molecular diagnosis. Cancer 1995;75:1410–7.
15. Tsuboi K, Hirayoshi K, Takeuchi K, et al. Expression of the c-myc gene in human gastrointestinal malignancies. Biochem Biophys Res Commun 1987;146: 699–704.
16. Takayama T, Ohi M, Hayashi T, et al. Analysis of K-ras, APC, and beta-catenin in aberrant crypt foci in sporadic adenoma, cancer, and familial adenomatous polyposis. Gastroenterology 2001;121:599–611.
17. Bourne HR, Sanders DA, McCormick F. The GTPase superfamily: conserved structure and molecular mechanism. Nature 1991;349:117–27.
18. Spirio LN, Samowitz W, Robertson J, et al. Alleles of APC modulate the frequency and classes of mutations that lead to colon polyps. Nat Genet 1998;20:385–8.
19. Lamlum H, Ilyas M, Rowan A, et al. The type of somatic mutation at APC in familial adenomatous polyposis is determined by the site of the germline mutation: a new facet to Knudson's 'two-hit' hypothesis. Nat Med 1999;5:1071–5.
20. Korinek V, Barker N, Morin PJ, et al. Constitutive transcriptional activation by a beta-catenin-Tcf complex in APC-/- colon carcinoma. Science 1997;275:1784–7.

21. Morin PJ, Sparks AB, Korinek V, et al. Activation of beta-catenin-Tcf signaling in colon cancer by mutations in beta-catenin or APC. Science 1997;275:1787–90.

22. Goss KH, Groden J. Biology of the adenomatous polyposis coli tumor suppressor. J Clin Oncol 2000;18:1967–79.

23. van de Wetering M, Sancho E, Verweij C, et al. The beta-catenin/TCF-4 complex imposes a crypt progenitor phenotype on colorectal cancer cells. Cell 2002;111: 241–50.

24. Peifer M, Polakis P. Wnt signaling in oncogenesis and embryogenesis—a look outside the nucleus. Science 2000;287:1606–9.

25. Mann B, Gelos M, Siedow A, et al. Target genes of beta-catenin-T cell-factor/lymphoid-enhancer-factor signaling in human colorectal carcinomas. Proc Natl Acad Sci U S A 1999;96:1603–8.

26. Kastan MB, Onyekwere O, Sidransky D, et al. Participation of p53 protein in the cellular response to DNA damage. Cancer Res 1991;51:6304–11.

27. Kuerbitz SJ, Plunkett BS, Walsh WV, et al. Wild-type p53 is a cell cycle checkpoint determinant following irradiation. Proc Natl Acad Sci U S A 1992;89: 7491–5.

28. Woods DB, Vousden KH. Regulation of p53 function. Exp Cell Res 2001;264: 56–66.

29. Lane DP. Cancer. p53, guardian of the genome. Nature 1992;358:15–6.

30. Rosty C, Young JP, Walsh MD, et al. Colorectal carcinomas with KRAS mutation are associated with distinctive morphological and molecular features. Mod Pathol 2013;26(6):825–34.

31. Soussi T. The p53 tumor suppressor gene: from molecular biology to clinical investigation. Ann N Y Acad Sci 2000;910:121–37 [discussion: 37–9].

32. Baker SJ, Preisinger AC, Jessup JM, et al. p53 gene mutations occur in combination with 17p allelic deletions as late events in colorectal tumorigenesis. Cancer Res 1990;50:7717–22.

33. Kikuchi-Yanoshita R, Konishi M, Ito S, et al. Genetic changes of both p53 alleles associated with the conversion from colorectal adenoma to early carcinoma in familial adenomatous polyposis and non-familial adenomatous polyposis patients. Cancer Res 1992;52:3965–71.

34. Kirsch DG, Kastan MB. Tumor-suppressor p53: implications for tumor development and prognosis. J Clin Oncol 1998;16:3158–68.

35. Russo A, Bazan V, Iacopetta B, et al. The TP53 colorectal cancer international collaborative study on the prognostic and predictive significance of p53 mutation: influence of tumor site, type of mutation, and adjuvant treatment. J Clin Oncol 2005;23:7518–28.

36. Hedrick L, Cho KR, Fearon ER, et al. The DCC gene product in cellular differentiation and colorectal tumorigenesis. Genes Dev 1994;8:1174–83.

37. Thiagalingam S, Lengauer C, Leach FS, et al. Evaluation of candidate tumour suppressor genes on chromosome 18 in colorectal cancers. Nat Genet 1996; 13:343–6.

38. Cho KR, Oliner JD, Simons JW, et al. The DCC gene: structural analysis and mutations in colorectal carcinomas. Genomics 1994;19:525–31.

39. Popat S, Houlston RS. A systematic review and meta-analysis of the relationship between chromosome 18q genotype, DCC status and colorectal cancer prognosis. Eur J Cancer 2005;41:2060–70.

40. Sun XF, Rutten S, Zhang H, et al. Expression of the deleted in colorectal cancer gene is related to prognosis in DNA diploid and low proliferative colorectal adenocarcinoma. J Clin Oncol 1999;17:1745–50.

41. Keino-Masu K, Masu M, Hinck L, et al. Deleted in Colorectal Cancer (DCC) encodes a netrin receptor. Cell 1996;87:175–85.
42. Eppert K, Scherer SW, Ozcelik H, et al. MADR2 maps to 18q21 and encodes a TGFbeta-regulated MAD-related protein that is functionally mutated in colorectal carcinoma. Cell 1996;86:543–52.
43. Miyaki M, Iijima T, Konishi M, et al. Higher frequency of Smad4 gene mutation in human colorectal cancer with distant metastasis. Oncogene 1999;18: 3098–103.
44. Abdel-Rahman WM, Mecklin JP, Peltomaki P. The genetics of HNPCC: application to diagnosis and screening. Crit Rev Oncol Hematol 2006;58:208–20.
45. Peltomaki P. Deficient DNA mismatch repair: a common etiologic factor for colon cancer. Hum Mol Genet 2001;10:735–40.
46. Schwitalle Y, Kloor M, Eiermann S, et al. Immune response against frameshift-induced neopeptides in HNPCC patients and healthy HNPCC mutation carriers. Gastroenterology 2008;134:988–97.
47. Weisenberger DJ, Siegmund KD, Campan M, et al. CpG island methylator phenotype underlies sporadic microsatellite instability and is tightly associated with BRAF mutation in colorectal cancer. Nat Genet 2006;38:787–93.
48. Shen L, Kondo Y, Rosner GL, et al. MGMT promoter methylation and field defect in sporadic colorectal cancer. J Natl Cancer Inst 2005;97:1330–8.
49. Das PM, Singal R. DNA methylation and cancer. J Clin Oncol 2004;22:4632–42.
50. van Engeland M, Derks S, Smits KM, et al. Colorectal cancer epigenetics: complex simplicity. J Clin Oncol 2011;29:1382–91.
51. Lao VV, Grady WM. Epigenetics and colorectal cancer. Nat Rev Gastroenterol Hepatol 2011;8:686–700.
52. Rosty C, Walsh MD, Walters RJ, et al. Multiplicity and molecular heterogeneity of colorectal carcinomas in individuals with serrated polyposis. Am J Surg Pathol 2013;37:434–42.
53. Laiho P, Kokko A, Vanharanta S, et al. Serrated carcinomas form a subclass of colorectal cancer with distinct molecular basis. Oncogene 2007;26:312–20.
54. Makinen MJ. Colorectal serrated adenocarcinoma. Histopathology 2007;50: 131–50.
55. O'Brien MJ, Yang S, Mack C, et al. Comparison of microsatellite instability, CpG island methylation phenotype, BRAF and KRAS status in serrated polyps and traditional adenomas indicates separate pathways to distinct colorectal carcinoma end points. Am J Surg Pathol 2006;30:1491–501.
56. Jass JR, Do KA, Simms LA, et al. Morphology of sporadic colorectal cancer with DNA replication errors. Gut 1998;42:673–9.
57. Buecher B, Cacheux W, Rouleau E, et al. Role of microsatellite instability in the management of colorectal cancers. Dig Liver Dis 2013;45(6):441–9.
58. Thibodeau SN, Bren G, Schaid D. Microsatellite instability in cancer of the proximal colon. Science 1993;260:816–9.
59. Lothe RA, Peltomaki P, Meling GI, et al. Genomic instability in colorectal cancer: relationship to clinicopathological variables and family history. Cancer Res 1993;53:5849–52.
60. Gryfe R, Kim H, Hsieh ET, et al. Tumor microsatellite instability and clinical outcome in young patients with colorectal cancer. N Engl J Med 2000;342: 69–77.
61. Sargent DJ, Marsoni S, Monges G, et al. Defective mismatch repair as a predictive marker for lack of efficacy of fluorouracil-based adjuvant therapy in colon cancer. J Clin Oncol 2010;28:3219–26.

62. Zaanan A, Flejou JF, Emile JF, et al. Defective mismatch repair status as a prognostic biomarker of disease-free survival in stage III colon cancer patients treated with adjuvant FOLFOX chemotherapy. Clin Cancer Res 2011;17:7470–8.
63. Sinicrope FA, Foster NR, Thibodeau SN, et al. DNA mismatch repair status and colon cancer recurrence and survival in clinical trials of 5-fluorouracil-based adjuvant therapy. J Natl Cancer Inst 2011;103:863–75.
64. Popat S, Hubner R, Houlston RS. Systematic review of microsatellite instability and colorectal cancer prognosis. J Clin Oncol 2005;23:609–18.
65. Ogino S, Meyerhardt JA, Irahara N, et al. KRAS mutation in stage III colon cancer and clinical outcome following intergroup trial CALGB 89803. Clin Cancer Res 2009;15:7322–9.
66. Kim GP, Colangelo LH, Wieand HS, et al. Prognostic and predictive roles of high-degree microsatellite instability in colon cancer: a National Cancer Institute-National Surgical Adjuvant Breast and Bowel Project Collaborative Study. J Clin Oncol 2007;25:767–72.
67. Ribic CM, Sargent DJ, Moore MJ, et al. Tumor microsatellite-instability status as a predictor of benefit from fluorouracil-based adjuvant chemotherapy for colon cancer. N Engl J Med 2003;349:247–57.
68. Kelley RK, Venook AP. Prognostic and predictive markers in stage II colon cancer: is there a role for gene expression profiling? Clin Colorectal Cancer 2011;10:73–80.
69. Lievre A, Bachet JB, Boige V, et al. KRAS mutations as an independent prognostic factor in patients with advanced colorectal cancer treated with cetuximab. J Clin Oncol 2008;26:374–9.
70. Benvenuti S, Sartore-Bianchi A, Di Nicolantonio F, et al. Oncogenic activation of the RAS/RAF signaling pathway impairs the response of metastatic colorectal cancers to anti-epidermal growth factor receptor antibody therapies. Cancer Res 2007;67:2643–8.
71. Van Cutsem E, Peeters M, Siena S, et al. Open-label phase III trial of panitumumab plus best supportive care compared with best supportive care alone in patients with chemotherapy-refractory metastatic colorectal cancer. J Clin Oncol 2007;25:1658–64.
72. Jimeno A, Messersmith WA, Hirsch FR, et al. KRAS mutations and sensitivity to epidermal growth factor receptor inhibitors in colorectal cancer: practical application of patient selection. J Clin Oncol 2009;27:1130–6.
73. Di Nicolantonio F, Martini M, Molinari F, et al. Wild-type BRAF is required for response to panitumumab or cetuximab in metastatic colorectal cancer. J Clin Oncol 2008;26:5705–12.
74. Siena S, Sartore-Bianchi A, Di Nicolantonio F, et al. Biomarkers predicting clinical outcome of epidermal growth factor receptor-targeted therapy in metastatic colorectal cancer. J Natl Cancer Inst 2009;101:1308–24.
75. Bokemeyer C, Van Cutsem E, Rougier P, et al. Addition of cetuximab to chemotherapy as first-line treatment for KRAS wild-type metastatic colorectal cancer: pooled analysis of the CRYSTAL and OPUS randomised clinical trials. Eur J Cancer 2012;48:1466–75.
76. Bokemeyer C, Bondarenko I, Hartmann JT, et al. Efficacy according to biomarker status of cetuximab plus FOLFOX-4 as first-line treatment for metastatic colorectal cancer: the OPUS study. Ann Oncol 2011;22:1535–46.
77. Vale CL, Tierney JF, Fisher D, et al. Does anti-EGFR therapy improve outcome in advanced colorectal cancer? A systematic review and meta-analysis. Cancer Treat Rev 2012;38:618–25.

78. De Roock W, Claes B, Bernasconi D, et al. Effects of KRAS, BRAF, NRAS, and PIK3CA mutations on the efficacy of cetuximab plus chemotherapy in chemotherapy-refractory metastatic colorectal cancer: a retrospective consortium analysis. Lancet Oncol 2010;11:753–62.

79. Soeda H, Shimodaira H, Watanabe M, et al. Clinical usefulness of KRAS, BRAF, and PIK3CA mutations as predictive markers of cetuximab efficacy in irinotecan- and oxaliplatin-refractory Japanese patients with metastatic colorectal cancer. Int J Clin Oncol 2012. [Epub ahead of print].

80. Mao C, Yang ZY, Hu XF, et al. PIK3CA exon 20 mutations as a potential biomarker for resistance to anti-EGFR monoclonal antibodies in KRAS wild-type metastatic colorectal cancer: a systematic review and meta-analysis. Ann Oncol 2012;23:1518–25.

81. Barratt PL, Seymour MT, Stenning SP, et al. DNA markers predicting benefit from adjuvant fluorouracil in patients with colon cancer: a molecular study. Lancet 2002;360:1381–91.

82. Bertagnolli MM, Niedzwiecki D, Compton CC, et al. Microsatellite instability predicts improved response to adjuvant therapy with irinotecan, fluorouracil, and leucovorin in stage III colon cancer: Cancer and Leukemia Group B Protocol 89803. J Clin Oncol 2009;27:1814–21.

83. Kim ST, Lee J, Park SH, et al. Clinical impact of microsatellite instability in colon cancer following adjuvant FOLFOX therapy. Cancer Chemother Pharmacol 2010;66:659–67.

84. O'Connell MJ, Lavery I, Yothers G, et al. Relationship between tumor gene expression and recurrence in four independent studies of patients with stage II/III colon cancer treated with surgery alone or surgery plus adjuvant fluorouracil plus leucovorin. J Clin Oncol 2010;28:3937–44.

85. Clark-Langone KM, Wu JY, Sangli C, et al. Biomarker discovery for colon cancer using a 761 gene RT-PCR assay. BMC Genomics 2007;8:279.

86. Gray RG, Quirke P, Handley K, et al. Validation study of a quantitative multigene reverse transcriptase-polymerase chain reaction assay for assessment of recurrence risk in patients with stage II colon cancer. J Clin Oncol 2011;29:4611–9.

87. Webber EM, Lin JS, Evelyn PW. Oncotype DX tumor gene expression profiling in stage II colon cancer. Application: prognostic, risk prediction. PLoS Curr 2010;2.

88. Maak M, Simon I, Nitsche U, et al. Independent validation of a prognostic genomic signature (coloprint) for patients with stage ii colon cancer. Ann Surg 2013;257:1053–8.

89. Tan IB, Tan P. Genetics: an 18-gene signature (ColoPrint(R)) for colon cancer prognosis. Nat Rev Clin Oncol 2011;8:131–3.

90. Salazar R, Roepman P, Capella G, et al. Gene expression signature to improve prognosis prediction of stage II and III colorectal cancer. J Clin Oncol 2011;29:17–24.

91. Hyslop T, Waldman SA. Molecular staging of node negative patients with colorectal cancer. J Cancer 2013;4:193–9.

92. Hurwitz H, Fehrenbacher L, Novotny W, et al. Bevacizumab plus irinotecan, fluorouracil, and leucovorin for metastatic colorectal cancer. N Engl J Med 2004;350:2335–42.

93. Cohen MH, Gootenberg J, Keegan P, et al. FDA drug approval summary: bevacizumab plus FOLFOX4 as second-line treatment of colorectal cancer. Oncologist 2007;12:356–61.

94. Kozloff M, Yood MU, Berlin J, et al. Clinical outcomes associated with bevacizumab-containing treatment of metastatic colorectal cancer: the BRiTE observational cohort study. Oncologist 2009;14:862–70.

95. Golubovskaya VM, Kweh FA, Cance WG. Focal adhesion kinase and cancer. Histol Histopathol 2009;24:503–10.

96. Dunn KB, Heffler M, Golubovskaya VM. Evolving therapies and FAK inhibitors for the treatment of cancer. Anticancer Agents Med Chem 2010;10:722–34.

97. Heffler M, Golubovskaya V, Conroy J, et al. Fak and has inhibition synergistically decrease colon cancer cell viability and affect expression of critical genes. Anticancer Agents Med Chem 2013;13:584–94.

98. Rossi S, Di Narzo AF, Mestdagh P, et al. MicroRNAs in colon cancer: a roadmap for discovery. FEBS Lett 2012;586:3000–7.

99. Tokarz P, Blasiak J. The role of microRNA in metastatic colorectal cancer and its significance in cancer prognosis and treatment. Acta Biochim Pol 2012;59:467–74.

100. Schetter AJ, Okayama H, Harris CC. The role of microRNAs in colorectal cancer. Cancer J 2012;18:244–52.

101. Luo X, Burwinkel B, Tao S, et al. MicroRNA signatures: novel biomarker for colorectal cancer? Cancer Epidemiol Biomarkers Prev 2011;20:1272–86.

102. Oberg AL, French AJ, Sarver AL, et al. miRNA expression in colon polyps provides evidence for a multihit model of colon cancer. PLoS One 2011;6:e20465.

103. Ryan BM, Robles AI, Harris CC. Genetic variation in microRNA networks: the implications for cancer research. Nat Rev Cancer 2010;10:389–402.

104. Link A, Balaguer F, Shen Y, et al. Fecal MicroRNAs as novel biomarkers for colon cancer screening. Cancer Epidemiol Biomarkers Prev 2010;19:1766–74.

105. Shibuya H, Iinuma H, Shimada R, et al. Clinicopathological and prognostic value of microRNA-21 and microRNA-155 in colorectal cancer. Oncology 2010;79:313–20.

106. Kulda V, Pesta M, Topolcan O, et al. Relevance of miR-21 and miR-143 expression in tissue samples of colorectal carcinoma and its liver metastases. Cancer Genet Cytogenet 2010;200:154–60.

107. Nielsen BS, Jorgensen S, Fog JU, et al. High levels of microRNA-21 in the stroma of colorectal cancers predict short disease-free survival in stage II colon cancer patients. Clin Exp Metastasis 2011;28:27–38.

108. Schetter AJ, Leung SY, Sohn JJ, et al. MicroRNA expression profiles associated with prognosis and therapeutic outcome in colon adenocarcinoma. JAMA 2008;299:425–36.

Translational Research in Endocrine Surgery

Scott K. Sherman, MD, James R. Howe, MD*

KEYWORDS

- Endocrine cancer • Heritable cancer syndromes
- Pancreatic neuroendocrine tumors • Thyroid surgery • MEN2

KEY POINTS

- Basic science research has identified the genes responsible for several hereditary endocrine tumor syndromes, and has elucidated the cell-signaling pathways critical to development of endocrine cancer.
- Genetic testing for these mutations allows identification of at-risk individuals for screening before the onset of symptoms, and in some cases permits prophylactic surgery.
- Mutations in genes of the MAP-kinase signaling pathway (most commonly *RET* or *BRAF*) are found in most familial and sporadic thyroid cancers and cause constitutive proliferative signaling, leading to malignancy.
- Small-molecule kinase inhibitors block aberrant promalignant signaling in several endocrine cancers, and represent an active area of research with great potential. Improvements in progression-free survival have been reported with these drugs for thyroid, adrenal, and endocrine pancreatic cancer, but responses are usually not durable, and efforts to understand and overcome inhibitor resistance are ongoing.
- In pancreatic neuroendocrine tumors, drugs targeting somatostatin receptors alleviate symptoms, are useful for imaging, and can prolong life. Targeted radiotherapy directed toward these receptors and the development of additional receptor targets promise to improve the treatment of these tumors in the future.

INTRODUCTION

The past 30 years have seen astounding advances in the science of endocrine surgery. From early successes in mapping and cloning genes responsible for heritable endocrine cancer syndromes, to sequencing the human genome, to adoption of next-generation sequencing techniques, a broad understanding of genes responsible

Disclosures: S.K.S. was supported by NIH 5T32 #CA148062-03.
Department of Surgery, Carver College of Medicine, The University of Iowa, 200 Hawkins Drive, Iowa City, IA 52242, USA
* Corresponding author.
E-mail address: james-howe@uiowa.edu

for familial and sporadic endocrine cancers now exists. This development has enabled genetic testing of at-risk family members and even prophylactic surgery for some carriers of mutant genes. Parallel efforts to determine the function of these altered genes have defined cell-signaling pathways susceptible to treatment. High-throughput gene expression methodologies now give insight into entire networks of cellular processes perturbed in endocrine malignancy. The knowledge gained has led to development of small-molecule kinase inhibitors and other therapies that are able to specifically target the genes, pathways, and cells responsible for disease. New treatments based on rational drug development and targeted therapies continue to be the focus of aggressive investigation and ongoing clinical trials. Diagnosis and prognostication in endocrine cancer has likewise been improved using the results of mutation and gene-expression data. The aim of this article is to review advances in the basic science of endocrine cancer, and highlight how these discoveries are being translated into real-world tests and therapies that will affect the practice of endocrine surgery today and in the near future. Heritable and sporadic tumors of the thyroid, parathyroids, adrenals, and pancreas are emphasized. It is expected that familiarity with these breakthroughs and with the ongoing challenges in endocrine cancer surgery will enhance clinicians' ability to apply the latest scientific developments to the optimal care of their patients.

THYROID
Overview of Mitogen-Activated Protein Kinase

The mitogen-activated protein kinase (MAPK) cascade is a cellular signaling pathway now established as central to thyroid cancer. In this cascade, extracellular signals such as vascular endothelial growth factor (VEGF), platelet-derived growth factor (PDGF), and many others activate membrane-bound receptor tyrosine kinases, including RET, which cause RAS activation and induction of the RAS-RAF-MEK-ERK-MAP signaling cascade (**Fig. 1**).[1,2] Activation of the MAPK pathway influences diverse cellular processes including cell-cycle control, proliferation, differentiation, motility, and apoptosis.[3,4] The pathway is highly regulated through expression of multiple isoforms of component proteins and cross-talk with related pathways, such as phosphatidylinositol-3-kinase/Akt/mammalian target of rapamycin (PI3K/Akt/mTOR), Janus-kinase, PKC/NF-κB, and Wnt/β-catenin, each contributing to different functional roles in different tissues and contexts.[2,5,6] Apart from its physiologic role in thyroid differentiation, growth, and function, the MAPK pathway can also contribute to development of thyroid cancer by aberrant activation at several points. In sporadic and hereditary medullary thyroid cancer (MTC), mutant RET activates RAS, causing constitutive MAPK signaling,[7] while mutations in both RET and RAS are common in follicular thyroid cancer.[8] Downstream in the pathway, mutation in the BRAF serine/threonine kinase has emerged as the most common genetic abnormality in papillary thyroid cancer (PTC), and is also present in anaplastic thyroid cancer (ATC).[9,10] In total, mutation in some element of the MAPK pathway is present in more than 70% of thyroid cancers, marking this as the central cellular control element in thyroid oncogenesis.[11] Over the past 25 years, basic and translational research has defined the role of the MAPK pathway in thyroid cancer and has produced promising new diagnostic and therapeutic strategies for this heterogeneous disease.

RET Proto-Oncogene

Although the phenotype and autosomal dominant inheritance pattern of multiple endocrine neoplasia type 2 had been recognized for some time, it was not until

1987 that genetic linkage analysis mapped the causative locus for MEN2A to near the centromere of chromosome 10.[12,13] Other heritable MTC phenotypes, such as MEN2B and familial medullary thyroid cancer (FMTC), were subsequently linked to the same region.[14] A gene known to map to this part of chromosome 10 was the RET proto-oncogene. RET (REarranged during Transfection) was first identified as a human lymphoma oncogene capable of transforming cells in vitro.[15] A gene isolated from papillary thyroid cancer specimens (PTC) had the same effect and also mapped to chromosome 10.[16,17] Further investigation showed that this PTC oncogene was actually chimeric RET rearranged and fused with another gene to form the RET/PTC proto-oncogene.[18,19] In 1993, linkage narrowed the MEN2A locus to a small area near the RET proto-oncogene,[20] and RET was identified as the causative gene in MEN2A and FMTC, with 2 groups reporting heterozygous germline mutations in affected patients, but not in normal controls and unaffected family members.[21,22] Description of RET mutations in MEN2B kindreds followed soon thereafter.[23–25]

Genetic tests to presymptomatically identify affected individuals in families with MEN2 and FMTC became more directed after identification of these mutations.[26] Wells and colleagues[27] became the first to use a genetic test to recommend prophylactic surgery, performing total thyroidectomy and parathyroidectomy in asymptomatic patients within MEN2A families found to carry RET mutations. Of interest is that even in patients with normal calcitonin levels, all of the thyroidectomy specimens contained evidence of precancerous C-cell hyperplasia or overt MTC.

With RET identified as the mutation responsible for MEN2A, MEN2B, and FMTC, it became clear that disease features varied according to the specific mutations present. In 1994, Mulligan and colleagues[28] reported that MEN2A families with parathyroid hyperplasia and pheochromocytoma carried the C634R RET mutation much more frequently than families lacking these disease features. In 1996, the International RET Consortium pooled sequencing and clinical data from 477 MEN2 and FMTC families to catalogue the various mutations' phenotypic associations (**Table 1**).[29] These data revealed that codon-634 mutations accounted for 85% of MEN2A cases, and that the C634R mutation was significantly more likely to lead to hyperparathyroidism and pheochromocytoma. Families with the less aggressive FMTC had mutations in several codons including 634, but none carried the C634R mutation. Finally, 75 of 79 MEN2B families had the same M918T mutation. These results and others demonstrated the robustness of the genetic diagnoses, provided valuable information regarding which patients were at highest risk for additional disease features beyond MTC, and provided a strong rationale for very early surgery in the highest-risk patients to preempt development of metastatic MTC.[29,30]

Consensus guidelines grouping all known mutations into risk categories with recommendations for screening and age of thyroidectomy were developed in 2001,[31] and updated by the American Thyroid Association (ATA) in 2009.[32] For the highest-risk MEN2B mutations, thyroidectomy is recommended as soon as possible and ideally before 1 month of age, with central node dissection recommended if surgery is delayed beyond 1 year of age[32] (**Table 2**). For the next highest risk group, thyroidectomy is recommended before 5 years, and for some lesser high-risk mutations, patients and surgeons may consider delaying thyroidectomy to before age 10 in the setting of normal calcitonin and ultrasonography, less aggressive family history, and strict compliance with screening.[31,32] Certain MEN2A mutations, such as C609Y, lead to MTC usually only after age 20 to 40 years,[33] and thyroidectomy between ages 5 and 10 for these patients can be acceptable under the ATA guidelines.[32] Nevertheless, rare examples of MTC in very young patients with mutations thought to confer lower

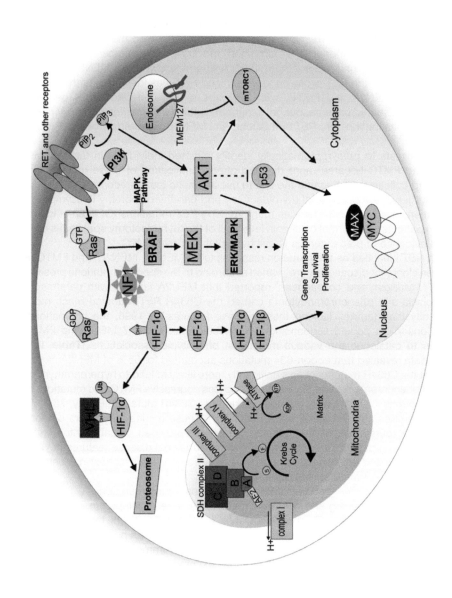

risk do exist,[31,32,34] and therefore early thyroidectomy (before age 5 years) remains a reasonable option for these groups.[31,32] With the high sensitivity and specificity of genetic testing, and the fact that 98% of MEN2 patients have a known *RET* mutation,[31] genetic testing is now the standard to determine prophylactic surgical therapy in MEN2.

RET in Sporadic MTC

RET mutations are found with high frequency in sporadic MTC. A study of 100 sporadic MTC patients with 10-year median follow-up identified somatic *RET* mutations in 43%, and found that their presence strongly correlated with lymph node and distant metastases (70% and 30% vs. 26% and 12% in *RET*-positive and *RET*-negative patients, $P<.0001$).[35] Of patients with mutations, 79% had the same M918T mutation found in most MEN2B cases. Sporadic *RET* mutations also independently predicted worse outcomes, with significantly reduced disease-free and overall survival.[35] In a separate study of 36 patients with sporadic and 21 with familial MTC, 75% of tumors had *RET* mutations and 16% had *RAS* mutations.[36] Knowledge of mutational status in sporadic MTC will likely become increasingly important for stratification in clinical trials, or in directing therapy toward specific pathways.

Overview of BRAF

RAF kinase is normally activated by RAS, and in turn activates MEK in the MAPK pathway (see **Fig. 1**). Three genes encode different isoforms of RAF (A-RAF, B-RAF, and C-RAF), and of these, *BRAF* has proved to be important in several human cancers.[6] In 2002, a genome-level screen for cancer-related mutations found activating somatic *BRAF* mutations in many human tumor cell types, including 59% of melanoma lines studied.[37] Although more than 30 *BRAF* mutations have been described, a single base-pair substitution (T1799A) replacing valine with glutamate at residue 600 (V600E) is both the most common and most potent mutation, leading to a 700-fold increased kinase activity, constitutive activation of the MAPK pathway, transformation of cells in vitro, and growth of tumors in mice in vivo.[4,37,38]

Fig. 1. Simplified overview of commonly mutated oncogenes, tumor suppressors, and pathways in endocrine cancer. In the mitogen-activated protein kinase (MAPK) pathway (*right center*), extracellular ligands activate receptor kinases such as RET, VEGFR, PDGFR, and others, initiating the RAS/RAF/MEK/ERK signaling cascade, resulting in gene transcription and proliferation. Activating mutations in these proteins lead to constitutive signaling. In the phosphatidylinositol-3-kinase (PI3K) cascade (*right side*), receptor activation causes activation of Akt, also affecting cellular survival and regulating apoptosis. Mammalian target of rapamycin (mTOR) signaling promotes survival, and is stimulated by Akt and repressed by TMEM127. In neurofibromatosis type 1, loss of NF1 function prevents termination of RAS signaling. In von Hippel–Lindau syndrome, VHL (*left top*) targets HIF proteins for ubiquitination (Ub) and proteasomal degradation. When HIF persists because of mutated VHL, continuous activation of hypoxia genes leads to angiogenesis and tumor development. In the mitochondrion (*left side*), defects in subunits of complex II, SDH A, B, C, and D, and assembly factor 2 (AF2) impair electron transport and induce a pseudohypoxic state. MAX (in nucleus) interacts with MYC and other transcription factors to repress cell growth, and loss of function allows proliferation. F, fumarate; OH-P, hydroxyproline residue; PIP2, phosphatidylinositol bisphosphate; PIP3, phosphatidylinositol trisphosphate; S, succinate. (*Adapted from* Fishbein L, Nathanson KL. Pheochromocytoma and paraganglioma: understanding the complexities of the genetic background. Cancer Genet 2012;205:1; with permission.)

Table 1
Frequency of common *RET* mutations in 477 families with MEN2A, MEN2B, and FMTC by codon and presence of medullary thyroid carcinoma (MTC), hyperparathyroidism (HPT), and pheochromocytoma (PCC)

	Codon, No. (%) of Families with Mutations							
	609	611	618	620	634	768	804	918
MEN2B	0	0	0	0	0	0	0	75 (100)
MEN2A(1)	0	0	5 (6)	2 (2)	84 (92)	0	0	0
MEN2A(2)	0	3 (3)	4 (4)	12 (13)	76 (80)	0	0	0
MEN2A(3)	1 (8)	2 (15)	1 (8)	0	9 (69)	0	0	0
FMTC	2 (7)	1 (3)	10 (33)	5 (17)	9 (30)	3 (10)	0	0
Other	2 (1.5)	7 (5)	18 (13)	13 (10)	93 (68)	1[a] (<1)	2[a] (1.5)	0

MEN2A(1): MTC+HPT+PCC; MEN2A(2): MTC+PCC; MEN2A(3): MTC+HPT.
[a] Families with medullary thyroid carcinoma (FMTC) but too few cases (≤3) per family to exclude other MEN2A disease features.
Data from Eng C, Clayton D, Schuffenecker I, et al. The relationship between specific RET proto-oncogene mutations and disease phenotype in multiple endocrine neoplasia type 2. International RET mutation consortium analysis. JAMA 1996;276:1575–9.

Soon after the initial report of *BRAF* mutations in human cancer, the V600E mutation was reported in a high percentage of human PTCs. Kimura and colleagues[39] found the *BRAF* mutation in 28 of 78 (36%) adult, non–radiation-exposed PTC specimens, whereas *RET* and *RAS* mutations accounted for only 16% of cases each. Concurrently, another group reported the V600E mutation in 24 of 35 (69%) PTC specimens in a screen of 476 samples from diverse types of primary tumors.[40] *BRAF* mutation was determined to occur more frequently in tall-cell and less commonly in follicular variants of PTC,[4] and a recent meta-analysis established a 45% overall prevalence of the V600E mutation in papillary thyroid cancer (1118 of 2470 published cases).[10] Whereas MTCs do not carry *BRAF* mutations, 24% to 40% of ATCs do, and *BRAF* mutations are common in poorly differentiated, recurrent, and radioiodine-resistant thyroid cancers.[4,9]

Table 2
Recommended age for prophylactic thyroidectomy by codon for selected *RET* mutations based on risk of medullary thyroid cancer (MTC)

Recommended Age for Thyroidectomy	MTC Risk Category[32]	Codons
Before 1 y (preferably before 1 mo)	D	883, 918, 922, compound 804[a]
Before 5 y	C	634
Consider surgery before 5 y	B	609, 611, 618, 620, 630
Consider delaying to before 5–10 y[b]	A	768, 790, 791, 804[a], 891

For additional mutations and details, see Refs.[31,32]
[a] Compound 804+(778, 805, 806, or 904) mutations have higher risk than isolated codon 804 mutations.[32]
[b] With less aggressive family history and appropriate negative screening.[32]
Adapted from Calva D, O'Dorisio TM, Sue O'Dorisio M, et al. When is prophylactic thyroidectomy indicated for patients with the RET codon 609 mutation? Ann Surg Oncol 2009;16:2237; with permission, and updated to reflect current American Thyroid Association guidelines.

Intense research in the past decade revealed much about the molecular, cellular, and clinical effects of *BRAF* mutation. Determination of the crystal structure of mutant BRAF protein showed how the V600E mutation, nestled between activating phosphorylation sites at T599 and S602, disrupts the hydrophobic interactions that stabilize the inactive form of the protein, and mimics the conformation of a phosphorylated state.[38] This change creates a pseudophosphorylated conformation, leading to constitutive pathway activation and tumorigenic behavior. Consistent with this model, invasiveness of thyroid cancer cell cultures expressing BRAF V600E was found to require signaling via the MAPK pathway.[41] Thyroid cells with the V600E mutation also show reduced markers of differentiation. Using inducible *BRAF* V600E mutant rat thyroid cell lines, Mitsutake and colleagues[42] showed suppressed expression of genes necessary for iodine handling and thyroid differentiation, such as thyrotropin receptor (*TSHR*), sodium-iodine symporter (*NIS*), and thyroglobulin (*Tg*), as well as increased chromosomal instability. In both rat and human thyroid cell lines, these phenotypes could be corrected by treatment with the MAPK inhibitor U0126.[41]

Despite the clear importance of the MAPK pathway, there is a growing understanding that *BRAF* mutations also influence related pathways. In thyroid cell culture with an inducible V600E mutation, Palona and colleagues[6] showed upregulation of matrix metalloproteinases and inhibitors of apoptosis. The upregulation was not blocked by inhibitors of the MAPK pathway, but instead depended on NF-κB. Similarly, Liu and Xing[5] showed that while a MEK kinase inhibitor led to reduced invasiveness and cell-cycle arrest in thyroid lines harboring *BRAF* mutations, this effect was potentiated by concurrent blockade of the NF-κB pathway. Wild-type BRAF must form homodimers or heterodimers with CRAF to signal, and it forms these dimers only in response to RAS signaling. By contrast, BRAF V600E is always active, and forms homodimers or heterodimers in the absence of RAS signaling, and can additionally activate MEK as a monomer.[43] Monomers and homodimers of mutant BRAF as well as heterodimers with wild-type RAF proteins may participate in MEK-independent signaling with the PI3K/AKT/mTOR, NF-κB, and other pathways.[44] Through both direct activity of mutant BRAF and feedback from the constitutively active MAPK pathway,[45] mutant BRAF may contribute to cross-talk effects in other pathways. These complex interactions belie the standard linear depiction of the MAPK pathway and have frustrated the development of some pathway inhibitor–based therapeutics.

BRAF in Clinical Risk

As data accumulated to elucidate the molecular effects of the *BRAF* V600E mutation in thyroid cancer, clinical data have similarly accrued to support a picture of uncontrolled promalignant signaling. Tumors with the *BRAF* V600E mutation show increased risk for recurrence, lymphatic and distant metastases, and unfavorable pathologic characteristics predictive of more aggressive disease. In one study, 76% (24 of 34) of *BRAF* V600E–positive (*BRAF+*) PTC primary tumors had positive sentinel lymph nodes, whereas only 17% (12 of 69) of *BRAF* V600E–negative (*BRAF−*) primary tumors did.[46] In another series, correlation of outcomes with retrospective *BRAF* testing of 190 PTC fine-needle aspiration (FNA) specimens showed that patients with *BRAF+* FNAs had higher rates of unfavorable pathologic characteristics, with more frequent recurrence (36% vs 12%), more lymph node metastases (39% vs 19%), and more capsular invasion (29% vs 16%) than *BRAF−* FNAs.[47] A long-term study of 203 PTC patients with median follow-up of more than 7 years found significant association between *BRAF+* status and recurrence (21 vs 7%, $P = .04$), but *BRAF* status itself was not an independent predictor of recurrence on multivariate analysis.[48] Pooling 2470 patients from 452 studies regarding *BRAF* mutational status and clinical outcomes in PTC, Tufano and colleagues[10] determined that *BRAF* mutation correlates with a higher risk of recurrence and metastasis. Overall, *BRAF* positivity was associated with significantly higher relative risk (RR) of tumor recurrence (24.9% vs 12.6%, RR 1.93), lymph node metastasis (54.1% vs 36.8%, RR 1.32), stage III or IV disease (35.4% vs 19.6%, RR 1.70), and extrathyroidal extension (46.2% vs 23.6%, RR 1.71) compared with *BRAF−* PTCs. There was no difference in distant metastasis (8.0% vs 7.9%). Testing for *BRAF* mutation informs risk estimates for resected thyroid cancer, and inclusion of *BRAF* status modestly improves performance of the AMES, MACIS, TNM, and ATA risk scores.[49] Likewise for thyroid papillary microcarcinoma (TPMC), a risk score incorporating *BRAF* status allowed identification of high-risk cancers that would not be identified by histology alone in a small study of 29 aggressive TPMCs matched to 30 nonaggressive cancers and validated in 40 others.[50] Although PTC has a favorable prognosis with greater than 90% survival at 10 years,[10] the *BRAF* V600E mutation puts patients at higher risk for recurrence, subjecting them to additional treatments and interventions, and likely causing worse quality of life, even if it does not cause decreased survival.

While knowledge of mutations in resected cancers improves prognostication, some have sought to apply molecular testing to prospective surgical decision making. Based on their results correlating *BRAF+* FNAs with higher recurrence risk even after correcting for unfavorable tumor characteristics, Xing and colleagues[47] suggested that preoperative knowledge of *BRAF* status by FNA could help surgeons choose whether to perform prophylactic central neck dissection. The place for lymphadenectomy in well-differentiated thyroid cancer remains controversial. Some retrospective studies have suggested incremental improvements in recurrence and survival, but these are balanced against higher rates of hypocalcemia and nerve injury.[51] Prospective studies to determine whether preoperative *BRAF* testing of FNA specimens is useful for predicting occult lymph node metastases have yielded conflicting results. One study (N = 51) found that *BRAF* positivity in excised tumors did not correlate with nodal metastases, but did not test for *BRAF* preoperatively and had a low rate of *BRAF* mutation (29%).[52] A larger study (N = 148) found that *BRAF+* FNA specimens were significantly associated with occult lymph node metastases after prophylactic central neck dissection, and concluded that *BRAF* status may be helpful in the decision whether to perform nodal dissection in a clinically node-negative neck.[53] Unless a prospective randomized trial with long-term follow-up is conducted, the optimal extent of nodal dissection will likely remain uncertain.

Chemotherapeutics Targeting BRAF and MAPK

Multiple proteins in the BRAF-MAPK pathway have been targeted for the treatment of thyroid cancer, and these pathways remain among the most active areas of pharmaceutical research. In 2008, a phase I trial showed promise for selumetinib/AZD6244, a selective MEK1/2 inhibitor, which included a patient with metastatic MTC with a prolonged period of stable disease.[54] In *BRAF*-mutated metastatic melanoma, a phase III trial of the MEK inhibitor trametinib demonstrated significantly prolonged progression-free and overall survival in the treatment group.[55] More recently, researchers completed an early phase trial of selumetinib in metastatic, radioiodine-refractory thyroid cancer.[56] Applying the preclinical observation that treatment with MEK inhibitors seemed to restore thyroid differentiation and iodine uptake in thyroid cells, they treated 20 patients with well-differentiated, metastatic, radioiodine-refractory, follicular-origin thyroid cancer with selumetinib. After 4 weeks iodine uptake was reassessed with ^{124}I positron emission tomography scans, and 12 of 20 patients had increased uptake. Of these patients, 8 had enough uptake to justify treatment with

^{131}I, and of these, 5 had partial responses and 3 had stable disease 6 months after treatment. Cancers with *RAS* mutations responded best to selumetinib (5 of 5), whereas only 1 of 9 cancers with *BRAF* V600E had enough uptake to warrant treatment with ^{131}I. Although limited in size, this rapid translation of cell culture and mouse data to human clinical trials may herald a new approach to kinase-inhibitor treatment in thyroid cancer.

Sorafenib, a multikinase inhibitor, has some activity in thyroid cancer, but early human use has shown low response rates. In 2008, sorafenib was shown to more potently inhibit thyroid cancer cells harboring the *RET/PTC1* gene rearrangement than those with *BRAF* V600E.[57] In a phase II trial of sorafenib for ATC, only 2 of 20 patients showed a partial response, and another 5 had stable disease; median progression-free survival was only 1.9 months.[58] Despite these modest results, there is growing evidence that response to treatment might be improved by prospective tumor genotyping, allowing improved selection of patients most likely to respond. In a trial of another multikinase inhibitor, Piscazzi and colleagues[1] analyzed results according to gene expression, finding no relationship between response to sunitinib treatment and tumor expression of traditional sunitinib targets VEGF receptor (VEGFR), c-KIT, and PDGF receptor (PDGFR). Response did correspond to expression of mutant *RET*, whereby mutation-positive patients enjoyed higher response rates than those with *BRAF* or *RAS* mutations, providing further enthusiasm for prospective genetic profiling of thyroid cancers in future trials. Yet another multiple tyrosine kinase inhibitor, cabozantinib/XL184, showed improved progression-free survival of 11.2 months, versus 4.0 months with placebo, in a phase III trial of the drug in progressive MTC.[59] Cabozantinib was approved by the Food and Drug Administration for the treatment of advanced MTC in November, 2012.

Kinase inhibitors specifically targeting BRAF have also been developed. One such is PLX4720, which inserts into the adenosine triphosphate (ATP)-binding site of mutant BRAF, stabilizing its inactive state. In vitro, the inhibitor blocks phosphorylation of downstream BRAF targets and leads to upregulation of suppressed markers of thyroid differentiation.[60] In a mouse model, Nehs and colleagues[61] injected V600E ATC cells into mouse thyroids and then treated the animals with PLX4720. Treated mice had resectable tumors after 7 days and lived to the end point of 50 days, whereas untreated mice were found to have unresectable tumors at 7 days and were euthanized by day 35 because of tumor burden. To more closely mimic the advanced stage at which ATC usually presents, this group next started inhibitor treatment at 28 days after administration of tumor cells to allow metastatic disease to become established, and still demonstrated tumor regression.[62] Based on these studies and data in melanoma with the similar but orally available BRAF inhibitor vemurafenib, Rosove and colleagues[63] reported a complete response to vemurafenib in a critically ill patient with metastatic *BRAF+* ATC, providing clinical evidence of the promise of this approach in human ATC.

In one of the most encouraging inhibitor trials to date, a phase III, manufacturer-sponsored trial of the RET inhibitor vandetanib recently showed efficacy in patients with advanced MTC.[64] Treatment with vandetanib was associated with median progression-free survival time of 30.5 months, versus 19.3 months for placebo (hazard ratio 0.46, 95% confidence interval 0.31–0.69), and objective response rates by RECIST criteria (Response Evaluation Criteria in Solid Tumors) of 45% versus 13% ($P<.001$, with high placebo response rate attributable to 93% cross-over to open-label vandetanib treatment among patients who progressed on placebo). Mild toxicities were common and serious toxicities occurred, including grade 3 or 4 diarrhea, hypertension, and QTc prolongation in 11%, 9%, and 8%, respectively, of treated patients. These results suggest that this drug will play a role in the treatment of MTC in the future.

Translational Research in Thyroid Nodules

An area of persistent clinical interest is the thyroid nodule with indeterminate cytology by FNA. Around 30% of all nodules have indeterminate FNA results, and of these around 30% harbor malignancy.[65] Because of the risk of malignancy, most patients with indeterminate nodules undergo surgery. Several novel methods have recently emerged to derive additional information from FNA specimens to select patients at low risk of malignancy who do not need surgery and to identify those likely to have cancer who will benefit from total thyroidectomy. McCoy and colleagues[66] studied 670 patients at a single institution in cohorts before and after the introduction of routine molecular testing of all nonbenign thyroid FNA specimens. These investigators reported that testing for mutations in *RET*, *RAS*, *BRAF*, and *PAX8/PPAR-γ* (a fusion of the thyroid transcription factor *PAX8* promoter with the peroxisome proliferator-activated receptor-γ1 gene, which is found in some follicular thyroid cancers[67]) identified mutations in 15% of indeterminate or nondiagnostic FNAs. Of 25 patients with positive molecular testing and no other indication for thyroidectomy, all were ultimately found to have some malignant changes, and 22 of 25 (88%) required total thyroidectomy based on current guidelines. With knowledge of the molecular testing results, 18 of these patients elected to undergo total thyroidectomy at their initial surgery. Concurrently, owing to the increased preoperative knowledge, the sensitivity of intraoperative frozen section dropped to only 1.7% and was abandoned at their institution. The investigators concluded that routine molecular testing (at an additional $104 per specimen) adds valuable knowledge, helps to select the correct initial surgery more often, and is cost-effective by limiting the need for later reoperation for completion thyroidectomy.[66] Overall, detecting a known malignant mutation on thyroid FNA has a positive predictive value for malignancy of nearly 100% for *BRAF*, *RET*, or *PAX8/PPAR-γ*, and 74% to 87% for *RAS*, and these patients should undergo total thyroidectomy.[65]

Although testing for mutations of known malignant potential can identify patients who should undergo total thyroidectomy, with its low negative predictive value it cannot rule out malignancy. An emerging approach to this challenge uses differences in microRNA (miRNA) expression to separate benign and malignant thyroid nodules. miRNA can distinguish benign from malignant thyroid FNA specimens with high accuracy; however, when applied to indeterminate nodules the negative predictive values remain below 90%, and are insufficient to recommend against surgery.[68] Nevertheless, potential discovery of additional informative miRNA or improvements in classification algorithms make this a promising avenue of research.

Another strategy assesses differential mRNA expression by quantitative polymerase chain reaction (PCR). In 2012, a multicenter validation study of a commercially available gene-expression assay for indeterminate thyroid FNA specimens reported results from 265 patients who underwent thyroidectomy.[69] The assay measures expression of 142 genes and uses a proprietary algorithm to classify specimens as benign or malignant. In this study, 32% of patients were ultimately found to have malignancy, and the gene expression classifier correctly identified 78 of these 85 (91.7%) as suspicious for malignancy. The negative predictive value of the test was 85% to 95%, depending on the Bethesda classification assigned to the specimen. These results were reported as evidence that the test could help avoid unnecessary thyroidectomies. At least one study funded by the company reported that the rate of surgery in indeterminate nodules classified as benign by the gene-expression test decreased to 7% among patients of participating endocrinologists, compared with 74% overall for indeterminate nodules before adoption of the test.[70] Despite the promise of these reports, the authors of the present review believe that it is premature to decide against surgery based on the results of Alexander and colleagues. All data collection and analysis in both studies was performed by the manufacturer, and the validation study employed a relatively small sample size of 265 patients. As such, these results could represent a best-case scenario of the test's performance. Furthermore, in the utilization study, the proportion of total tests classified as benign was not reported, making it impossible to determination the total rate of surgery.[70] An industry-sponsored study claiming cost-effectiveness of this $3200 test used a cost model that assumed very high 30% and 44% complication rates for hemithyroidectomy and total thyroidectomy, and did not account for the costs and impact on quality of life of missed cancer diagnoses.[71] Finally, while this test clearly adds information over cytology results alone, the unanswered question is whether negative predictive values of as low as 85% in the highest risk category (implying a 15% rate of malignancy) would be sufficient for most surgeons to recommend against surgery. A larger, independent validation of the test should be done,[72] and studies of reduced thyroidectomy rates after application of the test must include appropriate follow-up to determine how many patients not having surgery based on a negative test result ultimately develop cancer or undergo thyroidectomy at a later time.

Until completion of such studies, the authors of the present review agree with the management algorithm of Nikiforov and colleagues[73] for solitary thyroid nodules with indeterminate cytology, which was based on analysis of 1056 FNA specimens. Indeterminate FNAs have a cancer risk of 14% to 54% and should undergo molecular testing with a limited and less expensive panel (*BRAF*, *RAS*, *RET*, and *PAX8/PPAR-γ*). Patients with positive results should undergo total thyroidectomy because of the high risk of malignancy (87%–95%). Patients with follicular lesions or atypia of undetermined significance and negative testing have a risk of malignancy of 6% and may consider observation, repeat FNA, or diagnostic lobectomy, whereas those with follicular neoplasm/suspicion for follicular neoplasm or suspicion for malignancy have a risk of malignancy of 14% to 28% and should undergo diagnostic lobectomy.[73]

PARATHYROID/MEN1

Parathyroid abnormalities encompass both benign and malignant disease, and hyperparathyroidism is a feature of MEN1 and MEN2A syndromes. Parathyroid carcinoma remains exceedingly rare, but is strongly associated with the tumor-suppressor *HRPT2/CDC73*. Germline *HRPT2* mutations cause familial hyperparathyroidism/jaw-tumor syndrome, and somatic mutation of *HRPT2* is found in more than 75% of sporadic parathyroid carcinomas.[74–76] Some patients with seemingly sporadic parathyroid carcinoma will be found to have germline *HRPT2* mutations, making genetic testing of patients with parathyroid carcinoma potentially helpful by identifying related gene carriers who will benefit from serum calcium screening.[75] Parafibromin, the protein product of *HRPT2*, acts as a cell-cycle regulator in the Wnt pathway through interaction with β-catenin, and is involved in histone modification during transcription.[77] Loss of immunohistochemical staining for parafibromin is highly suggestive of parathyroid carcinoma, and in the future may aid in the diagnosis of malignant parathyroid tumors.[78,79]

Hyperparathyroidism (HPT) occurs in a minority of MEN2A patients, with the risk strongly influenced by the specific *RET* mutation present (see **Table 1**).[29] The incidence of HPT in MEN2A is known to be 20% to 35%,[80] and is much more common with mutations of codon 634, although HPT also occurs in 1% to 5% of patients with codon 609, 611, 618, and 620 mutations.[81] By contrast, HPT is the most common manifestation of MEN1, with nearly 100% of carriers affected by the age of 50 years **(Table 3)**.[31] The *MEN1* gene was first mapped to chromosome 11 by linkage in 1988,[82] and cloned in 1997.[83,84] The menin tumor-suppressor protein encoded by *MEN1* interacts with many different proteins including transcription factors and cell-cycle regulatory proteins, can bind DNA directly, and although it seems to play a role in chromatin remodeling and genomic stability, its exact function remains unclear.[85–87] Unlike MEN2 mutations, which cluster at particular codons, *MEN1* mutations are highly variable, with more than 1100 distinct germline mutations described and the most common occurring in only 4.5% of families (as opposed to 85% of MEN2A families having *RET* codon-634 mutations).[29,86] Also unlike MEN2, in MEN1, individuals show similar manifestations of the disease within affected families, but have considerable variation between families, even those sharing the same mutation.[86] Thus while genetic testing for *MEN1* mutations is available, identifying carriers does not suggest a specific prophylactic surgical therapy, as in MEN2, but rather identifies those who require screening for development of different manifestations of the disease. Lairmore and colleagues[88] found that genetic testing for MEN1 helped identify biochemical changes 5 to 10 years before the development of clinically apparent tumors, allowing for early surgical intervention in some cases. Those at risk for MEN1 by family history or confirmed through genetic testing should begin serum calcium screening before the age of 10 years to detect development of HPT.[89] In sporadic HPT, keen attention to family history suggestive of MEN1 (pituitary adenoma, pancreatic neuroendocrine tumor, hyperparathyroidism, thymic carcinoid, cutaneous angiofibroma, ependymoma, nodular adrenocortical hyperplasia, or multiple lipomas) helps identify patients who may benefit from genetic testing and 4-gland exploration.[88,90]

The importance of the *MEN1* gene to parathyroid disease is highlighted by the frequency of somatic *MEN1* mutation in sporadic parathyroid adenomas. Cromer and colleagues[91] performed whole-exome sequencing on 8 sporadic parathyroid adenomas and corresponding genomic DNA, identifying 29 somatic mutations in the

Table 3
Selected autosomal dominant endocrine cancer syndromes and penetrance of phenotypic features

Syndrome	Gene(s)	Overall Penetrance of Disease Feature[a]			
		MTC	**HPT**	**PCC/PGL**	**PNET**
MEN1	*MEN1*	NA	100% at age 50[31]	<1%[31]	53% at age 50[133]
MEN2A	*RET*	90%–100%[31,80]	20–35%[b,80]	40%[b,80]	NA
MEN2B	*RET*	100%[14,31]	Rare[14]	19%–53%[158–160]	NA
FMTC	*RET*	100% by definition	0% by definition	0% by definition	NA
vHL	*VHL*	NA	NA	10–20%[b,92,102]	10%–17%[161]
TSC	*TSC1, TSC2*	NA	NA	NA	1%[152]
NF1	*NF1*	NA	NA	6%[95]	<10%[152]

Abbreviations: FMTC, familial medullary thyroid cancer; HPT, hyperparathyroidism; MEN, multiple endocrine neoplasia; MTC, medullary thyroid cancer; NA, not applicable; NF1, neurofibromatosis type 1; PCC/PGL, pheochromocytoma/paraganglioma; PNET, pancreatic neuroendocrine tumor; TSC, tuberous sclerosis complex; vHL, von Hippel–Lindau syndrome.
[a] Reported penetrance tends to increase with age/length of follow-up.
[b] Individual risk is highly dependent on particular mutation present.

adenomas. Screening of 185 additional sporadic parathyroid adenomas for these mutations by direct sequencing revealed *MEN1* mutations in 35.2% of the validation cohort, whereas only 1 of the other mutations (occurring in 1 of 185 patients) was found. Thus, although the exact mechanisms by which *RET* and *MEN1* lead to parathyroid disease remain unknown, somatic *MEN1* mutation is a frequent event in sporadic and heritable parathyroid disease.

PHEOCHROMOCYTOMA/PARAGANGLIOMA

In addition to MEN2A, other autosomal dominant heritable disorders predispose patients to develop pheochromocytomas or paragangliomas (PCC/PGL), including neurofibromatosis type 1 (NF1), von Hippel–Lindau syndrome (vHL), and familial paraganglioma syndromes.[85] Genetic testing for these conditions is available but, as with MEN1, no specific prophylactic surgical procedure exists. Genetic testing therefore allows screening and early discovery of tumors, as well as prevention of anesthesia complications by preoperative α-blockade in patients who might have PCCs. Overall, approximately 25% of PCCs display malignant characteristics, and approximately one-third of all PCCs are associated with a known germline mutation.[92]

Patients with NF1 are at increased risk for PCC. Although the *NF1* gene has been known for some time,[93,94] because of its large size (300 kb, 57 exons), complexity (36 different pseudogenes and multiple splice variants), and diversity of mutations causing the disorder, NF1 continues to be diagnosed based on clinical phenotype rather than genetic testing.[95] Around 6% of NF1 patients will develop PCC.[95] Among NF1 patients developing PCC, 67% show loss of the nonmutated *NF1* region in tumor specimens, suggesting that PCCs in NF1 require a "second hit" for tumor development.[95] *NF1* is also the most common somatically mutated gene in sporadic PCC (26% of sporadic tumors), with loss of heterozygosity of the wild-type allele in 91% of these.[96] Neoplasia in NF1 follows pathways familiar from other endocrine cancers. One function of the *NF1* protein product neurofibromin is in RAS/MAPK signaling, where it interacts with RAS to stimulate the RAS guanosine triphosphatase, which terminates its signal (see **Fig. 1**).[97] Lack of functional neurofibromin thereby allows the RAS signal to persist, activating the MAPK and PI3K/AKT/mTOR pathways. Activation of mTOR in *NF1*-mutated tumors is influenced by inactivation of tuberin, the product of the tuberous sclerosis complex gene *TSC2*.[98] As such, development of tumors in neurofibromatosis is intimately related to the mechanisms underlying tumors in MEN2 and tuberous sclerosis.[85]

After identification of the gene causing vHL in 1993,[99] it became possible to screen at-risk patients based on genetic testing for PCCs, cerebellar hemangioblastomas, retinal angiomas, renal cell carcinomas, pancreatic neuroendocrine tumors, endolymphatic sac tumors, and cystadenomas of the pancreas, epididymis, and broad ligament, which characterize the disease.[85,100] Although less common than the hallmark central nervous system and retinal hemangioblastomas (60%–80% of patients) and renal clear cell carcinomas (70% lifetime risk),[101] PCCs occur in 10% to 20% of vHL patients.[92] In 573 vHL patients, Ong and colleagues[102] found PCCs to be significantly more common (penetrance ~60% by 50 years vs 5% to 20% in other groups) and occurring earlier (mean 21.7 vs 27.8 years, $P = .012$) in patients with missense mutations of surface residues of the VHL protein, compared with those with deletions, truncations, or missense mutations of core residues. This genotypic distinction between mutations with low and high risk of PCC correlates closely with the earlier clinical designation of vHL types 1 and 2[102]. VHL protein interacts with elongin as part of an E3 ubiquitin ligase complex, and also directly with hypoxia-inducible factor (HIF) subunits

1 and 2α to target them for degradation (see **Fig. 1**).[102] Mutant proteins may fail to cause degradation of HIF proteins, leading to promalignant signaling, but as some patients with mutations that do not disrupt HIF interactions still develop PCC, additional mechanisms, such as failure of normal apoptosis of adrenal progenitor cells, may be responsible for PCC features of vHL syndrome.[101,102]

Germline mutations in each of the 4 succinate dehydrogenase complex subunits and of a gene required for flavination and function of the complex (*SDHA*, *SDHB*, *SDHC*, *SDHD*, *SDHAF2*, collectively called SDHx) predispose to autosomal dominant familial paraganglioma syndrome, with distinct phenotypes and inheritance. The SDH genes form mitochondrial complex II, which is involved in both the tricarboxylic acid cycle and electron transport chain.[92] *SDHD* was first identified as a cause of familial paraganglioma syndrome,[103] and *SDHD* mutations were soon reported in sporadic PGLs and hereditary and sporadic PCCs.[104,105] Inheritance of *SDHD* is autosomal dominant, but with a maternal-imprinting effect, such that patients inheriting the maternal copy display no symptoms, whereas those receiving a paternal allele have partial penetrance.[103] In affected patients, somatic loss of the maternal chromosome 11, containing the wild-type allele, is required for tumor development.[106] After identification of the *SDHD* mutation, reports of mutations causing the syndrome in the A,[107] B,[108] and C[109] SDH subunits, as well as in the SDH assembly factor 2 (*SDHAF2*) gene, followed.[110] No imprinting effect is observed in *SDHB* and *SDHC*, and inheritance is autosomal dominant, whereas *SDHAF2* shows paternal inheritance similar to *SDHD*.[108,109,111] As with HIF-stabilization in vHL syndrome, the SDHx mutations inactivate the SDH complex, leading to a defect in electron transport, accumulation of succinate, and induction of a pseudohypoxic state with consequent persistence of HIF factors. In turn, this induces angiogenesis and other proliferative and preneoplastic signaling (see **Fig. 1**).[107]

Features of PCC/PGL syndromes depend on the mutation present and the tumor's location. PGL tumors in the head and neck rarely produce active catecholamines, whereas up to 50% of their abdominal PCCs/PGLs do.[85,112] Malignant PCCs occur more commonly in families with *SDHB* mutations, whereas *SDHD* PCCs are more often benign.[113] In malignant PCC/PGL, *SDHB* mutations also portend a worse prognosis, and are associated with lower 5-year survival when compared with tumors without *SDHB* mutations.[114] Mutations of the other SDHx genes rarely lead to PCCs, and these syndromes are marked mostly by head and neck PGLs.[113]

Two additional PCC-related tumor suppressor genes, *TMEM127* and *MAX*, were identified in hereditary PCC kindreds without known mutations (see **Fig. 1**). Qin and colleagues[115] reported autosomal dominant inheritance of 6 distinct germline *TMEM127* mutations in 7 families, representing 30% of familial and 3% of apparently sporadic PCCs out of 102 screened. While the function of *TMEM127* remains unknown, it seems to behave as a tumor suppressor and negative regulator of mTORC1. It colocalizes with mTORC1, and siRNA knockdown of TMEM127 increases mTORC1 signaling, which is likewise observed with *NF1* mutations.[115] Screening of 642 sporadic PCCs found *TMEM127* mutations in only 6 patients (0.9%), making *TMEM127* the least common PCC susceptibility gene.[116] *MAX* mutations causing loss of protein expression were discovered in 3 kindreds by exome sequencing,[117] and then confirmed to affect 1.12% of 1694 sporadic and hereditary PCC patients without a known mutation.[118] MAX functions in dimerization of MYC/MAX/MXD1 transcription factors, where it helps to repress cell growth, and may influence the mTOR pathway.[117] Like *SDHAF2* and *SDHD*, transmission of familial *MAX* mutation is preferentially paternal, with tumors of affected patients expressing only the paternal allele either through uniparental disomy or loss of heterozygosity for chromosome 14q.[117]

Despite the host of mutations predisposing to PCCs and PGLs, there is an increasing understanding that the affected genes cluster into only a few pathways and relate to other forms of neuroendocrine cancer. Burnichon and colleagues[119] analyzed PCC/PGL specimens from 190 patients, performing microarray gene-expression testing and analysis for germline and somatic mutations by comparative genomic hybridization and direct sequencing. The investigators found that differences in gene expression allowed unsupervised hierarchical cluster analysis to correctly assign 67 of 69 hereditary tumors to 1 of 3 clusters concordant with their known mutations (*SDHx*, *VHL*, and *NF1/RET/TMEM127*). Analysis of 78 sporadic tumors that grouped to these same clusters uncovered somatic mutations of *RET* and *VHL* in 17, loss of *SDH* heterozygosity in 2 of 2 sporadic tumors that clustered with familial *SDHx* tumors, and loss of heterozygosity of the *VHL* locus in 16 of 16 tumors clustering with familial vHL tumors. Genes differentially expressed in the different clusters corresponded to mTOR and MAPK-pathway targets in the *NF1/RET/TMEM127* cluster, and to hypoxia-induced factors in the *SDHx* and *VHL* clusters. This distinction between tumors with induction of genes for pseudohypoxia response versus genes for proliferative signaling likely represents a fundamental biological difference in these tumors that will influence the targeting of personalized tumor therapies in the future.

ADRENOCORTICAL CARCINOMA

Adrenocortical carcinoma (ACC) remains a rare and deadly cancer, and has seen only limited improvements in therapy over time. The FIRM-ACT trial, which randomized patients with advanced ACC to treatment with mitotane plus either streptozocin (Sz+M) or etoposide, doxorubicin, and cisplatin (EDP+M), established EDP+M as the standard of care, owing to its higher objective response rate (23.2% vs 9.2%, $P<.001$) and similar toxicity.[120] Despite higher response rates with EDP+M, overall survival remained disappointing, with no significant difference between the two treatment groups (median 14.8 vs 12.0 months, $P = .07$).

In light of the poor performance of current treatments, several groups have analyzed ACC gene expression to find new therapeutic targets. Gene-expression arrays identified 2- to 6-fold overexpression of fibroblast growth factor receptor 1 (*FGFR1*) and 14- to 100-fold overexpression of insulin-like growth factor II (*IGF2*) as key components of ACC relative to benign adenomas and normal adrenal cortex.[121] Prior to this, *IGF2* was recognized to play a role in ACC. Patients with Beckwith-Widemann syndrome (BWS) are prone to ACC,[122] and the chromosomal region 11p15.5 that is altered in BWS contains *IGF2*, and is also altered in sporadic ACC.[123] At this parentally imprinted locus, duplications, deletions, gene methylation, chromosomal loss, and uniparental disomy cause variations in the effective copy number of *IGF2*, with increased gene dosage driving proliferation and malignancy in neural crest–derived tissues.[122,124] High expression of *IGF2* also correlates with earlier recurrence in ACC.[125] Based on these observations, small-molecule inhibitors of FGFR1 and IGF2's receptor, IGFR1, are currently in clinical trials, with results for the IGFR1 inhibitor OSI-906 expected in 2013.[124]

Trials of other small-molecule kinase inhibitors in ACC are ongoing. After failures of gefitinib, imatinib, and sorafenib to produce responses in advanced ACC, a phase II trial of the multikinase inhibitor sunitinib reported stable disease at 12 weeks in 5 of 35 treated patients (14%), with improved overall survival in responders.[126] A major problem with these kinase inhibitors is that similar to findings in other cancers, inhibition of one kinase protein may be overcome by compensatory upregulation of others.[45,124,127] Lin and colleagues[128] provided an example of this in ACC cell culture, finding that monotherapy with sunitinib effectively blocked phosphorylation of its targets VEGFR, PDGFR, and RET, but their downstream MAPK targets MEK and ERK actually showed increased phosphorylation. Combination therapy with sunitinib and the ERK inhibitor PD98059 resulted in greater proliferation inhibition (68% with both vs 23% and 19% inhibition with sunitinib or PD98059 alone). These results suggest that personalized therapy with gene-expression analysis leading to specific targeting of upregulated pathways could one day improve therapeutic response rates, but the additive toxicities of combination therapy remain an important practical obstacle to *in vivo* application.

Functional Adrenal Adenomas

As in other areas of endocrine dysfunction, exome sequencing has proved to be a powerful tool for identifying specific mutations in both familial and sporadic functional adrenal adenomas. Three genes, *KCNJ5*, *ATP1A1*, and *ATP2B3*, were recently found to cause aldosterone-producing adenomas (APAs). Somatic mutation of *KCNJ5* occurs in 30% to 40% of APAs, and germline mutations have been reported in a dominantly inherited syndrome of hyperaldosteronism and bilateral adrenal hyperplasia.[129–131] The *KCNJ5* gene encodes a potassium channel that causes depolarization and excessive aldosterone release when mutated.[129] Mutations in the Na^+/K^+ ATPase *ATPA1* and the Ca^{2+} ATPase *ATP2B3* likewise cause depolarization with aldosterone release, and somatic mutations in these genes occur in 7% of APAs.[130] Of note, a screen of 380 APAs found *KCNJ5* mutations in 49% of females but only 19% of males ($P<.001$)[131] while 17 of 21 (81%) ATPase mutations occurred in males.[130] Knowledge of these APA-causing mutations has not yet altered surgical management, but medical therapies targeting these genes could someday reduce the need for adrenalectomy in these patients.

PANCREATIC NEUROENDOCRINE TUMORS

Pancreatic neuroendocrine tumors (PNETs) present with distant disease in more than 60% of cases, and for unknown reasons their incidence has nearly doubled over the past 30 years.[132] In addition to sporadic cases, PNETs occur in vHL, NF1, MEN1, and tuberous sclerosis syndromes (see **Table 3**). Translational research in neuroendocrine cancer has shown progress in defining cell-surface receptor targets for imaging and treatment and in unraveling the genetic alterations present in this disease.

For pancreatic tumors associated with MEN1 and other heritable syndromes, optimal timing of surgery remains problematic. Functional (gastrinomas, insulinomas, glucagonomas, somatostatinomas, and so forth) and nonfunctional PNETs have a penetrance of 30% to 50% by age 40 years in MEN1 patients, and are a major cause of mortality.[31,133] Because surgical elimination of all at-risk tissue is not possible, intervention focuses on controlling symptoms and preempting metastatic malignant disease. Symptomatic functional tumors should be resected to prevent complications of their secreted hormones.[31] In nonfunctional and asymptomatic tumors, size has emerged as the best indication for intervention. Early reports indicated no association between tumor size and outcomes[134]; more recently, however, larger, nonfunctional pancreatic tumors were found to be significantly associated with poorer survival and higher rates of metastasis in a long-term study of more than 500 MEN1 patients.[133] Whereas only 10% of patients with tumors smaller than 10 mm had synchronous metastases, 18% with tumors 20 to 30 mm in size had synchronous metastases, and patients with tumors larger than 30 mm had a 43% rate of synchronous metastasis. The investigators therefore recommended resection when tumors become larger than 20 mm or are rapidly growing, as the risks from metastases outweigh the risks of pancreatic surgery at that point.

Receptor-Directed Treatment Strategies

Prognosis in sporadic PNETs has improved in recent years, with a Dutch registry showing all-stage 5-year survival for low-grade PNETs increasing from 51% during 1990 to 2000 to 65% from 2000 to 2010.[135] Recognition of the benefits of surgery for even metastatic disease may account for some of this improvement,[136] but treatments targeting somatostatin receptors have also played an important role.[135] Somatostatin analogues (SSAs) have been investigated since the 1970s in the control of hormonal symptoms of functional neuroendocrine tumors.[137] Although SSAs were initially studied for their relief of symptoms of carcinoid and other hormone overproduction syndromes, it is now understood that neuroendocrine tumor tissues actually overexpress somatostatin receptors.[138,139] Somatostatin receptors were first cloned in 1992.[140] Of the 5 human subtypes, most SSAs bind principally to type 2 (SSTR2) and type 5 (SSTR5) receptors.[141] SSTR signal transduction is complex, involving many pathways with abundant cross-talk, and is also dependent on cellular context.[142] Of interest in PNETs, SSTR2-mediated inhibition of the MAPK pathway and accumulation of cyclic adenosine monophosphate has been reported in the PNET-derived BON-1 cell line, and causes reduced release of chromogranin A.[143]

In 1998 a long-acting SSA (octreotide LAR) was introduced, allowing more stable drug delivery and treatment compliance. Octreotide benefits patients with functional and nonfunctional tumors, and treatment achieves disease stabilization in 50% to 60% of patients, with occasional partial or complete responses.[144] The PROMID study provided validation of the benefits of SSAs in a randomized trial, allocating 90 patients with metastatic functional and nonfunctional midgut NETs to treatment with octreotide LAR or placebo.[145] Octreotide LAR demonstrated improved median progression-free survival of 14.3 vs 6.0 months ($P<.0001$), with a low death rate that prevented evaluation of overall survival.[145]

SSTR overexpression in neuroendocrine tissues makes these receptors useful not only for their signaling effects but also as specific markers of tumor cells. This property has been exploited by coupling SSA molecules such as octreotide to radioactive isotopes, which permit tumor imaging and tumor-directed peptide receptor radionuclide therapy (PRRT). SSTR-based imaging is now recommended along with computed tomography (CT) for the staging of all tumors.[144] Variations in the specific SSTR ligand, the radiochelator, the imaging isotope used, and the combination of emission data with CT imaging have all improved the performance of SSTR-based imaging.[146] Somatostatin receptor scintigraphy (SRS) with ^{111}In-octreotide was the first to show widespread utility, but is being supplanted by positron-emitting isotopes, such as [68]Ga.[146] Although imaging with ^{111}In may miss clinically important primary or metastatic tumors in around 25% to 40% of cases, Gabriel and colleagues[147] reported sensitivity of 97% in 84 NET patients imaged with ^{68}Ga-DOTA-Tyr3-octreotide, versus 52% with SRS and 61% with CT.[148]

Lesions positive by SSTR-directed imaging may be treatable by PRRT. In this modality, the low-energy imaging radioligand is exchanged for β-emitting ^{90}Y or ^{177}Lu, with a somatostatin analogue directing the isotope to tumor cells.[149] Using ^{177}Lu-DOTA-octreotate in a series of 310 patients with advanced gastroenteropancreatic NETs, complete or partial responses were reported in 30% of patients overall and in 42% of nonfunctional PNETs.[150] Median overall survival was 46 months from treatment and 128 months from diagnosis. Although the relative benefits of

PRRT over chemotherapy and small-molecule therapies require continuing investigation, PRRT stands out by its ability to shrink tumors in a significant proportion of patients.

The success of SSAs raises the question of whether additional receptors might be helpful for combination treatment for tumors that do not respond to SSA therapy, or for tumors that do not express high levels of SSTRs. Imaging with radiolabeled gastric inhibitory polypeptide (GIP) has successfully visualized GIP receptor (GIPR)-expressing adrenal tumors,[151] and recent work by the authors' group has found that both GIPR and oxytocin receptors are overexpressed in neuroendocrine tumors relative to normal tissue.[139] GIPR has expression similar to SSTR2 in PNETs,[139] suggesting that these and other new receptor targets could provide expanded treatment options for PNETs.

Genetic Alterations in Sporadic PNETs

While SSTR-directed therapies have shown success, the reasons for SSTR overexpression remain unclear. Unlike in MTC where mutations in RET lead to constitutive activation, providing a mechanism for tumorigenesis, the overexpressed receptors in PNETs are not mutated, suggesting that their overexpression does not drive malignancy, but rather represents an upregulatory reaction to primary mutations in other genes.[152] Missiaglia and colleagues[153] advanced the understanding of these primary genetic defects, performing gene-expression profiling on 72 PNET tumor specimens with clinical and immunohistochemistry correlation. This study revealed that 85% of primary tumors had reduced staining for TSC2 or phosphatase and tensin homologue (PTEN) protein, with low expression correlating with decreased survival and increased metastasis. High expression of *FGF13*, which assists in p38 MAPK recruitment, also correlated with worse outcomes. *TSC2* and *PTEN* function to negatively regulate the PI3K/Akt/mTOR pathway, with mutations in either leading to increased proliferation and loss of hypoxia-induced growth inhibition (**Fig. 2**).

Jiao and colleagues[87] performed exome sequencing on 10 sporadic PNETs to discover somatically mutated genes, with verification in 58 additional tumors. This study showed that PNETs have a different mutational profile than pancreatic adenocarcinomas, with a low rate of mutation in *KRAS*, *TGF-β*, *CDKN2A*, and *TP53* (which are common in adenocarcinoma). Instead, the most commonly mutated genes in PNETs were *MEN1*, *DAXX/ATRX*, *TSC2*, and *PTEN* in 44%, 25%, 9%, and 7% of tumors, respectively. Death-associated domain protein and α-thalassemia/mental retardation syndrome X-linked (*DAXX/ATRX*) function in telomeric histone incorporation and chromatin remodeling, and had not been previously implicated in cancer. In the study by Jiao and colleagues,[87] mutations in these genes were associated with significantly improved survival in comparison with PNETs without *DAXX/ATRX* mutations. Subsequent studies found a perfect correlation between PNET *DAXX/ATRX* mutation and the telomerase-independent telomere maintenance (ALT) phenotype,[154] which can arise in cells with impairment of normal telomere maintenance and correlates with cell immortalization.[155] Along with the finding of *ATRX* mutations in additional cancer types with the ALT phenotype, this implies that *DAXX* and *ATRX* play important roles in telomere maintenance.[154] Testing for these mutations promises to provide important prognostic information, and further investigation of *DAXX/ATRX* function may uncover new insights into the pathogenesis of PNETs and other cancers.

Small-Molecule Therapies in Pancreatic Neuroendocrine Cancer

Recognition that genes in the mTOR pathway are mutated in at least 16% of PNETs and that the pathway's function may be impaired in up to 85% of tumors has spurred

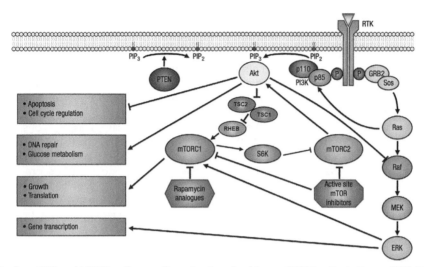

Fig. 2. mTOR and MAPK pathways. Receptor tyrosine kinases (RTKs) activate Ras or PI3K. Ras activates the MAPK cascade of Raf (including BRAF), MEK, and ERK kinases, leading to cell survival, gene transcription, and proliferation. Activated PI3K phosphorylates PIP2 to PIP3 (phosphatidylinositol bis- and trisphosphate). PTEN dephosphorylates PIP3 to PIP2, inhibiting its signal. PIP3 activates Akt, which causes dissociation of TSC2 from TSC1, releasing inhibition of RHEB (Ras Homologue Enriched in Brain), which then activates mTORC1. Rapamycin analogues such as everolimus inhibit mTOR proteins. Cross-talk between MAPK and PI3K pathways is indicated (Ras/PI3K, ERK/mTORC1, and Akt/Raf). ADP, adenosine diphosphate; ATP, adenosine triphosphate; GDP, guanosine diphosphate; GTP, guanosine triphosphate; HIF, hypoxia-inducible factor; SDH, succinate dehydrogenase. See also Maiese and colleagues.[162] (*From* Gadgeel SM, Wozniak A. Preclinical rationale for PI3K/Akt/mTOR pathway inhibitors as therapy for epidermal growth factor receptor inhibitor-resistant non-small-cell lung cancer. Clin Lung Cancer 2013;14(4):322–32; with permission.)

the use of mTOR inhibitors in PNETs.[87,153] The RADIANT-3 trial, a manufacturer-sponsored phase III trial, randomized 410 patients with advanced and progressing NETs of multiple primary sites to the mTOR inhibitor everolimus or best supportive therapy, and reported significantly improved progression-free survival in the everolimus arm (median 11.4 vs 5.4 months, $P<.001$).[156] Everolimus was effective in delaying progression, but tumor shrinkage occurred in only 5% of treated patients. No difference in overall survival was detected, possibly due to 73% cross-over to everolimus among patients initially randomized to placebo.

Pancreatic neuroendocrine tumors express VEGFR and PDGFR, which contribute to angiogenesis, and have provided a rationale for use of the multikinase inhibitor sunitinib in PNETs.[157] A manufacturer-sponsored phase III trial randomized 154 patients with advanced, progressive PNETs to sunitinib or placebo. The trial was halted when interim analyses detected a significant advantage in progression-free survival with sunitinib treatment (median 11.4 vs 5.5 months, $P<.001$). The effect on overall survival could not be estimated. Grade 1 and 2 side effects occurred in the majority of patients during treatment with either everolimus or sunitinib.[156,157] Grade 3 or 4 neutropenia and hypertension occurred in more than 10% of patients receiving sunitinib,[157] whereas a 7% rate of grade 3 or 4 stomatitis was the most frequent serious complication in patients taking everolimus.[156]

SUMMARY AND FUTURE DIRECTIONS

From genetic testing to targeted therapies, translational research in endocrine cancer has improved care and outcomes in endocrine surgery, but much work remains. Genetic markers will continue to help distinguish benign and malignant processes in cancers that are difficult to diagnose, such as indeterminate thyroid nodules and malignant parathyroid and adrenal tumors. However, adequate validation of new tests is essential to ensure that surgery is not delayed in those who will benefit from it and is avoided in those who will not. Further research in basic and clinical aspects of small-molecule kinase inhibitors will clarify the optimal uses for these agents, but the challenges of inhibitor resistance and paradoxic induction of related pathways remains a vexing problem. The plummeting cost of genetic sequencing promises dramatic advances in personalized, rational cancer therapy based on knowledge of the specific pathways affected. As individualized combination therapies proliferate, managing or avoiding toxicities of potent new drugs will assume even greater importance. Investigators and clinicians should feel encouraged by the strides made in translational research in endocrine cancer, and should continue to integrate these findings into practice to deliver superior patient outcomes.

REFERENCES

1. Piscazzi A, Costantino E, Maddalena F, et al. Activation of the RAS/RAF/ERK signaling pathway contributes to resistance to sunitinib in thyroid carcinoma cell lines. J Clin Endocrinol Metab 2012;97:E898.
2. Roskoski R Jr. ERK1/2 MAP kinases: structure, function, and regulation. Pharmacol Res 2012;66:105.
3. Caronia LM, Phay JE, Shah MH. Role of BRAF in thyroid oncogenesis. Clin Cancer Res 2011;17:7511.
4. Xing M. BRAF mutation in papillary thyroid cancer: pathogenic role, molecular bases, and clinical implications. Endocr Rev 2007;28:742.
5. Liu D, Xing M. Potent inhibition of thyroid cancer cells by the MEK inhibitor PD0325901 and its potentiation by suppression of the PI3K and NF-kappaB pathways. Thyroid 2008;18:853.
6. Palona I, Namba H, Mitsutake N, et al. BRAFV600E promotes invasiveness of thyroid cancer cells through nuclear factor kappaB activation. Endocrinology 2006;147:5699.
7. Kapiteijn E, Schneider TC, Morreau H, et al. New treatment modalities in advanced thyroid cancer. Ann Oncol 2012;23:10.
8. Santarpia L, Myers JN, Sherman SI, et al. Genetic alterations in the RAS/RAF/mitogen-activated protein kinase and phosphatidylinositol 3-kinase/Akt signaling pathways in the follicular variant of papillary thyroid carcinoma. Cancer 2010;116:2974.
9. Ricarte-Filho JC, Ryder M, Chitale DA, et al. Mutational profile of advanced primary and metastatic radioactive iodine-refractory thyroid cancers reveals distinct pathogenetic roles for BRAF, PIK3CA, and AKT1. Cancer Res 2009;69:4885.
10. Tufano RP, Teixeira GV, Bishop J, et al. BRAF mutation in papillary thyroid cancer and its value in tailoring initial treatment: a systematic review and meta-analysis. Medicine (Baltimore) 2012;91:274.
11. Knauf JA, Fagin JA. Role of MAPK pathway oncoproteins in thyroid cancer pathogenesis and as drug targets. Curr Opin Cell Biol 2009;21:296.

12. Mathew CG, Chin KS, Easton DF, et al. A linked genetic marker for multiple endocrine neoplasia type 2A on chromosome 10. Nature 1987;328:527.
13. Simpson NE, Kidd KK, Goodfellow PJ, et al. Assignment of multiple endocrine neoplasia type 2A to chromosome 10 by linkage. Nature 1987;328:528.
14. Lairmore TC, Howe JR, Korte JA, et al. Familial medullary thyroid carcinoma and multiple endocrine neoplasia type 2B map to the same region of chromosome 10 as multiple endocrine neoplasia type 2A. Genomics 1991;9:181.
15. Takahashi M, Ritz J, Cooper GM. Activation of a novel human transforming gene, ret, by DNA rearrangement. Cell 1985;42:581.
16. Fusco A, Grieco M, Santoro M, et al. A new oncogene in human thyroid papillary carcinomas and their lymph-nodal metastases. Nature 1987;328:170.
17. Donghi R, Sozzi G, Pierotti MA, et al. The oncogene associated with human papillary thyroid carcinoma (PTC) is assigned to chromosome 10 q11-q12 in the same region as multiple endocrine neoplasia type 2A (MEN2A). Oncogene 1989;4:521.
18. Grieco M, Santoro M, Berlingieri MT, et al. PTC is a novel rearranged form of the ret proto-oncogene and is frequently detected in vivo in human thyroid papillary carcinomas. Cell 1990;60:557.
19. Pierotti MA, Santoro M, Jenkins RB, et al. Characterization of an inversion on the long arm of chromosome 10 juxtaposing D10S170 and RET and creating the oncogenic sequence RET/PTC. Proc Natl Acad Sci U S A 1992;89:1616.
20. Lairmore TC, Dou S, Howe JR, et al. A 1.5-megabase yeast artificial chromosome contig from human chromosome 10q11.2 connecting three genetic loci (RET, D10S94, and D10S102) closely linked to the MEN2A locus. Proc Natl Acad Sci U S A 1993;90:492.
21. Mulligan LM, Kwok JB, Healey CS, et al. Germ-line mutations of the RET proto-oncogene in multiple endocrine neoplasia type 2A. Nature 1993;363:458.
22. Donis-Keller H, Dou S, Chi D, et al. Mutations in the RET proto-oncogene are associated with MEN 2A and FMTC. Hum Mol Genet 1993;2:851.
23. Hofstra RM, Landsvater RM, Ceccherini I, et al. A mutation in the RET proto-oncogene associated with multiple endocrine neoplasia type 2B and sporadic medullary thyroid carcinoma. Nature 1994;367:375.
24. Eng C, Smith DP, Mulligan LM, et al. Point mutation within the tyrosine kinase domain of the RET proto-oncogene in multiple endocrine neoplasia type 2B and related sporadic tumours. Hum Mol Genet 1994;3:237.
25. Carlson KM, Dou S, Chi D, et al. Single missense mutation in the tyrosine kinase catalytic domain of the RET protooncogene is associated with multiple endocrine neoplasia type 2B. Proc Natl Acad Sci U S A 1994;91:1579.
26. Chi DD, Toshima K, Donis-Keller H, et al. Predictive testing for multiple endocrine neoplasia type 2A (MEN 2A) based on the detection of mutations in the RET protooncogene. Surgery 1994;116:124.
27. Wells SA Jr, Chi DD, Toshima K, et al. Predictive DNA testing and prophylactic thyroidectomy in patients at risk for multiple endocrine neoplasia type 2A. Ann Surg 1994;220:237.
28. Mulligan LM, Eng C, Healey CS, et al. Specific mutations of the RET proto-oncogene are related to disease phenotype in MEN 2A and FMTC. Nat Genet 1994;6:70.
29. Eng C, Clayton D, Schuffenecker I, et al. The relationship between specific RET proto-oncogene mutations and disease phenotype in multiple endocrine neoplasia type 2. International RET Mutation Consortium analysis. JAMA 1996;276:1575.

30. Skinner MA, DeBenedetti MK, Moley JF, et al. Medullary thyroid carcinoma in children with multiple endocrine neoplasia types 2A and 2B. J Pediatr Surg 1996;31:177.

31. Brandi ML, Gagel RF, Angeli A, et al. Guidelines for diagnosis and therapy of MEN type 1 and type 2. J Clin Endocrinol Metab 2001;86:5658.

32. Kloos RT, Eng C, Evans DB, et al. Medullary thyroid cancer: management guidelines of the American Thyroid Association. Thyroid 2009;19:565.

33. Calva D, O'Dorisio TM, Sue O'Dorisio M, et al. When is prophylactic thyroidectomy indicated for patients with the RET codon 609 mutation? Ann Surg Oncol 2009;16:2237.

34. Simon S, Pavel M, Hensen J, et al. Multiple endocrine neoplasia 2A syndrome: surgical management. J Pediatr Surg 2002;37:897.

35. Elisei R, Cosci B, Romei C, et al. Prognostic significance of somatic RET oncogene mutations in sporadic medullary thyroid cancer: a 10-year follow-up study. J Clin Endocrinol Metab 2008;93:682.

36. Agrawal N, Jiao Y, Sausen M, et al. Exomic sequencing of medullary thyroid cancer reveals dominant and mutually exclusive oncogenic mutations in RET and RAS. J Clin Endocrinol Metab 2013;98:E364.

37. Davies H, Bignell GR, Cox C, et al. Mutations of the BRAF gene in human cancer. Nature 2002;417:949.

38. Wan PT, Garnett MJ, Roe SM, et al. Mechanism of activation of the RAF-ERK signaling pathway by oncogenic mutations of B-RAF. Cell 2004;116:855.

39. Kimura ET, Nikiforova MN, Zhu Z, et al. High prevalence of BRAF mutations in thyroid cancer: genetic evidence for constitutive activation of the RET/PTC-RAS-BRAF signaling pathway in papillary thyroid carcinoma. Cancer Res 2003;63:1454.

40. Cohen Y, Xing M, Mambo E, et al. BRAF mutation in papillary thyroid carcinoma. J Natl Cancer Inst 2003;95:625.

41. Liu D, Hu S, Hou P, et al. Suppression of BRAF/MEK/MAP kinase pathway restores expression of iodide-metabolizing genes in thyroid cells expressing the V600E BRAF mutant. Clin Cancer Res 2007;13:1341.

42. Mitsutake N, Knauf JA, Mitsutake S, et al. Conditional BRAFV600E expression induces DNA synthesis, apoptosis, dedifferentiation, and chromosomal instability in thyroid PCCL3 cells. Cancer Res 2005;65:2465.

43. Poulikakos PI, Persaud Y, Janakiraman M, et al. RAF inhibitor resistance is mediated by dimerization of aberrantly spliced BRAF(V600E). Nature 2011; 480:387.

44. Bommarito A, Richiusa P, Carissimi E, et al. BRAFV600E mutation, TIMP-1 upregulation, and NF-kappaB activation: closing the loop on the papillary thyroid cancer trilogy. Endocr Relat Cancer 2011;18:669.

45. Lito P, Pratilas CA, Joseph EW, et al. Relief of profound feedback inhibition of mitogenic signaling by RAF inhibitors attenuates their activity in BRAFV600E melanomas. Cancer Cell 2012;22:668.

46. Kim J, Giuliano AE, Turner RR, et al. Lymphatic mapping establishes the role of BRAF gene mutation in papillary thyroid carcinoma. Ann Surg 2006;244:799.

47. Xing M, Clark D, Guan H, et al. BRAF mutation testing of thyroid fine-needle aspiration biopsy specimens for preoperative risk stratification in papillary thyroid cancer. J Clin Oncol 2009;27:2977.

48. Kim TY, Kim WB, Rhee YS, et al. The BRAF mutation is useful for prediction of clinical recurrence in low-risk patients with conventional papillary thyroid carcinoma. Clin Endocrinol (Oxf) 2006;65:364.

49. Prescott JD, Sadow PM, Hodin RA, et al. BRAF(V600E) status adds incremental value to current risk classification systems in predicting papillary thyroid carcinoma recurrence. Surgery 2012;152:984.

50. Niemeier LA, Kuffner Akatsu H, Song C, et al. A combined molecular-pathologic score improves risk stratification of thyroid papillary microcarcinoma. Cancer 2012;118:2069.

51. Rotstein L. The role of lymphadenectomy in the management of papillary carcinoma of the thyroid. J Surg Oncol 2009;99:186.

52. Dutenhefner SE, Marui S, Santos AB, et al. Braf, a tool in the decision to perform elective neck dissection? Thyroid 2012. [Epub ahead of print].

53. Joo JY, Park JY, Yoon YH, et al. Prediction of occult central lymph node metastasis in papillary thyroid carcinoma by preoperative BRAF analysis using fine-needle aspiration biopsy: a prospective study. J Clin Endocrinol Metab 2012;97:3996.

54. Adjei AA, Cohen RB, Franklin W, et al. Phase I pharmacokinetic and pharmacodynamic study of the oral, small-molecule mitogen-activated protein kinase kinase 1/2 inhibitor AZD6244 (ARRY-142886) in patients with advanced cancers. J Clin Oncol 2008;26:2139.

55. Flaherty KT, Robert C, Hersey P, et al. Improved survival with MEK inhibition in BRAF-mutated melanoma. N Engl J Med 2012;367:107.

56. Ho AL, Grewal RK, Leboeuf R, et al. Selumetinib-enhanced radioiodine uptake in advanced thyroid cancer. N Engl J Med 2013;368:623.

57. Henderson YC, Ahn SH, Kang Y, et al. Sorafenib potently inhibits papillary thyroid carcinomas harboring RET/PTC1 rearrangement. Clin Cancer Res 2008;14:4908.

58. Savvides P, Nagaiah G, Lavertu PN, et al. Phase II trial of sorafenib in patients with advanced anaplastic carcinoma of the thyroid. Thyroid 2013;23(5):600–4.

59. Shoffski P, Elisei R, Muller S, et al. An international, double-blind, randomized, placebo-controlled phase III trial (EXAM) of cabozantinib (XL184) in medullary thyroid carcinoma (MTC) patients (pts) with documented RECIST progression at baseline. J Clin Oncol 2012;30 [abstract].

60. Nucera C, Nehs MA, Nagarkatti SS, et al. Targeting BRAFV600E with PLX4720 displays potent antimigratory and anti-invasive activity in preclinical models of human thyroid cancer. Oncologist 2011;16:296.

61. Nehs MA, Nagarkatti S, Nucera C, et al. Thyroidectomy with neoadjuvant PLX4720 extends survival and decreases tumor burden in an orthotopic mouse model of anaplastic thyroid cancer. Surgery 2010;148:1154.

62. Nehs MA, Nucera C, Nagarkatti SS, et al. Late intervention with anti-BRAF(V600E) therapy induces tumor regression in an orthotopic mouse model of human anaplastic thyroid cancer. Endocrinology 2012;153:985.

63. Rosove MH, Peddi PF, Glaspy JA. BRAF V600E inhibition in anaplastic thyroid cancer. N Engl J Med 2013;368:684.

64. Wells SA Jr, Robinson BG, Gagel RF, et al. Vandetanib in patients with locally advanced or metastatic medullary thyroid cancer: a randomized, double-blind phase III trial. J Clin Oncol 2012;30:134.

65. Nikiforov YE, Yip L, Nikiforova MN. New strategies in diagnosing cancer in thyroid nodules: impact of molecular markers. Clin Cancer Res 2013;19(9):2283–8.

66. McCoy KL, Carty SE, Armstrong MJ, et al. Intraoperative pathologic examination in the era of molecular testing for differentiated thyroid cancer. J Am Coll Surg 2012;215:546.

67. Kroll TG, Sarraf P, Pecciarini L, et al. PAX8-PPARgamma1 fusion oncogene in human thyroid carcinoma [corrected]. Science 2000;289:1357.

68. Lodewijk L, Prins AM, Kist JW, et al. The value of miRNA in diagnosing thyroid cancer: a systematic review. Cancer Biomark 2012;11:229.

69. Alexander EK, Kennedy GC, Baloch ZW, et al. Preoperative diagnosis of benign thyroid nodules with indeterminate cytology. N Engl J Med 2012;367:705.

70. Duick DS, Klopper JP, Diggans JC, et al. The impact of benign gene expression classifier test results on the endocrinologist-patient decision to operate on patients with thyroid nodules with indeterminate fine-needle aspiration cytopathology. Thyroid 2012;22:996.

71. Li H, Robinson KA, Anton B, et al. Cost-effectiveness of a novel molecular test for cytologically indeterminate thyroid nodules. J Clin Endocrinol Metab 2011;96:E1719.

72. McShane LA, Conley BA, Cavenagh MM, et al. Criteria for use of omics-based predictors in NCI-sponsored clinical trials. J Clin Oncol 2012;30 [abstract 58].

73. Nikiforov YE, Ohori NP, Hodak SP, et al. Impact of mutational testing on the diagnosis and management of patients with cytologically indeterminate thyroid nodules: a prospective analysis of 1056 FNA samples. J Clin Endocrinol Metab 2011;96:3390.

74. Carpten JD, Robbins CM, Villablanca A, et al. HRPT2, encoding parafibromin, is mutated in hyperparathyroidism-jaw tumor syndrome. Nat Genet 2002;32:676.

75. Shattuck TM, Valimaki S, Obara T, et al. Somatic and germ-line mutations of the HRPT2 gene in sporadic parathyroid carcinoma. N Engl J Med 2003;349:1722.

76. Alvelos MI, Mendes M, Soares P. Molecular alterations in sporadic primary hyperparathyroidism. Genet Res Int 2011;2011:275802.

77. Mosimann C, Hausmann G, Basler K. Parafibromin/Hyrax activates Wnt/Wg target gene transcription by direct association with beta-catenin/Armadillo. Cell 2006;125:327.

78. Tan MH, Morrison C, Wang P, et al. Loss of parafibromin immunoreactivity is a distinguishing feature of parathyroid carcinoma. Clin Cancer Res 2004;10:6629.

79. Juhlin CC, Hoog A. Parafibromin as a diagnostic instrument for parathyroid carcinoma—Lone Ranger or part of the posse? Int J Endocrinol 2010;2010:324964.

80. Howe JR, Norton JA, Wells SA Jr. Prevalence of pheochromocytoma and hyperparathyroidism in multiple endocrine neoplasia type 2A: results of long-term follow-up. Surgery 1993;114:1070.

81. Frank-Raue K, Rybicki LA, Erlic Z, et al. Risk profiles and penetrance estimations in multiple endocrine neoplasia type 2A caused by germline RET mutations located in exon 10. Hum Mutat 2011;32:51.

82. Larsson C, Skogseid B, Oberg K, et al. Multiple endocrine neoplasia type 1 gene maps to chromosome 11 and is lost in insulinoma. Nature 1988;332:85.

83. Chandrasekharappa SC, Guru SC, Manickam P, et al. Positional cloning of the gene for multiple endocrine neoplasia-type 1. Science 1997;276:404.

84. Lemmens I, Van de Ven WJ, Kas K, et al. Identification of the multiple endocrine neoplasia type 1 (MEN1) gene. The European Consortium on MEN1. Hum Mol Genet 1997;6:1177.

85. Oberg K. The genetics of neuroendocrine tumors. Semin Oncol 2013;40:37.

86. Lemos MC, Thakker RV. Multiple endocrine neoplasia type 1 (MEN1): analysis of 1336 mutations reported in the first decade following identification of the gene. Hum Mutat 2008;29:22.

87. Jiao Y, Shi C, Edil BH, et al. DAXX/ATRX, MEN1, and mTOR pathway genes are frequently altered in pancreatic neuroendocrine tumors. Science 2011;331:1199.

88. Lairmore TC, Piersall LD, DeBenedetti MK, et al. Clinical genetic testing and early surgical intervention in patients with multiple endocrine neoplasia type 1 (MEN 1). Ann Surg 2004;239:637.

89. Akerstrom G, Stalberg P. Surgical management of MEN-1 and -2: state of the art. Surg Clin North Am 2009;89:1047.

90. Waldmann J, Lopez CL, Langer P, et al. Surgery for multiple endocrine neoplasia type 1-associated primary hyperparathyroidism. Br J Surg 2010; 97:1528.

91. Cromer MK, Starker LF, Choi M, et al. Identification of somatic mutations in parathyroid tumors using whole-exome sequencing. J Clin Endocrinol Metab 2012; 97:E1774.

92. Fishbein L, Nathanson KL. Pheochromocytoma and paraganglioma: understanding the complexities of the genetic background. Cancer Genet 2012; 205:1.

93. Barker D, Wright E, Nguyen K, et al. A genomic search for linkage of neurofibromatosis to RFLPs. J Med Genet 1987;24:536.

94. Seizinger BR, Rouleau GA, Ozelius LJ, et al. Genetic linkage of von Recklinghausen neurofibromatosis to the nerve growth factor receptor gene. Cell 1987;49:589.

95. Bausch B, Borozdin W, Mautner VF, et al. Germline NF1 mutational spectra and loss-of-heterozygosity analyses in patients with pheochromocytoma and neurofibromatosis type 1. J Clin Endocrinol Metab 2007;92:2784.

96. Welander J, Larsson C, Backdahl M, et al. Integrative genomics reveals frequent somatic NF1 mutations in sporadic pheochromocytomas. Hum Mol Genet 2012;21:5406.

97. Martin GA, Viskochil D, Bollag G, et al. The GAP-related domain of the neurofibromatosis type 1 gene product interacts with ras p21. Cell 1990; 63:843.

98. Johannessen CM, Reczek EE, James MF, et al. The NF1 tumor suppressor critically regulates TSC2 and mTOR. Proc Natl Acad Sci U S A 2005;102:8573.

99. Latif F, Tory K, Gnarra J, et al. Identification of the von Hippel-Lindau disease tumor suppressor gene. Science 1993;260:1317.

100. Curley SA, Lott ST, Luca JW, et al. Surgical decision-making affected by clinical and genetic screening of a novel kindred with von Hippel-Lindau disease and pancreatic islet cell tumors. Ann Surg 1998;227:229.

101. Maher ER, Neumann HP, Richard S. von Hippel-Lindau disease: a clinical and scientific review. Eur J Hum Genet 2011;19:617.

102. Ong KR, Woodward ER, Killick P, et al. Genotype-phenotype correlations in von Hippel-Lindau disease. Hum Mutat 2007;28:143.

103. Baysal BE, Ferrell RE, Willett-Brozick JE, et al. Mutations in SDHD, a mitochondrial complex II gene, in hereditary paraganglioma. Science 2000; 287:848.

104. Gimm O, Armanios M, Dziema H, et al. Somatic and occult germ-line mutations in SDHD, a mitochondrial complex II gene, in nonfamilial pheochromocytoma. Cancer Res 2000;60:6822.

105. Astuti D, Douglas F, Lennard TW, et al. Germline SDHD mutation in familial phaeochromocytoma. Lancet 2001;357:1181.

106. Hensen EF, Jordanova ES, van Minderhout IJ, et al. Somatic loss of maternal chromosome 11 causes parent-of-origin-dependent inheritance in SDHD-linked paraganglioma and phaeochromocytoma families. Oncogene 2004; 23:4076.

107. Burnichon N, Briere JJ, Libe R, et al. SDHA is a tumor suppressor gene causing paraganglioma. Hum Mol Genet 2010;19:3011.

108. Astuti D, Latif F, Dallol A, et al. Gene mutations in the succinate dehydrogenase subunit SDHB cause susceptibility to familial pheochromocytoma and to familial paraganglioma. Am J Hum Genet 2001;69:49.

109. Niemann S, Muller U. Mutations in SDHC cause autosomal dominant paraganglioma, type 3. Nat Genet 2000;26:268.

110. Hao HX, Khalimonchuk O, Schraders M, et al. SDH5, a gene required for flavination of succinate dehydrogenase, is mutated in paraganglioma. Science 2009;325:1139.

111. Bayley JP, Kunst HP, Cascon A, et al. SDHAF2 mutations in familial and sporadic paraganglioma and phaeochromocytoma. Lancet Oncol 2010;11:366.

112. Welander J, Soderkvist P, Gimm O. Genetics and clinical characteristics of hereditary pheochromocytomas and paragangliomas. Endocr Relat Cancer 2011; 18:R253.

113. Timmers HJ, Gimenez-Roqueplo AP, Mannelli M, et al. Clinical aspects of SDHx-related pheochromocytoma and paraganglioma. Endocr Relat Cancer 2009;16:391.

114. Amar L, Baudin E, Burnichon N, et al. Succinate dehydrogenase B gene mutations predict survival in patients with malignant pheochromocytomas or paragangliomas. J Clin Endocrinol Metab 2007;92:3822.

115. Qin Y, Yao L, King EE, et al. Germline mutations in TMEM127 confer susceptibility to pheochromocytoma. Nat Genet 2010;42:229.

116. Abermil N, Guillaud-Bataille M, Burnichon N, et al. TMEM127 screening in a large cohort of patients with pheochromocytoma and/or paraganglioma. J Clin Endocrinol Metab 2012;97:E805.

117. Comino-Mendez I, Gracia-Aznarez FJ, Schiavi F, et al. Exome sequencing identifies MAX mutations as a cause of hereditary pheochromocytoma. Nat Genet 2011;43:663.

118. Burnichon N, Cascon A, Schiavi F, et al. MAX mutations cause hereditary and sporadic pheochromocytoma and paraganglioma. Clin Cancer Res 2012;18:2828.

119. Burnichon N, Vescovo L, Amar L, et al. Integrative genomic analysis reveals somatic mutations in pheochromocytoma and paraganglioma. Hum Mol Genet 2011;20:3974.

120. Fassnacht M, Terzolo M, Allolio B, et al. Combination chemotherapy in advanced adrenocortical carcinoma. N Engl J Med 2012;366:2189.

121. Giordano TJ, Thomas DG, Kuick R, et al. Distinct transcriptional profiles of adrenocortical tumors uncovered by DNA microarray analysis. Am J Pathol 2003; 162:521.

122. Begemann M, Spengler S, Gogiel M, et al. Clinical significance of copy number variations in the 11p15.5 imprinting control regions: new cases and review of the literature. J Med Genet 2012;49:547.

123. Gicquel C, Bertagna X, Schneid H, et al. Rearrangements at the 11p15 locus and overexpression of insulin-like growth factor-II gene in sporadic adrenocortical tumors. J Clin Endocrinol Metab 1994;78:1444.

124. Kirschner LS. The next generation of therapies for adrenocortical cancers. Trends Endocrinol Metab 2012;23:343.

125. de Fraipont F, El Atifi M, Cherradi N, et al. Gene expression profiling of human adrenocortical tumors using complementary deoxyribonucleic acid microarrays identifies several candidate genes as markers of malignancy. J Clin Endocrinol Metab 2005;90:1819.

126. Kroiss M, Quinkler M, Johanssen S, et al. Sunitinib in refractory adrenocortical carcinoma: a phase II, single-arm, open-label trial. J Clin Endocrinol Metab 2012;97:3495.

127. Stommel JM, Kimmelman AC, Ying H, et al. Coactivation of receptor tyrosine kinases affects the response of tumor cells to targeted therapies. Science 2007;318:287.

128. Lin CI, Whang EE, Moalem J, et al. Strategic combination therapy overcomes tyrosine kinase coactivation in adrenocortical carcinoma. Surgery 2012;152: 1045.

129. Choi M, Scholl UI, Yue P, et al. K+ channel mutations in adrenal aldosterone-producing adenomas and hereditary hypertension. Science 2011;331:768.

130. Beuschlein F, Boulkroun S, Osswald A, et al. Somatic mutations in ATP1A1 and ATP2B3 lead to aldosterone-producing adenomas and secondary hypertension. Nat Genet 2013;45(4):440–4.

131. Boulkroun S, Beuschlein F, Rossi GP, et al. Prevalence, clinical, and molecular correlates of KCNJ5 mutations in primary aldosteronism. Hypertension 2012; 59:592.

132. Yao JC, Hassan M, Phan A, et al. One hundred years after "carcinoid": epidemiology of and prognostic factors for neuroendocrine tumors in 35,825 cases in the United States. J Clin Oncol 2008;26:3063.

133. Triponez F, Dosseh D, Goudet P, et al. Epidemiology data on 108 MEN 1 patients from the GTE with isolated nonfunctioning tumors of the pancreas. Ann Surg 2006;243:265.

134. Lowney JK, Frisella MM, Lairmore TC, et al. Pancreatic islet cell tumor metastasis in multiple endocrine neoplasia type 1: correlation with primary tumor size. Surgery 1998;124:1043.

135. Korse CM, Taal BG, van Velthuysen ML, et al. Incidence and survival of neuroendocrine tumours in the Netherlands according to histological grade: Experience of two decades of cancer registry. Eur J Cancer 2013;49(8):1975–83.

136. Mayo SC, de Jong MC, Pulitano C, et al. Surgical management of hepatic neuroendocrine tumor metastasis: results from an international multi-institutional analysis. Ann Surg Oncol 2010;17:3129.

137. Long RG, Barnes AJ, Adrian TE, et al. Suppression of pancreatic endocrine tumour secretion by long-acting somatostatin analogue. Lancet 1979;2:764.

138. O'Toole D, Saveanu A, Couvelard A, et al. The analysis of quantitative expression of somatostatin and dopamine receptors in gastro-entero-pancreatic tumours opens new therapeutic strategies. Eur J Endocrinol 2006;155:849.

139. Sherman SK, Carr JC, Wang D, et al. Gastric inhibitory polypeptide receptor is a promising target for imaging and therapy in neuroendocrine tumors. Surgery, in press.

140. Yamada Y, Post SR, Wang K, et al. Cloning and functional characterization of a family of human and mouse somatostatin receptors expressed in brain, gastrointestinal tract, and kidney. Proc Natl Acad Sci U S A 1992;89:251.

141. Kaemmerer D, Peter L, Lupp A, et al. Molecular imaging with (6)(8)Ga-SSTR PET/CT and correlation to immunohistochemistry of somatostatin receptors in neuroendocrine tumours. Eur J Nucl Med Mol Imaging 2011;38:1659.

142. Cervia D, Bagnoli P. An update on somatostatin receptor signaling in native systems and new insights on their pathophysiology. Pharmacol Ther 2007;116:322.

143. Ludvigsen E, Stridsberg M, Taylor JE, et al. Subtype selective interactions of somatostatin and somatostatin analogs with sst1, sst2, and sst5 in BON-1 cells. Med Oncol 2004;21:285.

144. Oberg K, Knigge U, Kwekkeboom D, et al. Neuroendocrine gastro-entero-pancreatic tumors: ESMO Clinical Practice Guidelines for diagnosis, treatment and follow-up. Ann Oncol 2012;23(Suppl 7):vii124.
145. Rinke A, Muller HH, Schade-Brittinger C, et al. Placebo-controlled, double-blind, prospective, randomized study on the effect of octreotide LAR in the control of tumor growth in patients with metastatic neuroendocrine midgut tumors: a report from the PROMID Study Group. J Clin Oncol 2009;27:4656.
146. Kwekkeboom DJ, Kam BL, van Essen M, et al. Somatostatin-receptor-based imaging and therapy of gastroenteropancreatic neuroendocrine tumors. Endocr Relat Cancer 2010;17:R53.
147. Gabriel M, Decristoforo C, Kendler D, et al. 68Ga-DOTA-Tyr3-octreotide PET in neuroendocrine tumors: comparison with somatostatin receptor scintigraphy and CT. J Nucl Med 2007;48:508.
148. Dahdaleh FS, Lorenzen A, Rajput M, et al. The value of preoperative imaging in small bowel neuroendocrine tumors. Ann Surg Oncol 2013;20(6):1912–7.
149. Zaknun JJ, Bodei L, Mueller-Brand J, et al. The joint IAEA, EANM, and SNMMI practical guidance on peptide receptor radionuclide therapy (PRRNT) in neuroendocrine tumours. Eur J Nucl Med Mol Imaging 2013;40(5):800–16.
150. Kwekkeboom DJ, de Herder WW, Kam BL, et al. Treatment with the radiolabeled somatostatin analog [177 Lu-DOTA 0, Tyr3]octreotate: toxicity, efficacy, and survival. J Clin Oncol 2008;26:2124.
151. Lacroix A, Bolte E, Tremblay J, et al. Gastric inhibitory polypeptide-dependent cortisol hypersecretion—a new cause of Cushing's syndrome. N Engl J Med 1992;327:974.
152. de Wilde RF, Edil BH, Hruban RH, et al. Well-differentiated pancreatic neuroendocrine tumors: from genetics to therapy. Nat Rev Gastroenterol Hepatol 2012;9:199.
153. Missiaglia E, Dalai I, Barbi S, et al. Pancreatic endocrine tumors: expression profiling evidences a role for AKT-mTOR pathway. J Clin Oncol 2010;28:245.
154. Heaphy CM, de Wilde RF, Jiao Y, et al. Altered telomeres in tumors with ATRX and DAXX mutations. Science 2011;333:425.
155. Henson JD, Neumann AA, Yeager TR, et al. Alternative lengthening of telomeres in mammalian cells. Oncogene 2002;21:598.
156. Yao JC, Shah MH, Ito T, et al. Everolimus for advanced pancreatic neuroendocrine tumors. N Engl J Med 2011;364:514.
157. Raymond E, Dahan L, Raoul JL, et al. Sunitinib malate for the treatment of pancreatic neuroendocrine tumors. N Engl J Med 2011;364:501.
158. Iihara M, Yamashita T, Okamoto T, et al. A nationwide clinical survey of patients with multiple endocrine neoplasia type 2 and familial medullary thyroid carcinoma in Japan. Jpn J Clin Oncol 1997;27:128.
159. Machens A, Brauckhoff M, Holzhausen HJ, et al. Codon-specific development of pheochromocytoma in multiple endocrine neoplasia type 2. J Clin Endocrinol Metab 2005;90:3999.
160. Yip L, Cote GJ, Shapiro SE, et al. Multiple endocrine neoplasia type 2: evaluation of the genotype-phenotype relationship. Arch Surg 2003;138:409.
161. Jensen RT, Berna MJ, Bingham DB, et al. Inherited pancreatic endocrine tumor syndromes: advances in molecular pathogenesis, diagnosis, management, and controversies. Cancer 2008;113:1807.
162. Maiese K, Chong ZZ, Shang YC, et al. mTOR: on target for novel therapeutic strategies in the nervous system. Trends Mol Med 2013;19:51.

Getting From the Bench to the Patient: Biotechnology Strategies

Hagop Youssoufian, MD, Jonathan Lewis, MD, PhD*

KEYWORDS

- Biotechnology • Translational research • Immunotherapy • Synthetic biology
- Palifosfamide

KEY POINTS

- Translational research in biotech is predicated on cross-functional disciplines poised for identifying druggable targets and advancing the most promising ones through a gauntlet of scientific and regulatory hurdles.
- Synthetic biology uses synthetic DNA to express both exon-coded and intron-coded protein sequences to design, test, and build DNA-based therapeutics involving an engineering philosophy.
- Translational medicine holds the promise of accelerating the development of meaningful therapeutic drugs to address unmet medical needs. It starts with a practical question around a clinical issue rather than a fundamental biologic question, a "how" rather than a "why."

THE BENCH-TO-BEDSIDE PROCESS
A New Era of Cancer Drug Development—Breaking Down the Walls: Academic, Government, and Industry Partnership

Translational medicine holds the promise of accelerating the development of meaningful therapeutic drugs to address unmet medical needs. It starts with a practical question around a clinical issue rather than a fundamental biologic question, a "how" rather than a "why." The ultimate translational outcome may well be a new drug, but it can also be a combination of drugs, a device, a biomarker, or myriad other outcomes. Although the initial idea is often based on an unmet clinical need, the tools of basic research, including omics (eg, genomics or proteomics) and mechanistic

Disclosures: Hagop Youssoufian is a former employee of ZIOPHARM Oncology, Inc (former President of Research and Development), and Jonathan Lewis is an employee of ZIOPHARM Oncology, Inc (Chief Executive Officer), and both are shareholders of the company. The opinions expressed in this publication are solely those of the authors and do not necessarily reflect the opinions of ZIOPHARM Oncology, Inc.
One First Avenue, Parris Building 34, Navy Yard Plaza, Boston, MA 02129, USA
* Corresponding author.
E-mail address: JLewis@ziopharm.com

experiments, serve to initiate validation of the idea in cell-based and pilot animal studies (T0) (**Figs. 1** and **2**).[1,2] Ideas that show promise for further development are then evaluated in T1 evaluation with in vivo proof-of-concept studies followed by first in human (FIH) and small phase 1 clinical studies to evaluate safety.[2,3] Successful T1 leads to an expanded phase of clinical trials to investigate the efficacy in the given indication (T2). Often mechanism of action and surrogate biomarkers are also co-investigated and developed at this stage. Transition of this stage to a larger clinical evaluation permits large-scale evaluation of safety and efficacy (T3) (see **Fig. 2**).[4] T4 steps of translational medicine involve transition to clinical practice and impact on large patient populations.[3] This process is often iterative and learning from the clinical use of a drug informs the development of the next generation of novel and improved therapeutics (see **Fig. 2**).[1,3,5]

The Biotech Advantage

Translational research and drug development is a long and risky process (see **Fig. 2**). The advantage of having a major drug, however, that can benefit patients drives investments from government and the private sector. On average, the drug discovery process has taken approximately 15 years[6] and costs at least $1 billion for each new drug approved.[6,7] This process cannot be done in silos and requires an integrated and seamless collaboration between academia, industry, and governmental agencies (see **Fig. 2**; **Fig. 3**).[1,2]

In the United States, academic institutions with funding from the National Institutes of Health (NIH) play a major role in the initial identification and characterization of basic early-stage T0 discoveries. Many promising basic discoveries, however, do not progress in the therapeutic development pipeline in academia because of the gap between early-stage bench research and implementation into clinical practice. This gap has been termed, *the valley of death* (see **Fig. 2**).[8]

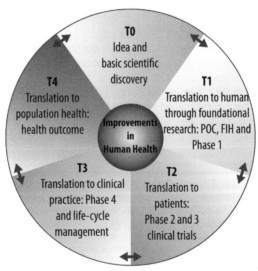

Fig. 1. Translational medicine is a long, iterative process that starts with a promising idea based on unmet clinical need and leads to benefits to improvements in human health. The clinical trial process is rigorous, and the ultimate goal is translation to population health. POC, proof of concept.

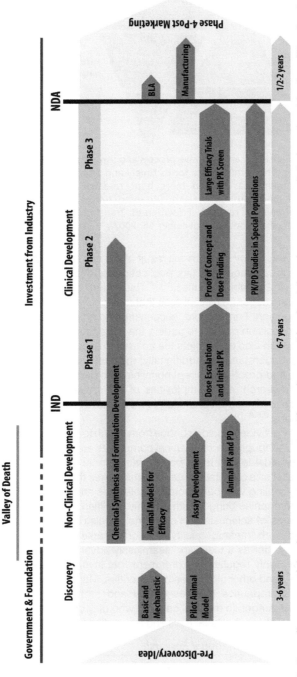

Fig. 2. Drug discovery and development process starts with prediscovery idea that is based on an unmet clinical need and leads to filing for the clinical application of compound. Translational medicine holds the promise of accelerating the development of meaningful therapeutic drugs to address unmet medical needs. It starts with a practical question around a clinical issue rather than a fundamental biologic question, a "how" rather than a "why." Collaboration between government, academia, and industry is key to success. BLA, Biologic License Application; NDA, New Drug Application.

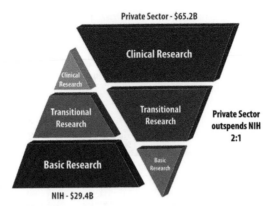

Fig. 3. Translational medicine is an expensive process and requires a partnership among academic, government and biotech/industry for its timely and effective execution. Traditionally, the NIH (government) has funded more basic research, and the private sector (industry) has funded more clinical research. (*Adapted from* Zerhouni E. Transforming health: NIH and the promise of research. Presented at: Transforming Health: Fulfilling the Promise of Research; Washington, DC, November 16, 2007.)

In many instances, this valley of death is a result of the traditional academic culture, with priorities of individual recognition (eg, publications and funding) and institutional net income through reimbursable activities.[2,9,10] This culture promotes the creation of basic research silos and separate clinical silos that may not be compatible with teamwork and team recognition. Furthermore, successful and efficient drug development requires robust early decision making regarding the therapeutic potential of developmental candidates, which also contradicts the academic need for basic research and depth in mechanistic understanding. Additionally, the costs associated with lead discovery, optimization, and proof-of-concept nonclinical studies; restraints in NIH funding for translational research; and complexities of the regulatory path required for maintaining patient safety limit the translation of many discoveries to clinical practice at academic institutions.[2,5,8–10]

The biotech industry provides a golden bridge from bench to bedside by providing the power of teamwork.[1] Although pharmaceutical companies are also highly adept practitioners of bench-to-bedside and team-based translational research, it is generally believed that the smaller size of biotech organizations makes them more nimble, faster, and more efficient in dealing with bureaucratic challenges and rapidly changing environments. Biotech companies bring together highly qualified, intensely goal-oriented and collaborative teams of scientists and clinicians, regulatory staff, biostatisticians, data managers, research nurses, quality support, marketing, and management personnel to work together as a team and seamlessly advance a drug development candidate through a highly regulated environment that involves the Food and Drug Administration (FDA)[11] and other global health authorities. Moreover, successful translation of promising therapeutics requires critical and strategic partnerships with physician-scientists at academic medical centers, who play critical roles in executing the FIH and phase 1 to phase 3 clinical trials and interacting with human subjects.[2]

Legislations that Enhance Translational Research

In 1971, President Nixon declared the war on cancer and signed the National Cancer Act. Since then, there has been a significant increase in research to improve the understanding of cancer biology and the development of more efficacious therapies.

This has resulted in considerable progress in translational research and in the treatment of certain cancer types, earliest and most significantly in childhood leukemia and testicular cancer.[12] Cancer remains, however, a major cause of death.[13] Several legislation statutes passed in the past 4 decades have addressed some of the limitations that are perceived to slow progress on the limited translation of promising drugs to clinical practice. For instance, due to widespread frustrations that discoveries made in academia were not being translated, the Bayh-Dole Act was put in place in 1980.[14] This act obligates the academic institutions (that receive federal/NIH funding) to partner with industry to translate innovative ideas. Additionally, to encourage biotechnology and pharmaceutical companies to develop drugs for the treatment of rare diseases, the Orphan Drug Act of January 1983 was put in place.[15,16] Moreover, in 1992, the Accelerated Approval Regulations were put in place to increase the speed of approval for novel or improved drugs that are intended to treat serious or life-threatening diseases.[17] More recently, in 2004, the Critical Path Initiative started to improve the drug and device development processes and to enhance the quality of data generated during the translational research.[18,19] As a consequence of all these measures, together with scientific and clinical advances, there was a record high of 39 new molecular entities approved by the FDA in 2012.[11]

Investment in Translational Research in Biotech

Biotech is one of the only industries that can create potential value in the absence of immediate revenue generation. Investors, who are major stakeholders in biotechnology companies, are investing initially in ideas, human capital, proved and novel approaches, and innovative strategies for drug development. Investors ascribe value based on net present value. Biotech companies bring together the following pillars that are critical to the success of translational research.

Idea

Translational research typically starts with a patient-centered idea that could provide a solution to an unmet medical need. The scientific discoveries and innovations at the *in silico*, molecular, cellular, and in vivo levels that are made based on this idea can result in effective solutions when they are put into practice. Biotech companies often bring together internal scientists and external clinical key opinion leaders to evaluate and bring forward the most promising ideas for translation.

Human subjects

Human subjects are the heroes in translational research and are essential in making the transition to clinical practice possible by agreeing to participate in an experimental clinical study. They participate in all phases of drug development—from phase 1 to phase 3 and beyond. Generally phase 1 and phase 2 studies are considered within the domain of translational research. Although FIH studies in other areas of medicine are often performed in healthy volunteers, most anticancer drugs are initially tested in patients with cancers who have often failed earlier stages of therapy. In this way, in addition to pharmacodynamics (PD) and pharmacokinetic (PK) studies, investigators have an opportunity to assess early signals of clinical activity in patients and begin to make biologic, PK, and clinical correlations as soon as possible. Nevertheless, the key endpoint of FIH studies remains an assessment of the safety profile of the experimental drug and the establishment of the maximally tolerated dose that should be used in future studies. Patients willingly provide their consent to serve as test subjects for drugs with unknown side effects. In addition to accepting this risk, these patients understand that they may not be (and often are not) the direct beneficiaries of any resulting discoveries, therapeutic or financial. Their motivation is by and large altruistic. Without their active participation, the opportunities for innovation and clinical breakthroughs would come to a standstill.

Study principal investigators

The studies' principal investigators (PIs) are often physician-scientists at academic medical centers who do not have any financial or personal conflicts of interest with the biotech company. PIs are personally responsible for conducting or supervising the conduct of the clinical research in human subjects and for protecting the rights, safety, and welfare of the subjects enrolled in the research. The PIs ensure that all in-human research is conducted in an ethical manner and in accordance with all federal, state, and local laws and regulations as well as institutional policies and that the subjects are fully informed of the research study and have clearly understood and then signed informed consent to participate in the study.

Nonclinical team

The main objectives of nonclinical studies for a candidate product are to identify and validate molecular targets for further clinical development, to understand the mechanism of action, and to determine the effect of the product on the body. This team performs cell-based and in vivo animal studies to determine what the most promising ideas for translation are. They also play an important role in understanding and defining nonclinical pharmacology-toxicology for both translation into the clinic and regulatory requirements. In addition, the members of this team carry out PD, PK, and pharmacology for absorption, distribution, metabolism, and excretion. Additionally, the nonclinical team performs studies to determine the mechanisms of action as well as the initial dose, schedule, and future dose increments that will be tested in humans. Potential dose-limiting and end-organ toxicities are identified and called to the attention of clinical investigators. PK studies in animal models that harbor tumors can yield valuable correlations between drug exposure (including the steady-state trough levels in the circulation and the area under the curve of the active drug) and safety or efficacy. These parameters can be readily monitored in subsequent FIH trials. Thus, the key goals of the nonclinical team are to delineate key toxicities in experimental models and anticipate and minimize harm to study subjects and to facilitate a more rational translational research plan.

Clinical operations and medical affairs

Clinical operations and medical affairs in many biotech and pharmaceutical companies are in charge of formulating the clinical development strategy for investigational drugs. Once an investigational drug has proved safe and efficacious in animal models and basic PK and PD parameters are established, it is necessary to translate these observations into the clinic. A medical team then engages in the designs of FIH and phase 1 clinical studies to identify a safe dose, the PK and PD of the investigational product, and the toxicity profile of the drug. Later stages of development involve the design of phase 2 and phase 3 clinical studies to identify initial signals of efficacy. The ultimate goal of this program is to obtain approval from the regulatory authorities to market the drug for the indication of choice. Depending on the disease targeted, these studies may involve comparison with drugs that have already been approved and constitute standard of care or with an inactive placebo.

Clinical operations

The clinical operations team is responsible for the successful execution of sponsored clinical studies in support of a regulatory filing (eg, NDA or Biologic License

Application). The clinical team plays a key role in the design of study protocols, including, but not limited to, input on the schedule of assessments, determination of the number of sites necessary to support enrollment, and advice on which countries to include. They are in charge of making certain that study staff members are appropriately qualified and trained to execute the study protocol. The clinical team ensures that protocol-defined tests and samples are acquired correctly and at appropriate time points as well as that study data are accurate and consistent with the sites' source documentation. Ultimately, clinical operations is accountable for (1) the quality of the study data, (2) overseeing the timely execution of study milestones, and (3) the management of the study budgets.

Chemistry, manufacturing, and control
The chemistry, manufacturing, and control (CMC) team is responsible for everything related to producing, analyzing, packaging, and delivering drugs for use in the clinical setting. The team evaluates physical and chemical properties of the drug to develop, optimize, and determine the proper scale for the manufacturing process. Whether it is a small or large molecule, the CMC team completes process development, chemical synthesis, and/or upstream processing for drug substance (eg, active pharmaceutical ingredient) manufacturing; formulation evaluation, dosage form development, and downstream purification are completed for drug product (eg, finished dosage form) manufacturing. The CMC team is also responsible for the development, qualification, and validation of all analytical methods used for process control or to analyze the drug for physical characteristics, potency, and purity at the time of release or during stability studies to establish retest/shelf-life dating.

Regulatory affairs
The regulatory function is absolutely vital in enabling the approval of safe and effective therapeutics so that they can become available worldwide. Regulatory affairs ensure regulatory compliance and prepare submissions and applications to agencies, such as the FDA, the European Medical Association, and other governmental agencies that oversee drug development (**Box 1**). These agencies are more likely to approve new molecular entities if (1) an unmet medical need is being addressed; (2) strong data for evidence of efficacy are demonstrated statistically and clinically; (3) safety concerns are minimal and the benefits to subjects outweigh the risks; (4) current good clinical practices and current good manufacturing practices are followed; and (5) medical key opinion leaders support the approval of the new drug. These approvals come after heavy investment in preclinical development and clinical trials as well as a commitment to ongoing safety monitoring. Ultimately, it is all about the data, which must be assembled in a highly rigorous and regulated manner.

Program management
Project managers often confront an overwhelming degree of complexity in extended, multifaceted projects, such as translational research and drug development. Program management leads cross-functional teams in all areas of drug development to advance therapies from early-stage development through commercial launch and life cycle management. Program managers lead without authority and manage through influence. They help to set metrics to ensure team responsibilities and that deadlines are met. They provide background information and context for issues and decisions. They collaborate with finance and line functions on budget activities as well as providing program visibility/transparency to senior management. In addition, they serve as a conduit for partnership communication and execution.

> **Box 1**
> **In the United States, the following regulatory steps form the pathway for obtaining approval from the FDA**
>
> - IND: Based on nonclinical studies, a product is identified as a viable candidate for further development, and then the sponsor initiates the appropriate studies to establish that the product will not expose humans to unreasonable risks. The IND allows the sponsor to ship the study drug to clinical investigators at many sites.
>
> - New Drug Application (NDA): NDA is the application for drug sponsors to formally apply to the FDA for approval of a new pharmaceutical for treatment of patients and sale and marketing in the United States. The data gathered during animal studies and human clinical trials under an IND become part of the NDA. The objectives of the NDA are to ensure that the drug is safe and efficacious for its intended use, its benefits outweigh its risk, the package insert labeling is appropriate, and the methods used for manufacturing maintain the drug's identity, strength, quality, and purity.
>
> - Biologic License Application: The Public Health Service Act requires the manufacturers of a biologic for sale to hold a license for that product. A Biologic License Application is submitted to the FDA and contains specific information on the chemistry, pharmacology (nonclinical and clinical), and manufacturing processes as well as the medical effects of the product. If the FDA requirements are met, the application is approved and a license is issued allowing marketing of the product.

DRUG DISCOVERY PROCESS AT ZIOPHARM ONCOLOGY
Translational Medicine in Practice

ZIOPHARM Oncology is a biotech company focused on the discovery and development of new cancer therapies in areas of unmet medical need. The authors team applies new knowledge and understanding in the molecular and cell biology of cancer to high unmet patient needs. The definitive goal is to develop safer, more precise therapeutics to ultimately improve care and quality of life for patients.

There are 2 examples of translational medicine that the authors are engaged in that are highlighted. First, palifosfamide (ZIO-201, isophosphoramide mustard [IPM]) is a small molecule in late-stage development, now in two phase 3 trials. Second, through a channel partnership with Intrexon Corporation, the authors are developing DNA therapeutics using synthetic biology. The translational bridge to the clinic for each of these strategies is reviewed.

Optimizing the Safety and Efficacy of a Highly Active DNA Cross-linking Small Molecule

Palifosfamide is a potent, bifunctional DNA alkylating agent with activity in multiple tumors.[20–22] Brock originally synthesized IPM.[23] This was followed by murine studies that determined its safety and showed that its efficacy was comparable to or better than ifosfamide.[23–26] Struck and his team at the Southern Research Institute in Birmingham, Alabama, did extensive work determining the 7-atom cross-linking mechanism and optimizing the preclinical performance of a nonformulated IPM. Preclinical studies of the activity of ZIO-201 and 2 halogenated analogs, ZIO-202 and ZIO-203, were critically evaluated in multiple xenograft models.[27] Struck and colleagues[27] demonstrated that ZIO-201 is active against cisplatin-resistant leukemia cells. ZIO-201 and cisplatin had similar activity in leukemia cells (P388) sensitive to cisplatin but ZIO-201 had an approximately 8-log cell kill greater antileukemia activity against cisplatin-resistant cells. The data also show that anticancer activities of ZIO-201, ZIO-202, and ZIO-203 are similar in human pancreas and prostate cancer xenografts and that many schedules were active. ZIO-201 was the most active, with the widest therapeutic window. It has also shown wide activity in multiple solid tumors (epithelial and sarcoma), lymphomas, and leukemias.[21,28]

Despite an intensive academic research program, however, optimization and stabilization of palifosfamide and its translation to the clinic did not begin until 2005 when ZIOPHARM worked with DEKK-TEK (a spin-off from Louisiana State University). The authors optimized the formulation of IPM as a stable tris salt system, and conducted several nonclinical and clinical studies. IPM is the stabilized active metabolite of ifosfamide and is in the same class as bendamustine, cyclophosphamide, and ifosfamide.[28] IPM evades typical resistance pathways[29] and is also active in aldehyde dehydrogenase–high cells,[21] which represent the resistant population of cancer stem cells. Unlike ifosfamide, IPM is not dependent on the cytochrome P450 system and aldehyde dehydrogenase for its activation, thereby having a consistent and predictable PK/PD relationship and lacking production of the toxic metabolites of acrolein and chloroacetalhehyde (**Fig. 4**) that have been associated with hemorrhagic cystitis and neurotoxicity.[29–32] More importantly, the plasma exposure at the biologically effective dose of IPM (150 mg/m^2 per dose or 450 mg/m^2 per cycle) corresponds to a higher concentration of active drug compared with the efficacious ifosfamide plasma exposure dose (4–8 g/m^2 per dose or 16–32 g/m^2 per cycle).[33–35]

Encouraging results in in vitro pharmacology, in vivo antitumor studies, and early-phase 1 clinical studies in patients with advanced cancers as well as an acceptable safety profile and therapeutic index provided the rationale and the basis for initiating clinical efficacy studies.[36] A randomized, open-label, multicenter phase 2 study (PICASSO) was conducted in patients with metastatic soft tissue sarcoma, a therapeutic area of significant unmet medical need. The primary objective of the PICASSO

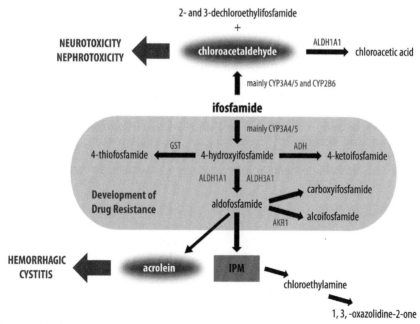

Fig. 4. Palifsofamide (IPM) is an active metabolite of ifosfamide that is independent of cytochrome P450 system and aldehyde dehydrogenase (ALDH) for its activation and evades the typical drug-resistance pathways.

study was to determine the safety and efficacy of IPM in combination with doxorubicin versus doxorubicin alone in a randomization schema. The study demonstrated that the IPM combination with doxorubicin was favorable over doxorubicin alone with a 3.4-month difference in median progression-free survival (95% CI, 0.191, 0.951) and a hazard ratio of 0.43. These data are consistent with an active drug in soft tissue sarcoma (**Fig. 5**).[37,38] The encouraging results observed in this study led to the initiation of PICASSO 3, a phase 3, multicenter, international, randomized, double-blind, placebo-controlled study of doxorubicin plus palifosfamide-tris versus doxorubicin plus placebo in subjects with first-line metastatic soft tissue sarcoma. This study is ongoing. The primary objective of the study is to evaluate the efficacy of the combination regimen, assessed by progression-free survival, overall survival, and quality of life as well as the safety and tolerability of the combination regimen. An additional ongoing phase 3, multinational, multicenter, randomized, controlled, open-label, adaptive study (MATISSE) is evaluating palifosfamide plus carboplatin and etoposide to determine the efficacy of this combination chemotherapy compared with carboplatin and etoposide alone in chemotherapy-naïve subjects with extensive-stage small cell lung cancer.

A recent analysis of PICASSO 3 revealed that the study did not meet its primary endpoint. Whatever the reason for this outcome, and true to the tenets of translational research, the future direction of palifosfamide may involve the fundamental understanding of kinetics, dose, and schedule together with progress in promising clinical proof-of-concept trials that can ultimately result in the effective translation of this molecule from the bench to the bedside for cancer patients.

Bringing Synthetic Biology into Clinical Practice

The announcement of the completion of the human genome project on April 14, 2003,[39] along with advancements in cancer biology and mechanistic understanding of the disease process and computer-based modeling and design principles as well as advances in genome synthesis technology, has created a new era for synthetic biology and disruptive gene therapy strategies that can revolutionize the entire drug discovery process.[40–43] These strategies are cost effective and time effective, which can reintroduce missing or depressed genes or gene products or factors to rewire cancer cells to self-destruct or attract mechanisms that can destroy them. Since 2011, ZIOPHARM Oncology in partnership with Intrexon Corporation (Blacksburg, Virginia) is using a regulatable synthetic biology platform with modular transgene design and assembly,[44,45] providing unique strategies for gene therapy in oncology. One of the authors key advantages is the ability to use synthetic DNA to express both exon-coded and intron-coded protein sequences. With the authors

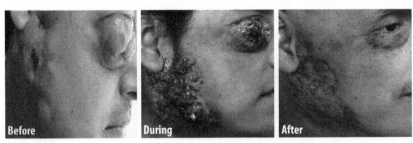

Fig. 5. Refractory rhabdomyosarcoma Sarcoma Partial Response to treatment, (*A*) tumor seen before, (*B*) during and (*C*) after two cycles of treatment.

enormous computational power, library of DNA, and large data and learning, they are able to design, test, and build DNA-based therapeutics with an engineering philosophy and guiding principles. The authors are developing systems that, like technology has done with computing, will lead to faster, better, cheaper translation and development.

Targets for Cancer Gene Therapy

The authors are working on many potential targets. The remainder of this article focuses on the authors initial immunotherapy strategy. One of the key hallmarks of cancer is tumor evasion from immune surveillance.[40] Tumor cells can evade immune detection by producing agents that suppress the activity of immune cells. Tumor cells also often fail to display antigens on their surface, effectively hiding from immune cells.[46,47] Furthermore, some tumor cells have enhanced expression of cell death factors, such as TRAIL (tumor necrosis factor-related apoptosis-inducing ligand) or Fas, that induce apoptosis of immune cells and dampen the immune response.[47,48] The understanding of how cytokines and signaling factors modulate immune surveillance has provided ideal targets for gene/immunotherapy in cancer.[49]

It is now apparent that interleukein 12 (IL-12) is one of the key cytokines in promoting immune surveillance of tumor cells.[50–52] IL-12 is a heterodimer (IL-12p70) consisting of disulfide-linked p35 and p40 chains and is produced by antigen-presenting cells, including dendritic cells (DCs) and macrophages.[50] IL-12 subsequently binds to the IL-12 receptor on natural killer cells and T cells and induces production of interferon gamma. Interferon gamma consequently promotes the expression of major histocompatibility complex antigens on tumor cells and antigen-presenting cells, which then augments stimulation of naïve T cells and differentiation into cytotoxic T cells (CTLs). Additionally, induction of antiangiogenic factors, such as interferon gamma–inducible protein 10 and monokines induced by interferon gamma in response to IL-12 and interferon gamma production, provide an additional mechanism of action for IL-12's antitumor activity.[50]

Because of the role of IL-12 in immune surveillance, it has been one of the high priority targets for cancer immunotherapy.[53] Since its discovery, several clinical trials have been performed to assess safety and efficacy of administering recombinant human (rh) IL-12 protein to patients with advanced cancers, including melanoma. Although immune and clinical responses were observed in some patients, systemic administration of rhIL-12 resulted in severe adverse events, including hypovolemic shock, leukopenia, hyperbilirubinemia, and elevated aspartate transaminase liver enzyme.[54–57] To minimize the systemic toxic effects, several subsequent trials introduced rhIL-12 subcutaneously or directly into the tumor. The results with intratumoral injection of IL-12 showed a considerably more positive profile of therapeutic effects with fewer severe adverse effects than what had been observed after systemic intravenous or subcutaneous administration.[58–61]

Inducible Ligand-regulated IL-12: From Bench to Bed-side

To limit the toxic side effects of continuous systemic or local delivery of IL-12 while maximizing therapeutic window, the authors are investigating the safety and efficacy of IL-12 DNA under the regulation of the RTS (RheoSwitch Therapeutic System) RheoSwitch gene expression platform. RTS represents a novel regulated gene expression system using INXN-1001, the activator ligand (**Fig. 6**). INXN-1001 is a small molecule and a member of the diacylhydrazine class of synthetic nonsteroidal ecdysone receptor ligands.[52] INXN-1001 is administered orally or potentially by other routes and binds to the RTS gene switch complex, resulting in transgene expression.[52]

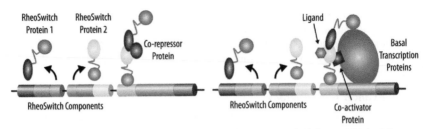

Fig. 6. The RheoSwitch Therapeutic System (Intrexon Corp, Blacksburg, Virgina) is a regulated promoter that is controlled by a small molecule oral activator (INXN-1001). The RTS consists of 2 fusion proteins that are expressed in a nonreplicative adenoviral vector that can be produced in host after adenoviral transduction. The binding of an oral activator (INXN-1001) stabilizes heterodimerization between the 2 fusion transcriptional coactivators and the components of the basal transcription machinery to induce expression of a target transgene.

Ad-RTS-hIL-12 is a novel synthetic gene construct in an adenovirus-based vector, with IL-12 expression only turned on when INXN-1001 triggers the RTS promoter.[52] Because the level of transgene expression (ie, protein production) is ligand concentration dependent, hIL-12 production can be modulated by the dose and frequency of oral INXN-1001 administration. The ability to turn transgene IL-12 expression on and off in vivo offers safety and potential therapeutic control to this treatment modality in that both the timing and level of IL-12 expression may be regulated by the dose and frequency of oral INXN-1001 administration, which may result in enhanced therapeutic index.[62] Potential IL-12-related adverse events may, therefore, be relieved by withdrawal of INXN-1001 administration.

Gelatin capsules of INXN-1001 in combination with the intratumoral administration of Ad-RTS-mIL-12 have been shown safe and effective in numerous nonclinical studies in melanoma, breast cancer, and colon and lung cancer, where the tumor IL-12 levels correlated with an increase of serum levels of interferon gamma.[63] These observations led to the filing of an Investigational New Drug (IND) application and studies in humans. In a phase 1 study, a standard 3 + 3 human dose-escalation schema in subjects with unresectable stage III/IV melanoma was performed to (1) assess the safety and tolerability of Ad-RTS-hIL-12 (1×10^{12} viral particles) along with orally administered INXN-1001; (2) explore viable biomarkers of efficacy; and (3) characterize the immune response to tumor antigens.

In this phase 1 study, with increasing levels of the INXN-1001, the authors observed a dose-dependent increase in serum levels of IL-12. Consistent with the expected mechanism of action of IL-12, the authors also observed dose-dependent increases in interferon gamma.[63] Based on these observations, the authors posit that IL-12 may be driving the DCs in tumor cells to preferentially present tumor antigens to helper T cells type 1 (T_H1), inducing local and systemic effects of tumor- specific $CD4^+$ T_H1 cells as well as $CD8^+$ CTLs (**Fig. 7**).

The authors preliminary phase 1 clinical observations with regulated Ad-RTS-hIL-12 are promising, show the initial safety of Ad-RTS-hIL-12, and provide a glimpse of its efficacy and mechanism of action. Importantly, the authors have observed some degree of clinical activity in 5 of 7 subjects in the 2 highest-dose cohorts, including 2 subjects who achieved the highest levels of Ad-RTS-hIL-12–induced interferon gamma.[63] Some of the subjects in this trial experienced a prominent inflammatory response with flattening of the injected lesion and a noninjected lesion and some have maintained a stable disease for more than 20 weeks. ZIOPHARM Oncology has now initiated two

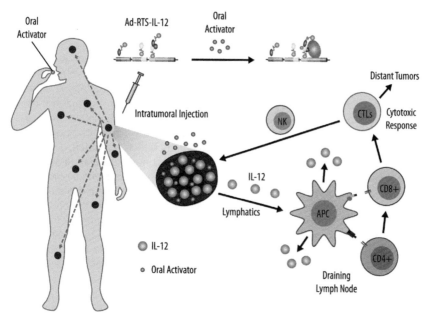

Fig. 7. Model for the mechanism of action of Ad-RTS-hIL-12–regulatable gene therapy. Intratumoral injection of viral particles of Ad-RTS-hIL-12 leads to a dose-dependent increase in levels of IL-12. IL-12 may then induce the DCs in tumor cells to preferentially present tumor antigens to antigen-presenting cells inducing local and systemic effects of specific antitumor CD4$^+$ T$_H$1 cells as well as CD8$^+$ CTLs.

phase 2 clinical studies to facilitate the translational path for this promising gene/immunotherapy strategy: one in melanoma and one in breast cancer.

The authors IL-12 studies validate the RTS expression platform for a controllable gene therapy approach. The modular nature of this strategy and the ability to effectively and efficiently introduce multiple genes of interest under the transcriptional control of the RTS platform has created immense opportunities for combinatorial cancer therapy and cancer immunotherapy. In coming years, the authors intend to efficiently and effectively bring synthetic biology products into practice for cancer therapy.

SUMMARY

Historically, the path to clinic has been long and complicated by various and relentless challenges. For example, in the past decade, several angiogenesis inhibitors have entered clinical practice. The concept for these inhibitors was initially published in 1971, when Dr Judah Folkman,[64,65] as surgeon at Harvard Medical School, reported that tumors cannot grow or spread without blood vessels and thus inhibition of angiogenesis can slow-down or treat cancer. Almost a decade later, in the early 1980s, vascular endothelial growth factor (also known as vascular permeability factor) was discovered and cloned.[66–68] Subsequently, Genetech, a company started in mid 1970s as a small biotechnology company with ambitions to become a major leader in oncology, developed an anti–vascular endothelial growth factor antibody and enabled transition of this compound into clinic. The phase 1 clinical trials in late-stage breast cancer patients were initiated in 1997. Through an arduous path and multiple initial failures, in 2004, this antibody (bevacizumab), labeled as Avastin, was the first angigogenesis inhibitor approved for treatment of colon cancer. Subsequently, Avastin has been approved for blood, breast, kidney, and brain cancers.

The authors have learned many lessons from the story of angiogenesis inhibitors from idea to clinic. The authors now know that translational medicine is an iterative process, relentlessly driven by data. This process does not end when a therapeutic reaches the clinic as the authors continue to learn from large populations of patients treated with approved drugs. There are many instances when the authors need to make the approved drugs even better or incorporate combination therapies to improve therapy or limit escape of tumors from treatment. The authors are adopting an engineering and computational strategy to enhance their approach.

In the new era of translational research with great technologic advancements, a better mechanistic understanding of cancer biology, in conjunction with a close partnership between academic and research institutions, government, and biotechnology/pharmaceutical companies, the authors predict that the path from bench to bedside will be less arduous. Biotech companies can move nimbly through the translational path by putting in place strategic planning to quickly identify, triage, communicate, and collaborate with academia and government to generate data that can drive the nonclinical, clinical, and CMC activities and hopefully bring the best ideas to patients in the form of new treatments.

REFERENCES

1. Bornstein SR, Licinio J. Improving the efficacy of translational medicine by optimally integrating health care, academia and industry. Nat Med 2011;17: 1567–9.
2. Qian M, Wu D, Wang E, et al. Development and promotion in translational medicine: perspectives from 2012 sino-american symposium on clinical and translational medicine. Clin Transl Med 2012;1:25.
3. Khoury MJ, Gwinn M, Yoon PW, et al. The continuum of translation research in genomic medicine: how can we accelerate the appropriate integration of human genome discoveries into health care and disease prevention? Genet Med 2007; 9:665–74.
4. Day M, Rutkowski JL, Feuerstein GZ. Translational medicine–a paradigm shift in modern drug discovery and development: the role of biomarkers. Adv Exp Med Biol 2009;655:1–12.
5. Keramaris NC, Kanakaris NK, Tzioupis C, et al. Translational research: from benchside to bedside. Injury 2008;39:643–50.
6. DiMasi JA, Hansen RW, Grabowski HG. The price of innovation: new estimates of drug development costs. J Health Econ 2003;22:151–85.
7. Malakoff D. Can treatment costs be tamed? Science 2011;331:1545–7.
8. Emmert-Buck MR. An NIH intramural percubator as a model of academic-industry partnerships: from the beginning of life through the valley of death. J Transl Med 2011;9:54.
9. Feldman AM. Does academic culture support translational research? Clin Transl Sci 2008;1:87–8.
10. Fox BA, Schendel DJ, Butterfield LH, et al. Defining the critical hurdles in cancer immunotherapy. J Transl Med 2011;9:214.
11. FDA. Available at: http://www.fda.gov/Drugs/default.htm. Accessed March 22, 2013.
12. Kersey JH. Fifty years of studies of the biology and therapy of childhood leukemia. Blood 1997;90:4243–51.

13. American Cancer Society facts and figures 2012. Available at: http://www.cancer.org/research/cancerfactsfigures/index. Accessed March 22, 2013.
14. Bayh-Dole act. Available at: http://www.b-d30.org/. Accessed March 22, 2013.
15. Orphan Drug Act. Available at: http://www.fda.gov/regulatoryinformation/legislation/federalfooddrugandcosmeticactfdcact/significantamendmentstothefdcact/orphandrugact/default.htm. Accessed March 22, 2013.
16. Henkel J. Orphan drug law matures into medical mainstay. FDA Consum 1999; 33:29–32.
17. Accelarated approval regulation. Available at: http://www.fda.gov/Drugs/ResourcesForYou/HealthProfessionals/ucm313768.htm. Accessed March 22, 2013.
18. Critical path initiative. Available at: http://www.fda.gov/scienceresearch/specialtopics/criticalpathinitiative/default.htm. Accessed March 22, 2013.
19. Woodcock J, Woosley R. The FDA critical path initiative and its influence on new drug development. Annu Rev Med 2008;59:1–12.
20. D'Adamo DR. Appraising the current role of chemotherapy for the treatment of sarcoma. Semin Oncol 2011;38(Suppl 3):S19–29.
21. Hingorani P, Zhang W, Piperdi S, et al. Preclinical activity of palifosfamide lysine (ZIO-201) in pediatric sarcomas including oxazaphosphorine-resistant osteosarcoma. Cancer Chemother Pharmacol 2009;64:733–40.
22. Jung S, Kasper B. Palifosfamide, a bifunctional alkylator for the treatment of sarcomas. IDrugs 2010;13:38–48.
23. Struck RF, Dykes DJ, Corbett TH, et al. Isophosphoramide mustard, a metabolite of ifosfamide with activity against murine tumours comparable to cyclophosphamide. Br J Cancer 1983;47:15–26.
24. Brock N, Gross R, Hohorst HJ, et al. Activation of cyclophosphamide in man and animals. Cancer 1971;27:1512–29.
25. Brock N, Hohorst HJ. Metabolism of cyclophosphamide. Cancer 1967;20:900–4.
26. Wagner T, Heydrich D, Jork T, et al. Comparative study on human pharmacokinetics of activated ifosfamide and cyclophosphamide by a modified fluorometric test. J Cancer Res Clin Oncol 1981;100:95–104.
27. Struck RF, Roychowdhury A, Maddry JA, et al. Development and anti-cancer testing of halogenated analogues. Proc Am Assoc Cancer Res 2006;47.
28. Maki RG. Ifosfamide in the neoadjuvant treatment of osteogenic sarcoma. J Clin Oncol 2012;30:2033–5.
29. Lewis LD, Meanwell CA. Ifosfamide pharmacokinetics and neurotoxicity. Lancet 1990;335:175–6.
30. Ingelman-Sundberg M, Sim SC, Gomez A, et al. Influence of cytochrome P450 polymorphisms on drug therapies: pharmacogenetic, pharmacoepigenetic and clinical aspects. Pharmacol Ther 2007;116:496–526.
31. Misiura K, Szymanowicz D, Kusnierczyk H, et al. Isophosphoramide mustard analogues as prodrugs for anticancer gene-directed enzyme-prodrug therapy (GDEPT). Acta Biochim Pol 2002;49:169–76.
32. Wrabetz E, Peter G, Hohorst HJ. Does acrolein contribute to the cytotoxicity of cyclophosphamide? J Cancer Res Clin Oncol 1980;98:119–26.
33. Lind MJ, Margison JM, Cerny T, et al. Comparative pharmacokinetics and alkylating activity of fractionated intravenous and oral ifosfamide in patients with bronchogenic carcinoma. Cancer Res 1989;49:753–7.
34. Lind MJ, Margison JM, Cerny T, et al. Prolongation of ifosfamide elimination half-life in obese patients due to altered drug distribution. Cancer Chemother Pharmacol 1989;25:139–42.

35. Lewis LD, Fitzgerald DL, Harper PG, et al. Fractionated ifosfamide therapy produces a time-dependent increase in ifosfamide metabolism. Br J Clin Pharmacol 1990;30:725–32.
36. Maki RG, Morgan RM, Lewis JL. Palifosfamide, a novel molecule for the treatement of soft tissue sarcoma. ESUN 2010.
37. Movva S, Verschraegen C. Systemic management strategies for metastatic soft tissue sarcoma. Drugs 2011;71:2115–29.
38. Verschraegen CF, Arias-Pulido H, Lee SJ, et al. Phase IB study of the combination of docetaxel, gemcitabine, and bevacizumab in patients with advanced or recurrent soft tissue sarcoma: the Axtell regimen. Ann Oncol 2012;23:785–90.
39. U.S. Department of Energy's Genomic Science Program, editor. U.S. Department of energy's genomic science program.
40. Hanahan D, Weinberg RA. Hallmarks of cancer: the next generation. Cell 2011; 144:646–74.
41. Cheng AA, Lu TK. Synthetic biology: an emerging engineering discipline. Annu Rev Biomed Eng 2012;14:155–78.
42. Ruder WC, Lu T, Collins JJ. Synthetic biology moving into the clinic. Science 2011;333:1248–52.
43. Ortiz R, Melguizo C, Prados J, et al. New gene therapy strategies for cancer treatment: a review of recent patents. Recent Pat Anticancer Drug Discov 2012;7:297–312.
44. Cress DE. The need for regulatable vectors for gene therapy for Parkinson's disease. Exp Neurol 2008;209:30–3.
45. Sowa G, Westrick E, Pacek C, et al. In vitro and in vivo testing of a novel regulatory system for gene therapy for intervertebral disc degeneration. Spine 2011; 36:E623–8.
46. Cordon-Cardo C, Fuks Z, Drobnjak M, et al. Expression of HLA-A, B, C antigens on primary and metastatic tumor cell populations of human carcinomas. Cancer Res 1991;51:6372–80.
47. Yoshikawa T, Saito H, Osaki T, et al. Elevated Fas expression is related to increased apoptosis of circulating CD8+ T cell in patients with gastric cancer. J Surg Res 2008;148:143–51.
48. Grimm M, Kim M, Rosenwald A, et al. Tumour-mediated TRAIL-Receptor expression indicates effective apoptotic depletion of infiltrating CD8+ immune cells in clinical colorectal cancer. Eur J Cancer 2010;46:2314–23.
49. Lizee G, Overwijk WW, Radvanyi L, et al. Harnessing the power of the immune system to target cancer. Annu Rev Med 2013;64:71–90.
50. Del Vecchio M, Bajetta E, Canova S, et al. Interleukin-12: biological properties and clinical application. Clin Cancer Res 2007;13:4677–85.
51. Tsung K, Norton JA. Lessons from Coley's toxin. Surg Oncol 2006;15:25–8.
52. Chan T. Therapeutic efficacy and systemic anti-tumor T cell immunity induced by RheoswitchAr-regulated IL-12 expression after intra-tumoral injection of adenovirus vector or vector-transduced dendritic cells.
53. US House Services, National Cancer Institute. Available at: http://ncifrederick. cancer.gov/research/brb/workshops/nci%20immunotherapy%20workshop% 207-12-07.pdf. 2007. Accessed March 22, 2013.
54. Car BD, Eng VM, Lipman JM, et al. The toxicology of interleukin-12: a review. Toxicol Pathol 1999;27:58–63.
55. Lacy MQ, Jacobus S, Blood EA, et al. Phase II study of interleukin-12 for treatment of plateau phase multiple myeloma (E1A96): a trial of the Eastern Cooperative Oncology Group. Leuk Res 2009;33:1485–9.

56. Waldner MJ, Neurath MF. Gene therapy using IL 12 family members in infection, auto immunity, and cancer. Curr Gene Ther 2009;9:239–47.
57. Rook AH, Zaki MH, Wysocka M, et al. The role for interleukin-12 therapy of cutaneous T cell lymphoma. Ann N Y Acad Sci 2001;941:177–84.
58. Van Herpen CM, Huijbens R, Looman M, et al. Pharmacokinetics and immunological aspects of a phase Ib study with intratumoral administration of recombinant human interleukin-12 in patients with head and neck squamous cell carcinoma: a decrease of T-bet in peripheral blood mononuclear cells. Clin Cancer Res 2003;9:2950–6.
59. Van Herpen CM, Looman M, Zonneveld M, et al. Intratumoral administration of recombinant human interleukin 12 in head and neck squamous cell carcinoma patients elicits a T-helper 1 profile in the locoregional lymph nodes. Clin Cancer Res 2004;10:2626–35.
60. Van Herpen CM, van der Laak JA, de Vries IJ, et al. Intratumoral recombinant human interleukin-12 administration in head and neck squamous cell carcinoma patients modifies locoregional lymph node architecture and induces natural killer cell infiltration in the primary tumor. Clin Cancer Res 2005;11:1899–909.
61. Van Herpen CM, van der Voort R, van der Laak JA, et al. Intratumoral rhIL-12 administration in head and neck squamous cell carcinoma patients induces B cell activation. Int J Cancer 2008;123:2354–61.
62. Komita H, Zhao X, Katakam AK, et al. Conditional interleukin-12 gene therapy promotes safe and effective antitumor immunity. Cancer Gene Ther 2009;16: 883–91.
63. Vergara-Silva A. Delivery of IL-12 shows promising clinical activity in unresectable stage III/IV melanoma. 2013.
64. Folkman J. Tumor angiogenesis: therapeutic implications. N Engl J Med 1971; 285:1182–6.
65. Folkman J, Merler E, Abernathy C, et al. Isolation of a tumor factor responsible for angiogenesis. J Exp Med 1971;133:275–88.
66. Senger DR, Asch BB, Smith BD, et al. A secreted phosphoprotein marker for neoplastic transformation of both epithelial and fibroblastic cells. Nature 1983; 302:714–5.
67. Senger DR, Galli SJ, Dvorak AM, et al. Tumor cells secrete a vascular permeability factor that promotes accumulation of ascites fluid. Science 1983;219: 983–5.
68. Leung DW, Cachianes G, Kuang WJ, et al. Vascular endothelial growth factor is a secreted angiogenic mitogen. Science 1989;246:1306–9.

Index

Note: Page numbers of article titles are in **boldface** type.

Surg Oncol Clin N Am 22 (2013) 903–916
http://dx.doi.org/10.1016/S1055-3207(13)00078-1
1055-3207/13/$ – see front matter © 2013 Elsevier Inc. All rights reserved.

surgonc.theclinics.com

United States Postal Service

Statement of Ownership, Management, and Circulation
(All Periodicals Publications Except Requestor Publications)

1. Publication Title	2. Publication Number	3. Filing Date
Surgical Oncology Clinics of North America	0 1 2 – 5 6 5	9/14/13

4. Issue Frequency	5. Number of Issues Published Annually	6. Annual Subscription Price
Jan, Apr, Jul, Oct	4	$274.00

7. Complete Mailing Address of Known Office of Publication *(Not printer)* *(Street, city, county, state, and ZIP+4®)*

Elsevier Inc.
360 Park Avenue South
New York, NY 10010-1710

Contact Person: Stephen Bushing
Telephone (Include area code): 215-239-3688

8. Complete Mailing Address of Headquarters or General Business Office of Publisher *(Not printer)*

Elsevier Inc., 360 Park Avenue South, New York, NY 10010-1710

9. Full Names and Complete Mailing Addresses of Publisher, Editor, and Managing Editor *(Do not leave blank)*

Publisher *(Name and complete mailing address)*

Linda Belfus, Elsevier, Inc., 1600 John F. Kennedy Blvd. Suite 1800, Philadelphia, PA 19103-2899

Editor *(Name and complete mailing address)*

Jessica McCool, Elsevier, Inc., 1600 John F. Kennedy Blvd. Suite 1800, Philadelphia, PA 19103-2899

Managing Editor *(Name and complete mailing address)*

Barbara Cohen-Kligerman, Elsevier, Inc., 1600 John F. Kennedy Blvd. Suite 1800, Philadelphia, PA 19103-2899

10. Owner *(Do not leave blank. If the publication is owned by a corporation, give the name and address of the corporation immediately followed by the names and addresses of all stockholders owning or holding 1 percent or more of the total amount of stock. If not owned by a corporation, give the names and addresses of the individual owners. If owned by a partnership or other unincorporated firm, give its name and address as well as those of each individual owner. If the publication is published by a nonprofit organization, give its name and address.)*

Full Name	Complete Mailing Address
Wholly owned subsidiary of	1600 John F. Kennedy Blvd., Ste. 1800
Reed/Elsevier, US holdings	Philadelphia, PA 19103-2899

11. Known Bondholders, Mortgagees, and Other Security Holders Owning or Holding 1 Percent or More of Total Amount of Bonds, Mortgages, or Other Securities. If none, check box ☐ None

Full Name	Complete Mailing Address
N/A	

12. Tax Status *(For completion by nonprofit organizations authorized to mail at nonprofit rates)* (Check one)
The purpose, function, and nonprofit status of this organization and the exempt status for federal income tax purposes:
☐ Has Not Changed During Preceding 12 Months
☐ Has Changed During Preceding 12 Months *(Publisher must submit explanation of change with this statement)*

PS Form 3526, September 2007 (Page 1 of 3 (Instructions Page 3)) PSN 7530-01-000-9931 PRIVACY NOTICE: See our Privacy policy in www.usps.com

13. Publication Title	14. Issue Date for Circulation Data Below
Surgical Oncology Clinics of North America	July 2013

15. Extent and Nature of Circulation		Average No. Copies Each Issue During Preceding 12 Months	No. Copies of Single Issue Published Nearest to Filing Date
a. Total Number of Copies *(Net press run)*		497	719
b. Paid Circulation (By Mail and Outside the Mail)	(1) Mailed Outside-County Paid Subscriptions Stated on PS Form 3541 (Include paid distribution above nominal rate, advertiser's proof copies, and exchange copies)	196	177
	(2) Mailed In-County Paid Subscriptions Stated on PS Form 3541 (Include paid distribution above nominal rate, advertiser's proof copies, and exchange copies)		
	(3) Paid Distribution Outside the Mails Including Sales Through Dealers and Carriers, Street Vendors, Counter Sales, and Other Paid Distribution Outside USPS®	89	92
	(4) Paid Distribution by Other Classes Mailed Through the USPS (e.g. First-Class Mail®)		
c. Total Paid Distribution (Sum of 15b (1), (2), (3), and (4))	▲	285	269
d. Free or Nominal Rate Distribution (By Mail and Outside the Mail)	(1) Free or Nominal Rate Outside-County Copies Included on PS Form 3541	49	25
	(2) Free or Nominal Rate In-County Copies Included on PS Form 3541		
	(3) Free or Nominal Rate Copies Mailed at Other Classes Through the USPS (e.g. First-Class Mail)		
	(4) Free or Nominal Rate Distribution Outside the Mail (Carriers or other means)		
e. Total Free or Nominal Rate Distribution (Sum of 15d (1), (2), (3) and (4))	▲	49	25
f. Total Distribution (Sum of 15c and 15e)	▲	334	294
g. Copies not Distributed (See instructions to publishers #4 (page 83))	▲	163	125
h. Total (Sum of 15f and g)	▲	497	419
i. Percent Paid (15c divided by 15f times 100)	▲	85.33%	91.50%

16. Publication of Statement of Ownership

☐ If the publication is a general publication, publication of this statement is required. Will be printed in the October 2013 issue of this publication. ☐ Publication not required

17. Signature and Title of Editor, Publisher, Business Manager, or Owner	Date
[signature] Stephen R. Bushing –Inventory/Distribution Coordinator	September 14, 2013

I certify that all information furnished on this form is true and complete. I understand that anyone who furnishes false or misleading information on this form or who omits material or information requested on the form may be subject to criminal sanctions (including fines and imprisonment) and/or civil sanctions (including civil penalties).

PS Form 3526, September 2007 (Page 2 of 3)

Moving?

Make sure your subscription moves with you!

To notify us of your new address, find your **Clinics Account Number** (located on your mailing label above your name), and contact customer service at:

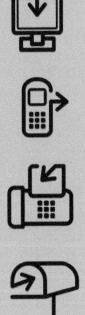

Email: journalscustomerservice-usa@elsevier.com

800-654-2452 (subscribers in the U.S. & Canada)
314-447-8871 (subscribers outside of the U.S. & Canada)

Fax number: 314-447-8029

Elsevier Health Sciences Division
Subscription Customer Service
3251 Riverport Lane
Maryland Heights, MO 63043

*To ensure uninterrupted delivery of your subscription, please notify us at least 4 weeks in advance of move.

Printed and bound by CPI Group (UK) Ltd, Croydon, CR0 4YY

03/10/2024

01040409-0011